Accession no.
36223587

D0336975

Health Studies

Health Studies
An Introduction

3rd edition

Edited by
Jennie Naidoo and Jane Wills

LIS LIBRARY

Date	Fund
8/12/15	nm-WAR

Order No

2672935

University of Chester

 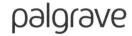

© Selection and Editorial Matter: Jennie Naidoo and Jane Wills 2015
Individual chapters © contributors 2015

All rights reserved. No reproduction, copy or transmission of this
publication may be made without written permission.

No portion of this publication may be reproduced, copied or transmitted
save with written permission or in accordance with the provisions of the
Copyright, Designs and Patents Act 1988, or under the terms of any licence
permitting limited copying issued by the Copyright Licensing Agency,
Saffron House, 6–10 Kirby Street, London EC1N 8TS.

Any person who does any unauthorized act in relation to this publication
may be liable to criminal prosecution and civil claims for damages.

The authors have asserted their rights to be identified as the authors of this
work in accordance with the Copyright, Designs and Patents Act 1988.

First edition 2001
Second edition 2008
Third edition 2015

First published 2001 by
PALGRAVE

Palgrave in the UK is an imprint of Macmillan Publishers Limited, registered
in England, company number 785998, of 4 Crinan Street, London, N1 9XW.

Palgrave Macmillan in the US is a division of St Martin's Press LLC,
175 Fifth Avenue, New York, NY 10010.

Palgrave is a global imprint of the above companies and is represented
throughout the world.

Palgrave® and Macmillan® are registered trademarks in the United States,
the United Kingdom, Europe and other countries.

ISBN: 978–1–137–34867–8

This book is printed on paper suitable for recycling and made from fully
managed and sustained forest sources. Logging, pulping and manufacturing
processes are expected to conform to the environmental regulations of the
country of origin.

A catalogue record for this book is available from the British Library.

A catalog record for this book is available from the Library of Congress.

Typeset by Aardvark Editorial Limited, Metfield, Suffolk.

Printed in China

Contents

List of figures   xii

List of tables   xiii

List of examples   xiv

Notes on contributors   xvii

Acknowledgements   xxi

Abbreviations   xxii

Introducing health studies   1
Jennie Naidoo and Jane Wills

What is health studies?   1

A focus on health   2

The disciplinary context of health studies   4

Investigating health   8

Synthesizing perspectives: food, nutrition, diet and obesity   11

Health promotion: an example of interdisciplinary practice   13

Health studies and employability   17

Using this book   19

References   20

1 Human biology and health   22
S.H. Cedar

Overview   23

Introduction   23

Part 1 The contribution of biology to health studies   24
    Cell theory   25
    Homeostasis   29
    Genes and genetics   30
    Ill health and disease   33

Part 2 Theoretical and research approaches   36
    Induction   38
    Deduction   38
    Proof and falsification   39
    Experimentation   40
    Techniques   41

Case study Biological explanations for obesity   43

Questions for further discussion   47

Further reading and resources   47
References   47

2   **History and health**   50
      Louise Hill Curth
      Overview   51
      Introduction   51
      Part 1 The contribution of history to health studies   53
            Developments in concepts of health and disease: six non-naturals 59
            Developments in medicine and healthcare   63
      Part 2 Theoretical and research approaches   66
            The development of the discipline   66
            The historical method: using sources, oral history   68
      Case study Food safety and bread in Victorian England   70
      Questions for further discussion   72
      Further reading and resources   72
      References   73

3   **Epidemiology and health**   78
      Nicola Crichton and Anne Mulhall
      Overview   79
      Introduction   79
      Part 1 The contribution of epidemiology to health studies   80
            The emergence of the evidence-based healthcare movement   83
            The link between ill health and socioeconomic conditions   85
            Concepts of health and disease in medical epidemiology   87
            Social epidemiology   89
      Part 2 Theoretical and research approaches   91
            The natural history of disease   92
            Identifying risk   93
            Classifying disease   93
            Diagnosing and treating disease   94
            Surveillance and the planning and evaluation of health services 94
            The methodologies used by epidemiology   96
      Case study Trends in obesity   104
      Questions for further discussion   108
      Further reading and resources   108
      References   109

4   **Health psychology**   113
      Jane Ogden
      Overview   114
      Introduction   114
      Part 1 The contribution of psychology to health studies   115

Health beliefs and behaviours   117
Communication in health settings   124
The experience of being ill and the example of pain   127
Part 2 Theoretical and research approaches   134
The health belief model   135
The protection motivation theory   136
The theory of planned behaviour   138
The stages of change model   140
The self-regulatory model   141
Developing interventions to change health-related behaviour   144
Case study The impact of beliefs on behaviour: the example of
obesity and diet   147
Questions for further discussion   149
Further reading   150
References   150

5   Sociology and health   155
Mat Jones and Norma Daykin
Overview   156
Introduction   156
Part 1 The contribution of sociology to health studies   157
Socioeconomic inequalities in health   159
Explaining health inequalities   161
Gender and health   165
Explaining gender inequalities in health   167
'Race', ethnicity and health   169
Part 2 Theoretical and research approaches   172
The sociology of lay–professional relationships: functionalist
approaches   173
Medicalization and social control   175
Marxist and political economy perspectives   176
Health professions and interprofessional relationships   178
Interactionist perspectives and the experience of illness   179
Sociology of the body   180
Social constructionist perspectives and beyond   181
Case study The social determinants and social construction of diet 183
Questions for further discussion   187
Further reading   187
References   188

6   Geography and health   196
Peter Anthamatten
Overview   197
Introduction   197
Part 1 The contribution of geography to health studies   199

Linking places to health through the natural environment   200
Linking places to health through the built environment   206
Linking places to health through the sociocultural environment   210
Part 2 Theoretical and research approaches   213
Health mapping   214
Geographic information systems   216
Case study Obesity and the built environment   219
Questions for further discussion   222
Further reading   223
References   224

7   Cultural studies and anthropology   228
Sarah Burch
Overview   229
Introduction   229
Part 1 The contribution of cultural studies and anthropology to
health studies   230
Cultural practices in relation to health   233
Health and illness across cultures   235
Lay knowledge and beliefs   240
Representations of health   243
Part 2 Theoretical and research approaches   248
Ethnography   251
Discourse and conversation analysis   253
Semiotics   255
Case study Breastfeeding and infant feeding across cultures   256
Questions for further discussion   259
Further reading   259
References   259

8   Politics and health   265
Clare Bambra, Katherine Smith and Lynne Kennedy
Overview   266
Introduction   266
Part 1 The contribution of political science to health studies   267
The political and the non-political   268
The political nature of health   270
Part 2 Theoretical and research approaches   274
Conservatism   275
Liberalism (and neoliberalism)   276
Socialism and social democracy   278
Nationalism (and fascism)   280
Feminism   281
Environmentalism   283
Case study The politics of 'fat'   284

Questions for further discussion   288
Further reading   288
References   289

9   Social policy and health   293
Bob Pitt and Liz Lloyd
Overview   294
Introduction   294
Part 1 The contribution of social policy to health studies   295
    The organization of welfare   296
    The changing role of the state in welfare   298
    Britain becomes a welfare state, 1945–50   299
    Challenging welfare, 1979–97   301
    Healthcare and New Labour, 1997–2010   302
    Coalition government health reforms since 2010   306
    Current health issues on the social policy agenda   306
Part 2 Theoretical and research approaches   312
    The development of the discipline   312
    From consensus to critique   313
    International and comparative social policy   314
    Research methods in social policy: in understanding health   318
    Research methods in social policy: policy analysis   320
    Research methods in social policy: the policy process   321
Case study A policy analysis of obesity in the UK   325
Questions for further discussion   328
Further reading and resources   328
References   329

**10 Organization and management of health and
      healthcare   334**
Vicki Taylor, Hilary Scott and Martin Walter
Overview   335
Introduction   335
Part 1 The contribution of management to health studies   337
    Understanding organizations   337
    Working across organizations   351
    Managing healthcare services   352
    Working in groups and teams   352
    Leadership   354
    Managing change   357
Part 2 Theoretical and research approaches   357
    Scientific management   358
    Bureaucracy and organizations   359
    The human relations approach to understanding people and
    organizations   360

Behavioural theory   361
Situation theory   361
Contingency theory   362
Motivation theories   362
Systems theory and the sociotechnical system approach   366
Chaos (or complexity) theory   368

Case study Formulating an obesity strategy   369

Questions for further discussion   371

Further reading   372

References   373

11   Health economics   377
     David Cohen

Overview   378

Introduction   378

Part 1 The contribution of economics to health studies   380
     Market forces and healthcare   381
     The allocation and distribution of healthcare 'off the market'   384

Part 2 Theoretical and research approaches   387
     Resources and money   387
     The output of healthcare   388
     The economic notion of cost   388
     The cost–benefit approach   389
     Techniques of economic appraisal   392

Case study The use of QALYs in the treatment of obesity   397

Questions for further discussion   398

Further reading   398

References   399

12   Ethics and law   401
     Peter Duncan

Overview   402

Introduction   402

Part 1 The contribution of ethics to health studies   404
     Aristotelianism   405
     Immanuel Kant and deontology   407
     J.S. Mill and utilitarianism   408
     Creating 'worthwhile lives': perspectives from ethics on 'the genetic
     revolution'   409
     The contribution of law to health studies   410
     The sources of law   412

Part 2 Theoretical and research approaches   414
     Theoretical and research approaches in ethics   415
     Theoretical and research approaches in law   417

The relationship between ethics and law: Is what we *must* do the
same as what we *ought* to do?   421
Dealing with the *must–ought* 'gap': consent and professional
conduct   423
Case study Banning 'junk food' advertising   424
Questions for further discussion   428
Further reading   428
References   428

Glossary   431
Index   442

List of figures

0.1   Disciplinary perspectives on food, nutrition and obesity   14

1.1   A typical animal cell   26
1.2   Organs and body systems   28

2.1   The humoural theory   57

3.1   Snow's map of Soho   81
3.2   Screening tests   95
3.3   Outline of a randomized controlled trial   100
3.4   Outline of the design of a case control study   102
3.5   Prevalence of obesity (BMI > 30 kg/m^2) among adults in England by gender, 1993–2012   105

4.1   The biopsychosocial model of health and illness   116
4.2   Ley's model of compliance   124
4.3   The gate control theory of pain   129
4.4   The health belief model   135
4.5   The protection motivation theory   137
4.6   The theory of planned behaviour   138
4.7   Model of behaviour change   141
4.8   Self-regulatory model of illness behaviour   142

6.1   The disease cycle   201
6.2   The demographic transition model   205
6.3   Prevalence of overweight, ages 20+, age standardized, both sexes, 2008   215
6.4   A geospatial analysis of John Snow's cholera map   218

9.1   Spheres of welfare: the mixed economy   298
9.2   The policy process   322

10.1   The NHS Outcomes Framework   339
10.2   Structure of the NHS   342
10.3   The healthcare leadership model   356
10.4   A congruency model of organizational behaviour   366

11.1   Supply, demand and market equilibrium   381
11.2   The cost–benefit framework   389

List of tables

3.1	Cause-and-effect relationships	99
3.2	Checklist for assessing the validity of RCTs	101
3.3	Common rates used in epidemiology	103
3.4	Estimating increased risk for the obese of developing associated diseases, taken from international studies	107
5.1	Life expectancy at birth by gender and NS-SEC class, 1982–86, 1992–96 and 2002–06	160
7.1	A comparison of a traditional homeopathic healer versus a modern allopathic physician	238
7.2	A comparison between a public information campaign and advertising a commercial product	244
8.1	Neoliberal and social justice approaches to health	278
9.1	Key changes in health policy, 1997–2010	303
9.2	Comparative welfare regimes	315
10.1	PESTLE analysis of environmental pressures	344
10.2	Environmental turbulence and the NHS	345
10.3	Categories of low-profile symbols in organizations	348
10.4	Analysis of organizational culture	348
10.5	Levels of organizational culture	349
10.6	A classification of teams	353
10.7	Categories that should form the basis for leadership in the NHS	356

List of examples

1.1   Application of biology to contemporary health issues   24
1.2   Chromosomal and genetic disorders   31
1.3   UK Biobank   33
1.4   Examples of research in biological sciences   36
1.5   Stem cells and regenerative medicine   36
1.6   Inductive reasoning and the example of eugenics   39
1.7   Clinical interventions: the double-blind trial   41

2.1   The application of history to the study of contemporary health issues   53
2.2   The body as a machine: the contribution of dissection and anatomy   63
2.3   Changes in the management of infectious diseases   64
2.4   Examples of historical health research   66
2.5   Foucault and history   67
2.6   Almanacs as a historical source   68

3.1   The application of epidemiology to contemporary health issues   80
3.2   John Snow and the Broad Street pump   81
3.3   Screening for prostate cancer   84
3.4   Lay interpretations of risk   86
3.5   Lay epidemiology and the health risks of Poly Implant Prostheses (PIP) breast implants   86
3.6   The social construction of illness   90
3.7   Examples of research in epidemiology   91

4.1   The application of health psychology to contemporary health issues   115
4.2   Impact of beliefs and behaviours on health: the example of stress   121
4.3   Health consultations   125
4.4   The gate control theory of pain   128
4.5   Examples of research in health psychology   134

5.1   Application of sociology to contemporary health issues   157
5.2   Changing patterns of risk in HIV/AIDS   169
5.3   'Race', ethnicity and health   170
5.4   Examples of research in sociology and health   172
5.5   Medicine as a threat to health   175
5.6   Professionalization in the NHS   178

6.1   The application of geography to the study of contemporary health issues   199
6.2   Environmental change and dengue fever   203
6.3   Environmental justice   208

6.4	Spatial access to healthcare	212
6.5	Examples of research in the geography of health	213
7.1	The application of cultural studies and anthropology to contemporary health issues	230
7.2	Food as culture	233
7.3	Cultural perceptions of mental health	236
7.4	Meanings of hypertension	237
7.5	Traditional healers and people with epilepsy	239
7.6	The menopause and hormone replacement therapy: understandings of risk	242
7.7	Accounts of pain	243
7.8	HIV/AIDS and the internet	246
7.9	SARS in the media	247
7.10	Examples of research in cultures and health	248
7.11	Ethnography and concepts of health among the Cree in Quebec	252
8.1	The application of politics to contemporary health issues	267
8.2	Politics and the NHS	269
8.3	Health and human rights	273
8.4	Politics in medical publications	273
8.5	Examples of research in politics and health	274
8.6	Socialist approaches to improving the health of populations	279
8.7	Patriarchy and health	282
9.1	The application of social policy to contemporary health issues	295
9.2	The Beveridge Report	300
9.3	Fair and equitable access to treatment: in vitro fertilization (IVF) provision in the UK	307
9.4	Stafford Hospital	310
9.5	Examples of research in health policy	312
9.6	Migrant health and care workers	317
9.7	Using textual analysis to understand policy	318
9.8	Policy-making: the example of a smoking ban in workplaces and public places	323
10.1	The application of organization and management to contemporary health issues	337
10.2	Organizational structures	340
10.3	Examples of health management research	357
10.4	The Hawthorne experiments	360
10.5	Job design	365
11.1	The application of economics to contemporary health issues	380
11.2	The relativity of need: the case of Viagra	385
11.3	Examples of research in health economics	387
11.4	The case of treatment for bone marrow cancer	391
11.5	The development of the QALY	395

12.1	The application of ethics and law to contemporary issues in health and healthcare	404
12.2	The dilemma of life	405
12.3	Kant and the dilemma of life	407
12.4	J.S. Mill and the dilemma of life	408
12.5	The use of genetic and reproductive technologies	410
12.6	Examples of research in ethics and law and health	414
12.7	Conceptual and theoretical examination in ethics	416
12.8	Judicial review and Lewisham Hospital, London	419

Notes on contributors

Peter James Anthamatten is Assistant Professor of Geography and Environmental Sciences at the University of Colorado, Denver, US, where he coordinates the GIS programme and teaches courses on mapping, health geography and public health classes. His research focuses on the relationship between children's health and the built environment, specifically how their environments relate to physical activity and other obesity-related behaviours. Prior to this, Peter worked in pedagogy to develop materials for teaching geography. He co-authored, with Helen Hazen, *An Introduction to the Geography of Health* (2011).

Clare Bambra is Professor of Public Health Geography, Durham University, UK. Her research focuses on the influence of welfare states and political structures on international variations in public health and health inequalities. Clare also examines labour markets and the relationships between work, worklessness and health. She is author of *Work, Worklessness and the Political Economy of Health* (2011).

Sarah Burch is the Director of Research & Scholarship in the Faculty of Health, Social Care & Education at Anglia Ruskin University, UK. She is also an Associate Lecturer with the Open University. Prior to this, she worked in a range of public sector organizations, principally with older and disabled people. Sarah's main teaching and research interests include gerontology, disability, childhood studies, gender and health policy. Her current research relates to promoting the wellbeing of older people.

S.H. Cedar lectures in biomedical sciences, physiological processes and new technologies at London South Bank University, UK. Her philosophy of healthcare teaching is based on understanding the principle of homeostasis, which, when maintained by the individual, defines health and after ill health enables the body to return to its normal functioning during healing or clinical intervention. This philosophy informs her book *Biology for Health: Applying the Activities of Daily Living* (2012), which explains the processes that maintain these daily activities in homeostasis. Dr Cedar researches in the area of stem cell biology, regeneration and ageing and in the ethics underlying these treatments.

David Cohen is Professor of Health Economics at the University of South Wales, UK. He came to the UK in 1972 after receiving a degree in economics from McGill University in his native Canada. David has published widely on many health economics issues, been a member of numerous committees and working parties and acted as specialist adviser to WHO and the House of Commons Select Committee on Welsh Affairs. He has been a member of many research commissioning panels, including the MRC Health Services and Public Health Research Board and the NIHR Health Technology Assessment and Service Delivery and Organisation Programmes.

Nicola Crichton is Pro Dean Research and Professor of Health Statistics at London South Bank University, UK. She has been teaching epidemiology, statistics and research methods for more than 20 years. Nicola has a wide range of research publications resulting from collaborations with a variety of health professionals. In addition, she has written statistical information points and texts on understanding statistical ideas specifically for a nursing audience.

Louise Hill Curth is Reader in Medical History and Head of the Centre for Medical History at the University of Winchester, UK. An early modern English historian, she has published extensively on early modern popular medical beliefs and practices for humans and animals. Her publications include *The Care of Brute Beasts: A Social and Cultural Study of Veterinary Medicine in Early Modern England* (2010), '*A plaine and easie waie to remedie a horse': Equine Medicine in Early Modern England* (2013) and *English Almanacs, Astrology and Popular Medicine* (2013). Louise is currently working on a monograph on early modern astrological medicine.

Norma Daykin, an academic researcher in applied health research, began researching the health impacts of arts 10 years ago, starting with a study of cultural notions of creativity and their impact on musicians, artists and participants in arts for health projects. Her research has explored the impact of visual and performing arts, particularly music, in a wide range of health and social care contexts. Norma is co-executive editor of *Arts and Health*. In 2008, she received the inaugural Royal Society for Public Health Award for Arts and Health Research, for her significant and innovative contribution to music and health research.

Peter Duncan is a freelance lecturer, writer and consultant working in the fields of health promotion and public health, and Visiting Senior Research Fellow at King's College London, UK. His research interests are focused on the theory, history and ethics of public health and health promotion. Peter's publications include *Critical Perspectives on Health* (2007) and *Values, Ethics and Health Care* (2010).

Mat Jones is a Senior Lecturer in Health, Community and Policy Studies at the University of the West of England, Bristol, UK. He combines a lecturing role in the fields of social science, health studies and public health with a wide range of externally commissioned research. Mat specializes in mixed method studies of complex community health initiatives, particularly centred on food, health and sustainability in school settings. It also encompasses wider agendas on health inequalities, wellbeing and social inclusion. His current academic interests include the relationship between gardening, cultural spaces and the public sphere in late modernity.

Lynne Kennedy was Lecturer in Public Health Nutrition at the University of Liverpool, UK. She had over 15 years' experience in health promotion, with special interests in food and health policy, and the politics of food. Lynne has now retired.

Liz Lloyd is a social gerontologist with particular interest in health and social care policies and practices related to ageing and care. Her recent research has included significant life events in old age, care at the end of life and maintaining dignity in later life. She is currently the Principal Investigator (UK) in an international project Healthy Ageing in Residential Places. Liz has published widely on ageing and the ethics of care, including *Ageing, Health and Care: A New International Approach* (2012).

Anne Mulhall was an independent research consultant. Her previous posts included Senior Scientific Officer at Queen Charlotte's Hospital, London, and Deputy Director of the Nursing Practice Research Unit, University of Surrey, UK. Her particular interests were evidence-based practice, the dissemination and implementation of research, ethnography, epidemiology and infection control. Anne has written three books on nursing research. Anne has now retired.

Jennie Naidoo has recently retired from her post as Principal Lecturer in Public Health and Health Promotion at the University of the West of England, UK, where she was a member of an interdisciplinary team delivering the MSc Public Health programme. Her background is in sociology and health promotion practice. Jennie has co-authored several bestselling textbooks on health promotion and public health.

Jane Ogden is a Professor in Health Psychology at the University of Surrey, UK, where she teaches psychology, nutrition and dietetics, and carries out research into areas such as eating behaviour and obesity, communication and women's health. She has published six books, including *Health Psychology: A Textbook* (2nd edn, 2000) and *The Psychology of Eating: From Healthy to Disordered Behaviour* (2nd edn, 2010), both bestsellers in their field. Jane has just published her first book for parents, *The Good Parenting Food Guide* (2014), which aims to help parents encourage their children to eat well without making food into a problem.

Bob Pitt is Senior Lecturer in the Department of Health and Social Sciences at the University of the West of England, UK. He has experience teaching social policy to a diverse range of UK and international students at undergraduate and postgraduate level including health professionals and social workers. Bob's background is in community work and community education, where he has worked on oral history and reminiscence projects with older people in Bristol. His research interest is on the educational journeys of adults returning to learn in further and higher education.

Hilary Scott worked in health and other public services at local, regional and national levels for more than 30 years. After several years as an NHS chief executive, she was appointed Deputy Health Service Ombudsman and then worked on the programme to reform the complaints and clinical negligence procedures at the Department of Health. She was an independent consultant for many years, helping organizations speak with people who have been affected by an error, or had cause to make a complaint, in a thoughtful and straightforward way. Hilary has now retired.

Katherine E. Smith is a Reader at the Global Public Health Unit in the School of Social and Political Science at the University of Edinburgh, UK. Her research focuses on analysing policies affecting public health (especially health inequalities) and better understanding the relationships between public health research, policy, advocacy and lobbying. Katherine recently brought some of this work together in *Beyond Evidence-based Policy in Public Health: The Interplay of Ideas* (2013), part of a new book series, Palgrave Studies in Science, Knowledge and Policy, which she co-edits with Professor Richard Freeman.

Vicki Taylor has worked in public health since 1985 in a range of different roles at local, regional and national levels, and is now Director of the Roundhouse Consultancy MK Ltd, which specializes in public health development, leadership and management. She is an assessor for the UK Public Health Register. Vicki provides support for the Public Health Wales Public Health Practitioner's Scheme and has previously supported public health practitioner development schemes in England. Vicki is series editor and author for the Transforming Public Health series on core public health competences and public health practitioner standards.

Martin Walter was employed in the NHS in laboratory work, computing, management and staff training for some 33 years. From 1988, he was Senior Lecturer at London South Bank University, teaching health services management studies to both UK and international students. He then worked as a freelance lecturer and consultant, and has now retired.

Jane Wills is Professor of Health Promotion at London South Bank University and has over 20 years' experience teaching and researching public health and health promotion. She co-authored, with Jennie Naidoo, the bestselling *Foundations for Health Promotion* (3rd edn, 2009), and has acted as adviser to the Department of Health, Royal Society of Public Health and several public health departments on workforce development and strategy. She is an experienced facilitator and expert educator in numerous skills areas, including social marketing and behaviour change, communication and evidence-informed practice. Jane's current research interests include what works to enable practitioners to support individuals to change.

Acknowledgements

The editors would like to thank all the contributing authors for their willingness to contribute again to this book. As always, thanks go to our families for their patience and support.

The authors and publisher would like to thank the following organizations for permission to reproduce copyright material:

The American Psychological Association for permission to reproduce Figure 4.7 'Model of Behaviour Change' from Prochaska and DiClemente (1982) 'Transtheoretical therapy: toward a more integrative model of change', *Psychotherapy: Theory Research and Practice* 19(3): 276–88.

The Health and Social Care Information Centre for permission to reproduce Figure 3.5 'Prevalence of obesity (BMI > 30 kg/m^2) among adults in England by gender, 1993–2012', from HSE (2012) Trend Tables.

The Leadership Academy for permission to reproduce Figure 10.3. The Healthcare Leadership Model and associated graphics are ©NHS Leadership Academy, 2013. All rights reserved.

The World Health Organization for permission to reproduce Figure 6.3 'Prevalence of overweight, ages 20+, age standardized, both sexes, 2008', Global Health Observatory map gallery, available at http://gamapserver.who.int/mapLibrary/Files/Maps/Global_Overweight_BothSexes_2008.png (2013).

Contains public sector information licensed under the Open Government Licence v3.0.

Abbreviations

A&E	accident and emergency
AIDS	acquired immune deficiency syndrome
BMI	body mass index
BSE	bovine spongiform encephalopathy
CCG	clinical commissioning group
CLBP	chronic lower back pain
CPS	Crown Prosecution Service
DH	Department of Health
DHSS	Department of Health and Social Services
DNA	deoxyribonucleic acid
EIDs	emerging infectious diseases
FTO	fat mass and obesity-associated gene
GDP	gross domestic product
GI	glycaemic index
GI tract	gastrointestinal tract
GIS	geographic information systems
GMC	General Medical Council
GNP	gross national product
GP	general practitioner
GPS	geographic positioning system
HFSS	high fat, salt and sugar (foods)
HIV	human immunodeficiency virus
HSCIC	Health and Social Care Information Centre
HSE	Health Survey for England
ICD	International Classification of Diseases
IVF	in vitro fertilization
LLSI	limiting long-standing illness
MRSA	methicillin-resistant Staphylococcus aureus
NCMP	National Child Measurement Programme
NHS	National Health Service
NICE	National Institute of Health and Clinical Excellence
NMC	Nursing and Midwifery Council
NS-SEC	National Statistics Socio-Economic Classification
ONS	Office for National Statistics
PCT	primary care trust
PESTLE	political, economic, sociocultural, technological, legal and environmental
PFI	public finance initiative
PTSD	post-traumatic stress disorder

QAA	Quality Assurance Agency for Higher Education
QALY	quality adjusted life year
RCT	randomized controlled trial
SARS	severe acute respiratory syndrome
UN	United Nations
WHO	World Health Organization

Introducing health studies

Health studies has the virtue of being a broad and interdisciplinary subject area that allows students to focus on the central topic of health without being confined to any one discipline. This book demonstrates how different disciplines construct health in different ways and have different ways of studying what health is and how it may be understood. This third edition of *Health Studies* has been revised and updated to ensure its continuing relevance and a new chapter on geography has been included.

This introductory book will help the reader to:

- Become familiar with a variety of perspectives on health issues

- Explore different constructions of health and its management for individuals and populations

- Relate these perspectives to the ways in which health and social care services could and should be organized

- Use these different perspectives to explore key health issues and contemporary challenges

- Understand the different research methodologies and methods that may be used to study health

- Be guided to areas that merit further study.

What is health studies?

Health studies is a field of enquiry that draws on theoretical perspectives from a wide range of **disciplines** or branches of knowledge. In some cases, it encompasses a study of health through a relatively traditional foundation course in social sciences. Elsewhere, interdisciplinary health studies courses emphasize, through a focus on specific topics, the many ways in which health may be understood and studied through the use of different academic disciplines. While there may be few apparent academic links between departments of economics, psychology or management, the concept of 'health' is studied in many different programmes and curricula, ranging from health studies, health sciences and health and wellbeing, to more vocational programmes such as health promotion and nursing. Some programmes select a combination of subject disciplines. It is the breadth of analysis and evidence that distinguishes health studies from being simply the application of any particular subject discipline to health.

As a unifying concept to facilitate interdisciplinary understanding, health studies has several unique strengths:

1. Health studies focuses on health but without any a priori ranking of different disciplines. Health studies therefore allows for creative exploration and collaboration around health needs and healthcare.

2. Health studies encourages interventions to take place in different disciplines, professions and organizations simultaneously. This achieves a synergistic effect – the whole effect being greater than the sum total of the different component parts.

3. Health studies allows creativity and exploration to flourish. Creativity is fostered when the accepted truths or ways of working are challenged by different perspectives within an overall attitude of mutual knowledge and respect.

A focus on health

This book is about the study of **health**. Most students probably have a clear idea of what they will be studying when they look at health. Yet, as individuals, groups and societies, our understanding of health differs and varies according to the context and situation. For example, a young female nursing student might tap into different meanings of health according to whether she is conducting experiments in the laboratory with her tutor group (biology), discussing dieting with her friends (cultural), trying to persuade a patient to quit smoking (psychology and health promotion) or lobbying for better transport to and from university (social policy, environmental science and geography). All these different meanings of health are valid within their own context. However, some definitions are more popular and more widely used than others. Historically and culturally, an objective, biological construction of health, derived from science and medicine, has dominated Western countries' concepts of health. But this dominant definition of health may be challenged by social understandings that see health as socially produced, and by holistic approaches that take biological, psychological and social factors into account.

Health can be defined as an objective and a subjective phenomenon. In objective terms, health is the normal functioning of biological entities. Normal functioning is assessed via the measurement of physical bodies, organs or systems, for example body mass index (BMI) measurements and blood pressure rates. Health may also be defined in relation to populations, for example disease prevalence rates. Health is also defined in subjective terms, which in turn are affected by one's nationality, age, gender and social class. For example, most children see health as 'eating the right things' and 'being fit', whereas older people define health more in terms of 'being able to cope' and continue to do daily tasks and activities.

Health can also refer to a number of different categories or entities, ranging from the cellular or organ focused (e.g. healthy hearts), the individually focused (e.g. healthy body and healthy mind), the socially focused (e.g. healthy societies with high levels of social capital and wellbeing) to the environmentally focused (e.g. sustainable housing and renewable energy sources). This diversity of meaning ensures that the concept of health is relevant to a wide range of disciplines and practitioners. However, it may also lead to confusion and misunderstanding if people attempt to use their definition of health in different contexts and situations.

One solution would be to have an overarching definition of health that encompasses all the different disciplinary and contextual meanings of health. Attempts have been made to do this. A holistic view of health was encapsulated in the World Health Organization's (WHO, 1946) definition:

> Health is a state of complete physical, mental and social well-being, not merely the absence of disease or infirmity.

In this definition, health may seem idealistic and unattainable but its frequent quotation reflects its symbolic significance in highlighting the importance of a multidimensional positive view of health. Other definitions suggest that health can be viewed in terms of resilience and the capacity of individuals, families and communities to cope successfully with risk or adversity. The following pronouncement from the WHO (1984, p. 1) emphasizes the dynamic and aspirational nature of health and its many social and environmental correlates:

> [Health is] the extent to which an individual or group is able, on the one hand, to realise aspirations and satisfy needs; and on the other hand, to change or cope with the environment. Health is, therefore, seen as a resource for everyday life, not the objective of living; it is a positive concept emphasising social and personal resources, as well as physical capacities.

The WHO Constitution from 1946 also states that health is a human right: 'The enjoyment of the highest attainable standard of health is one of the fundamental rights of every human being.' Violations of this right, such as violence against women or harmful traditional practices such as female genital mutilation, result in ill health. Vulnerability to ill health can also be reduced by the assertion of other rights to, for example, water, food and nutrition, information and education.

A consequence of the diversity of definitions of health is that the scope of health studies is vast, and although there is no consensus on what disciplines should be included or excluded, it will certainly include far more than a medical study of illness or disease or training in the care of the sick. Inevitably, this book presents a selection of disciplines that contribute to health studies. In the absence of a commonly accepted syllabus, the rationale for inclusion was to demonstrate the breadth of health studies and include what we perceive to be key contributory disciplines. A brief synopsis of the disciplines included in this book follows.

The disciplinary context of health studies

Many disciplines contribute to our knowledge and understanding of health. They also offer a range of perspectives about what is important in relation to health. Each of the twelve chapters in this book focuses on a specific discipline and its contribution to health within the broad subject area of health studies. Each chapter explains why the discipline is important to the study of health and provides a critical understanding of the conceptual and methodological insights offered by the discipline. Reading the book as a whole will demonstrate that simplistic and arbitrary separations of disciplines are unsatisfactory to explain the complexity of health. For example, life course epidemiology demonstrates sociobiological pathways whereby adverse childhood socioeconomic position is associated with postnatal lung function and subsequently with poor adult lung function through its effects on immune function and the likelihood of exposure to infectious agents. Repeated childhood infections may result in adverse educational attainment and lower adult socioeconomic position (Ben-Shlomo et al., 2014). Likewise, Conrad and Jacobson (2003) offer a fascinating and complex discussion of the overlap and links between biological and social perspectives using the example of cosmetic surgery. Cosmetic surgery may be used by women to enhance their social position as well as to conform to media-created notions of beauty. The area of biogenetics raises fundamental questions about the practicalities and realistic expectations of genetically tailored cures for diseases and the ethics of ownership and access to such knowledge, and the funding and management of the global project. While biogenetics is firmly embedded within the disciplines of biology and physiology, its impact and usefulness will depend on many factors that are addressed by different disciplines, for example social policy, economics, organizational studies and ethics. These examples of projects that span biology and social sciences demonstrate how, in real life, health issues are interdisciplinary. In order to understand and engage with these issues, and achieve results, people need to be able to transcend disciplinary boundaries and become familiar with using interdisciplinary perspectives.

Health is regarded as a key issue by each of these different disciplines. For each, health, or some particular aspect of health, has come under investigation, albeit in different ways. Thus, health studies is deemed by the Quality Assurance Agency for Higher Education (QAA) to be both 'multidisciplinary' and 'interdisciplinary'. These terms, along with the term 'interprofessional', are used interchangeably. Health studies can be seen as **multidisciplinary**, in that the insights and understanding of various discrete disciplines are combined to focus on a particular problem or experience, such as obesity. **Interdisciplinary** denotes relationships between and among the disciplines and implies added value by integration. Interdisciplinary study enables different perspectives on an issue such as obesity, just as one sees different facets of a crystal by turning it. The term **transdisciplinary** is increasingly used to describe the development of conceptual frameworks that use concepts, methods and questions that transcend traditional disciplinary boundaries to answer key issues. Working across disciplinary boundaries can be challenging for the student, as it means being able and willing to go beyond one's 'home' discipline and accept other disciplines' constructions of health as valid, meaningful and helpful.

In Western societies, health is frequently associated with the presence or absence of disease or illness. This derives from the dominance of medicine that offers a framework of scientific knowledge and understanding of the body. The body is understood to be an objective biological structure composed of different component parts and connecting pathways. Health and disease are objective states that are capable of being scientifically proven. Health is the normal functioning of the biological components of the body, whereas disease is manifested through signs and symptoms in parts of the body indicating a pathological abnormality. Someone has a disease if tests can verify the presence of a disease process such as a compromised immune system. The scientific biological concept of health is explored by S.H. Cedar in Chapter 1.

The scientific view of health has not always been the case. Health has been defined differently in different historical epochs. In ancient times, the Greeks defined *hygieia* (health) and *euexia* (soundness) as the ideal balance between the four bodily 'humours' of blood, phlegm, yellow bile and black bile. In the sixteenth and seventeenth centuries, scientists began increasingly to view the body as a machine that could be reduced to its component parts. This paradigm shift was underwritten by Descartes' (1596–1650) famous treatise, which proposed that the body and the soul are separate. 'Cartesian dualism', as this is called, allowed the corporeal body to be freed up for exploration through the methods of scientific study. This legitimized the exploration of the human body through dissection, something that had already been described by Vesalius in 1543. There followed a general trend towards empiricism (the idea that knowledge derives from observation or experiments rather than from theory). Historical concepts of health are discussed in Chapter 2 by Louise Hill Curth.

Epidemiology, the study of patterns of disease within populations, is particularly linked to public health. Epidemiological data contribute to the health agenda by identifying and prioritizing particular health problems according to their contribution to mortality and morbidity. Analysing patterns of disease and correlating these with the distribution of risk factors in populations can help identify the causes of ill health and disease. Once causes and risk factors have been identified, strategies to address these factors and thereby improve the health of populations can be planned and implemented. Epidemiology uses the techniques of scientific enquiry and quantitative study designs to identify relationships between risk factors and resulting diseases, and is the subject of Chapter 3 by Nicola Crichton and Anne Mulhall.

Epidemiological data confirm a link between socioeconomic status and health and the existence of social inequalities in health. However, knowing someone's socioeconomic status or risk factors cannot predict either their objective state of health or their subjective perception of health. Subjective perceptions are affected by people's knowledge, attitudes and behaviour, and this field of enquiry is studied in psychology. Psychological explanations for health acknowledge that mental functioning affects behaviour and both may be influenced by wider social factors. Health psychology aims to understand and explain the role of psychological factors in the cause, progression and consequence of health and illness. Many health promotion and disease prevention programmes focus on trying to persuade people to change their behaviour and make healthier choices. These programmes are informed by theoretical models of behaviour change and personality traits drawn from the discipline of psychology. In Chapter 4, Jane Ogden explores what contributes to people's behaviour and how the views of patients may differ from those of health professionals.

While the impact of social class on health has been extensively researched and documented, there is increasing recognition and documentation of the effect on health of other structural factors such as gender, sexuality and ethnicity. Social factors are not just important predictors of health status, they can also be powerful agents of health improvements. McKeown's (1976) historical analysis showed that socioeconomic factors, such as improved sanitation, nutrition and general improvements in living conditions, were more significant in improving health than medical advances or health services. Supranational economic policies, globalization and the commodification of influences on health also impact on health (www.who.int/social_determinants). Sociology is concerned not just with objective phenomena, but also with the social construction of meaning. This branch of sociology has investigated topics such as the social construction of the body and the meanings we give to medical surveillance. In Chapter 5, Mat Jones and Norma Daykin discuss the contribution of sociology to health studies, focusing particularly on the evidence and debates concerning health inequalities in modern society.

A person's geographical location also affects their health. Chapter 6 shows how the study of geography can explore ecological approaches that focus on how the natural, built and social environments impact on health. Peter Anthamatten explores how health issues such as the emergence of infectious diseases may be linked to farming and irrigation practices, and how the influence of global warming on human health is of growing importance and concern. The geographical approach to the study of health considers how changing relationships between people and their environments influence human health and suggests that health is not merely a biological interaction between a pathogen and human host, but a process that is situated among social factors.

It is common nowadays to think of health and ill health as an individual experience – personal and unique. However, these individual perceptions and experiences are in turn shaped and moulded by cultural norms, concepts and meanings that are evident in language and popular media representations. Individual perceptions and experiences draw on shared meanings that are current in the common culture of our social group or wider society. For example, a disease like cancer is often seen as an uncontrolled invasion of our body and self by an alien entity (Sontag, 1989). Wellness is frequently expressed through independence and control. The growing interest in the body reflects our emphasis on the individual and it is through our bodies that we express and shape our identity. In Chapter 7, Sarah Burch uses culture, expressed through language and visual signs, as a focus through which to explore health and illness.

The protection and promotion of health and the detection and treatment of illness are key functions of modern democratic governments. Government responsibility in this area is reflected in legislation and policy-making to protect and promote people's health, and the provision of health and social care services. Politics – the study of how power and ideological commitment are organized in society to achieve changes in policy – is therefore relevant to health. Health and healthcare services are contested issues, with political parties adopting different ideological stances on the extent of entitlement and how services are resourced. Typically, socialist groups have promoted a more interventionist role for government, leading to the charge of being a 'nanny state'. Conservative groups have been more laissez faire and 'hands off', leading to the charge that they have let big businesses promote wealth to the detriment of health. In Chapter 8, Clare Bambra, Katherine Smith and Lynne Kennedy examine the political context and processes in which decisions about healthcare policies and services are made and implemented, and explore some of the ideological views underpinning different political stances.

Social policies can promote health in diverse ways, ranging from protecting individual incomes and access to personal health and welfare services, to promoting sustainability and regeneration in neighbourhoods. However, health has to compete against other priorities, such as economic growth, in the policy-making arena. The need to rationalize the rising costs of healthcare has been a major feature of most health policy through the developed world. In Chapter 9, Bob Pitt and Liz Lloyd discuss different views on service provision and the emergence of a welfare state in the UK. Recent challenges to the welfare state, from both the left and right political parties, are identified and discussed. Health policy is a complex process involving different groups, agendas and lobbying. Chapter 9 examines the policy-making process from initiation and development, through implementation to evaluation and monitoring.

Policy is translated on the ground into everyday practices and routines. Practitioners who are concerned with treating ill people and/or promoting and protecting health are typically employees in large organizations. Practitioners' professional and academic knowledge and skills are mediated by their employing organization and its priorities, rules of conduct and resource constraints. In Chapter 10, Vicki Taylor, Hilary Scott and Martin Walter discuss organization and management issues and their impact on health. This chapter illustrates how and why health services change and looks at the organization of healthcare and why national systems may differ in their degree of centralization or local autonomy. The marketization of the NHS has led to a new focus on management, monitoring and audit within the NHS, and a growing appreciation of the importance of sound organization and management skills in practice.

Deciding priorities in terms of health-related government spending is difficult. Many different factors need to be taken into account: epidemiological patterns of disease and illness; whether or not effective strategies and treatments are available; the acceptability of such strategies and treatments; and the capacity to provide services and treatment according to need. Health economics has developed as a discipline in response to the need to make reasonable decisions about spending and rationing of resources in the health field, and is the subject of Chapter 11 by David Cohen. In the past two decades, economists have been active in deciding priorities in resource allocation. While cost reduction is a major incentive, efficiency is a broader criterion in which resources are used to maximize specific outcomes. The discourse in health economics of cost utility, cost–benefit analysis and quality adjusted life years suggests an objective and rational approach and one where the objectives are agreed. David Cohen argues that health economics is the only ethical approach to resource allocation and 'hard decisions'. Complex decisions can, he argues, be reduced to objective and quantifiable comparisons of cost and benefit. However, there is always more demand than capacity, leading to continuing debate about whether NHS services should be available according to need or the ability to pay.

Rationing dilemmas are just one example of the kinds of ethical and legal problems that face health professionals. Increasingly, health workers and services are being held responsible for the services they provide and this means they can be held to be negligent if, for example, they do not provide the appropriate quality or level of care. The advances in technological medicine mean that healthcare workers are faced with decisions about the nature and value of life and under what circumstances it is ethical to end or sustain life. In Chapter 12, Peter Duncan explains why it is important that anyone studying health explores ethical and legal concepts and issues, and has a framework for exploring the value base underlying their own actions. While practitioners working in the field of health are typically seen as altruistic, their practice cannot always be assumed to be wholly beneficial, and there are many cases where it is debateable whether one is doing good or harm. Recent examples include euthanasia and research involving the cloning of cells. The extent to which people should be allowed their autonomy in choosing lifestyles, given their impact on health and health services, is also debated within this chapter. The field of ethics and law provides a means of debating such issues, drawing on core ethical principles to try to unpick the complexities of modern health issues.

Investigating health

Most further and higher education is provided in terms of different academic disciplines, for example economics, psychology, politics. These academic disciplines are discrete areas of knowledge characterized by specific theoretical concerns and allegiance to particular types of methodology. An academic discipline centres on a particular definition of what is deemed worthy of knowing and what constitutes truth or reality, whether this is the causal relationship between a factor and an outcome (science) or the language and meanings that are used by individuals and are attributed to a particular phenomenon (social science). This is referred to as **ontology**. There are also different views about what represents knowledge and how that knowledge is produced and how it can be explored or measured. Each discipline has accepted ways of knowing or finding out about truth or reality, referred to as **epistemology**. Each of the disciplines presented in this book is located within different **paradigms** or ways of seeing the world. Each, therefore, poses different sorts of questions and requires different methods for answering them. Part 2 of each chapter discusses theoretical and methodological perspectives and you will find extended discussions of different methodologies ranging from scientific methods (Chapter 1), epidemiological study designs (Chapter 3) to social constructionism (Chapter 4).

Traditionally, a scientific approach tries to identify the cause of the phenomenon being studied, for example an illness, and aims to produce predictive models that say that in certain circumstances X will happen. It does this through the observation and measurement of variables, ideally in the context of a randomized controlled investigation. Epidemiology, physiology, economics and psychology all use this kind of approach and use scientific methodologies. Geographers use maps to show spatial patterns and analyse information. This scientific approach is associated with the philosophy of **positivism**. Positivism assumes that there are objective, external realities that can be known and understood, using appropriate scientific methodologies. Social and natural sciences have a common logical framework, which tries to understand the relationship or association between different variables. The quest to understand *why* something happens varies according to different disciplinary values. For example, a physiologist may be interested in the physical reactions that take place under stress, while a psychologist might be interested in why certain situations are perceived as stressful.

According to **social constructionism**, there is no single, fixed reality, but people have many different descriptions and accounts of health. We all try to interpret our experiences and learn to understand 'what health is' (for us). Thus, we can begin to understand health as a social product, influenced and formed by class, political processes and values, historical antecedents, gender, family life and so on. People's 'worlds of meaning' are also shaped by, and reflected in, all the customs and practices of the culture and society they live in. We can begin to understand this by looking at accounts of health and illness in discourses, narratives and media representations. The chapters on sociology, cultural studies, history and politics explore this approach to understanding.

Sociology and social policy may subscribe to science and social constructionism, using a scientific approach and quantitative data while advocating a critical stance towards such data. For example, the mortality rates of different social groups tell us that mortality is linked to employment status but do not reveal the mechanisms linking the two. Such data may also obscure the impact of other factors that may be equally important, such as gender or ethnicity. This may lead us to further questions: Why is data on social class more widely available than data on gender or ethnicity? How do data sets construct social class? Is social class primarily an economic or social concept?

While a scientific approach is appropriate for some questions, other questions demand a different approach. Exploring people's core values, ideals and principles calls for **interpretivist** methodologies that investigate the meanings people construct and maintain. In-depth investigation of small numbers of people, key events or written accounts are more rewarding if this kind of information is sought, although it cannot be claimed that such information is generalizable to whole populations. In their different ways, management, history, ethics and law, sociology, social policy, cultural studies and politics all use these kinds of methodologies.

Disciplines are also characterized by having accepted valid and systematic principles that guide inquiry or research known as **methodologies.** A distinction is often drawn between quantitative and qualitative methodologies. At its simplest, it has been argued that quantitative methodologies use numbers, whereas qualitative methodologies use words. Quantitative methodologies typically adopt a positivist approach, assuming that there is an objective reality waiting to be discovered, whereas qualitative methodologies typically adopt an interpretive approach, assuming that reality is socially constructed by people and society. It has also been argued that this distinction is unhelpful, and should be replaced by a focus on the aims of the research that distinguishes between exploratory and confirmatory research. Exploratory research seeks to find out new knowledge and insights about areas of interest, whereas confirmatory research sets out to test existing theories or hypotheses. Exploratory research tends to be qualitative, whereas confirmatory research tends to be quantitative. **Methods** are the specific research techniques used to collect and analyse data. Surveys and questionnaires are examples of research methods used in quantitative studies. Observations, interviews and focus groups are examples of methods used in qualitative studies.

Each chapter of the book focuses on different questions of importance in relation to health and Part 2 of each chapter discusses some of the methodologies and research approaches used to investigate health issues. What you may notice is the wide range of issues that are researched in relation to health. Reading through this book, you may find that some perspectives appeal to you more than others. Depending on your background, experiences and values, you may find some approaches immediately resonate more powerfully. The content of some perspectives will be more compelling and interesting than others, and you may also be more sympathetic to certain kinds of investigations or methodologies. Take, for example, the disciplines of sociology and biology – two contrasting academic disciplines that approach the study of health differently. Sociology is a social science that focuses on the study of social life; how society works, and how people function as social beings; and in relation to health it explores the social construction of health through the application of concepts such as social capital, liberty, democracy and equality. The focus is on communities of people and what enhances their collective health and wellbeing, as an objective and subjective concept. It may explore this from positivist through to interpretivist paradigms, from objective reality, for example studies of effects of income on health status, to socially constructed reality, for example what health means to individuals. Biology is a natural science that studies people as biological entities, with a focus on internal biological systems and components. It sees health as the normal functioning of individual physical beings. It explores such issues within a positivist paradigm, focusing on biological systems that have an objective reality we can discover.

Synthesizing perspectives: food, nutrition, diet and obesity

The value of health studies is that by drawing on many disciplines, it can provide a fuller account of health and begin to challenge existing boundaries of knowledge that lead to partial understandings of health. In order to illustrate the usefulness of the interdisciplinary approach, this book uses the example of food, nutrition, obesity and health as a contemporary health issue.

Nutrition is a key to healthy living, and food and diet embody many cultural and identity factors for people. The widespread adoption throughout the population of unhealthy or inadequate diets that lead to disease or premature death takes on social and national significance. Obesity prevalence has risen dramatically and rapidly over the past 20 years. The WHO (2013) reports that global obesity rates have more than doubled since 1980, and the current worldwide prevalence is estimated to be around 500 million people. An estimated 35% of adults over the age of 20, more than 2 billion people, are reported to be overweight. Obesity affects dimensions of human health in many different ways, leading to psychological costs, such as low self-image and confidence and social stigma, as well as physical costs, such as reduced mobility and poorer quality of life, in addition to premature death from heart attack, type 2 diabetes, pulmonary disorders and some cancers. The worldwide health impacts of obesity now rival those of smoking. The WHO (2013) suggests that 20% of the global burden of disease is due to obesity.

Diet (overeating) and exercise (not enough physical activity) are the two main factors implicated in obesity. Overconsumption of fast foods that are high in fats, salt and sugar and a lack of food consisting of complex carbohydrates, fruit and vegetables are characterized as the diet responsible for the rise in obesity. Low- and middle-income countries are also experiencing dramatically increasing rates of obesity as a result of lifestyle changes, for example urbanization, industrialization and the extension of fast-food outlets, less physical activity particularly due to energy-saving technological changes, and the increased consumption of cheap foods rich in fat and vegetable oils.

During the twentieth century, food production shifted from small farmers to large, centralized agricultural complexes with more emphasis on foods that appeal to mass markets, which comprise cheap ingredients, sugar and highly processed foods. Additionally, the processes of globalization and the integration of economies and societies have directly contributed to dietary changes in poor countries through the production and trade of international goods, foreign involvement in retailing and processing food, and global marketing campaigns (Lang and Heasman, 2004).

Addressing the issue of food and nutrition demands answers to a range of questions:

- What is a healthy diet and is this culturally or historically relative?

- Do people know what constitutes a healthy diet?

- How is obesity defined and measured?

- How easy is it to access foods for a healthy diet?

- What influences individual food choices?

- Is what people eat an entirely individual matter or should governments be concerned?

- What accounts for the rise in overweight and obesity?

- Can people be healthy at every/any size?

- What interventions are effective in promoting healthy eating and addressing obesity?

- What are the economic costs of the rise in overweight and obesity?

- How has globalization contributed to the rise in obesity?

In Figure 0.1, we show how the questions that need to be answered in order to tackle a complex issue such as obesity or nutrition sit within different disciplinary paradigms. These may range from a risk factor analysis of individual lifestyles that give rise to obesity, an economic cost–benefit analysis for the health service, to organizational change analyses suggesting how organizations and workplaces can be more health promoting. What is important for readers is to understand how and why different explanations and interpretations are offered and that these build on, and reinforce, each other. A biomedical perspective is concerned with classification and measurement and the relationship between food and health. The classification of obesity as a disease, although not all people who are obese or overweight are ill, and disputes over the use of BMI measurements to identify obesity reflect the dominance and limitations of this paradigm (Gard and Wright, 2005). On the other hand, social constructionist perspectives are concerned with the meanings and values attached to food and the ways these are reproduced and represented.

We also know that the ability to choose, access and purchase a healthy diet is not the same for all groups, and a social science perspective shows how food and dietary behaviour are affected by socioeconomic status. To arrive at a comprehensive overview of a topic like obesity requires inputs from many different disciplines.

Each chapter illustrates the perspective that discipline offers on obesity with a concluding case study. These include explanations for the rise in obesity from biological, psychological and environmental perspectives; critical analyses of the construction of obesity as a social, political and policy issue; and examples of interventions addressing the rise in obesity, for example the promotion of breast-feeding and its cultural implications and the ban on junk food advertising.

Interdisciplinary health studies is more than just a mixing of different disciplines. The bringing together of insights, knowledge and skills drawn from different disciplines has led to the creation of new areas of knowledge and practice that seek to protect and promote health in innovative and effective ways. Health promotion is a good example of this fertile merging of disciplinary knowledge and draws on epidemiology, psychology, sociology, cultural studies and politics (among other disciplines) to understand and promote the health of populations. The next section discusses health promotion in greater depth in order to illustrate the power and productivity of interdisciplinary health studies.

Health promotion: an example of interdisciplinary practice

Many different professions use interdisciplinary definitions of health. For example, health visitors typically use a combination of physical, psychological and social perspectives to promote the health and wellbeing of children and families. Health promotion is a good example of interdisciplinary practice because it is built on several different academic disciplines and taps into many varied perspectives on health. This brief discussion of health promotion will use healthy eating as an example of a health issue.

A focus on the ways in which health can be enhanced or promoted illustrates the contribution of many of the different disciplines outlined in this book. The term 'prevention', for example, suggests that it is possible to intervene in a causal process and implies that there are particular risks to health we can detect and manage. The identification of risk in preventive health tends to derive from epidemiological data referring to large populations showing that exposure to a particular factor is associated with an increased probability of the relevant disease occurring. For example, obesity is a risk factor for type 2 diabetes, hypertension and coronary artery disease (WHO, 2013). Risk factors such as eating a high-fat or salt diet are then translated into health programmes and become the targets for intervention. Protective factors may also be identified through epidemiological analysis, leading to strategies designed to

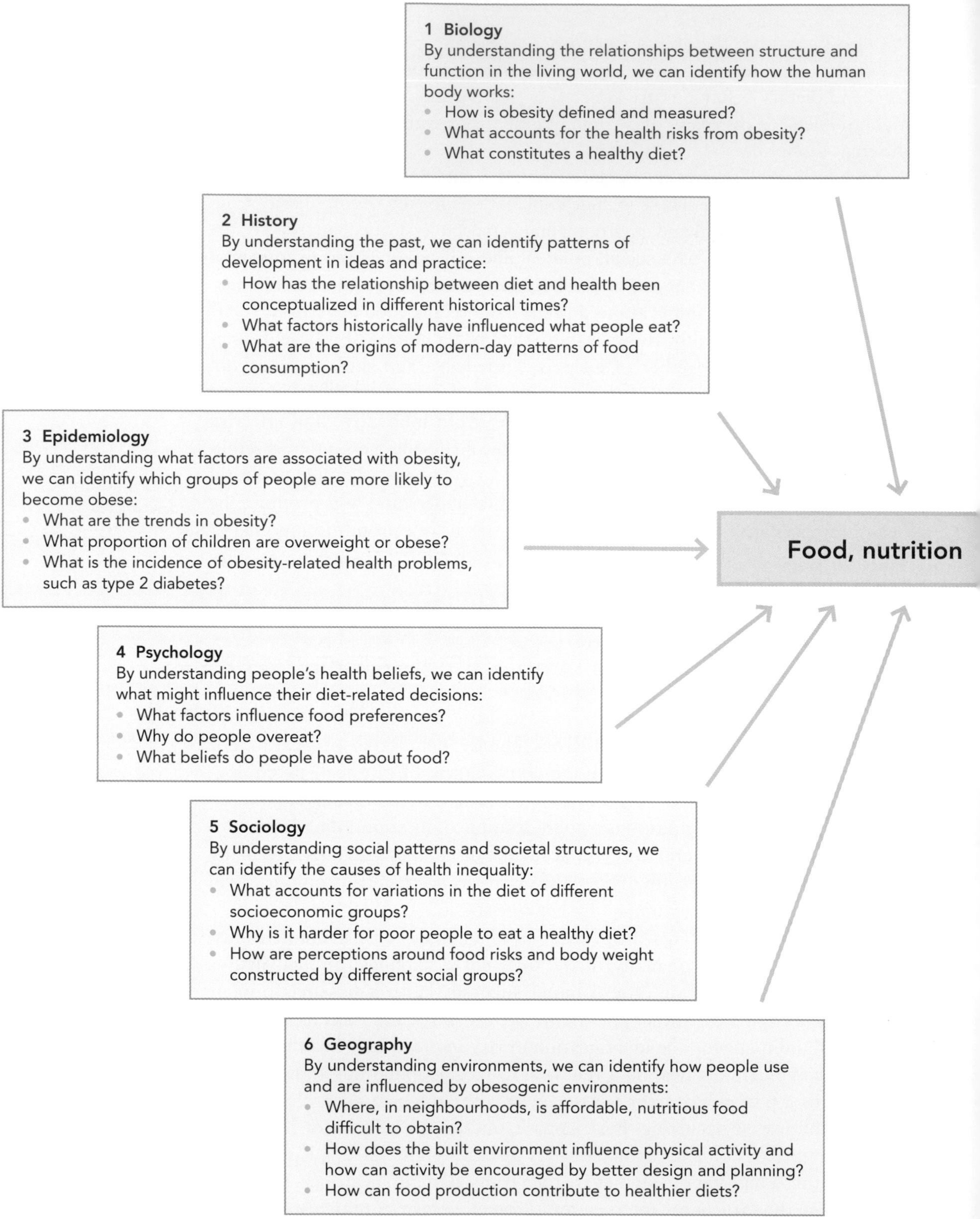

1 Biology
By understanding the relationships between structure and function in the living world, we can identify how the human body works:
- How is obesity defined and measured?
- What accounts for the health risks from obesity?
- What constitutes a healthy diet?

2 History
By understanding the past, we can identify patterns of development in ideas and practice:
- How has the relationship between diet and health been conceptualized in different historical times?
- What factors historically have influenced what people eat?
- What are the origins of modern-day patterns of food consumption?

3 Epidemiology
By understanding what factors are associated with obesity, we can identify which groups of people are more likely to become obese:
- What are the trends in obesity?
- What proportion of children are overweight or obese?
- What is the incidence of obesity-related health problems, such as type 2 diabetes?

4 Psychology
By understanding people's health beliefs, we can identify what might influence their diet-related decisions:
- What factors influence food preferences?
- Why do people overeat?
- What beliefs do people have about food?

5 Sociology
By understanding social patterns and societal structures, we can identify the causes of health inequality:
- What accounts for variations in the diet of different socioeconomic groups?
- Why is it harder for poor people to eat a healthy diet?
- How are perceptions around food risks and body weight constructed by different social groups?

6 Geography
By understanding environments, we can identify how people use and are influenced by obesogenic environments:
- Where, in neighbourhoods, is affordable, nutritious food difficult to obtain?
- How does the built environment influence physical activity and how can activity be encouraged by better design and planning?
- How can food production contribute to healthier diets?

Food, nutrition

Figure 0.1 **Disciplinary perspectives on food, nutrition and obesity**

12 Ethics and law
By understanding what we (individuals and society) value, and whether there are universal moral rules, we can identify principles that can be applied to decision-making, related to why, how and when to intervene in dietary choices:
- What are society's views on the responsibility of obese people for their condition?
- When and why (if ever) should the state intervene in people's food choices?
- What principles should govern food production and trade?

11 Economics
By understanding economic principles, we can identify rational criteria on which to base decision-making related to resource allocation:
- What are the economic effects of obesity on families, health and social care services and society in general?
- What are the most cost-effective ways of preventing, managing and treating obesity?
- What is the comparative burden of obesity with other conditions and how would this be measured?

10 Organization and management
By understanding the ways in which the public sector is organized, we can identify how to deliver more effective and accessible services:
- How can different organizations work together to coordinate food strategies?
- How are food and health policies and obesity strategies developed and implemented?
- What might influence organizations to mainstream food and health concerns?

and obesity

9 Social policy
By understanding the links between ideology, policy process and service provision, we can identify how a range of pressing social concerns may be addressed by government:
- Why is obesity on the current policy agenda?
- How are concerns about obesity framed in current policy?
- How has the role of the state in promoting and protecting the nation's diet changed?

8 Politics
By understanding the processes of conflict resolution, we can explore how the exercise of power influences food choices:
- How has globalization affected food choices and consumption?
- How do different ideologies construct issues of choice and responsibility in relation to food?
- How much influence do food companies have over food policies?

7 Cultural and anthropology studies
By understanding how concepts of health are produced and represented, we are more able to read and decode everyday cultural experiences:
- What contemporary meanings are attached to fatness and thinness?
- What is the popular representation of obesity in the media?
- How do different groups understand a healthy diet?

implement such factors throughout the relevant populations. Eating plenty of vegetables and fruit and daily exercise are examples of protective factors.

The focus on risk factors for disease reflects the clinical approach that emphasizes the importance of the individual patient and the biochemical basis of pathogenesis. The focus of prevention has thus been on manipulating individual risks and has largely ignored the socioeconomic dimension of disease. Eating behaviour is an individual behaviour pattern, but the consumption of fruit and vegetables is also linked to social class, gender, age and ethnicity. Surveys of eating habits, such as the annual Health Survey for England and the National Diet and Nutrition Survey (available at www.noo.org.uk/data_sources/adult), consistently show that there is a strong inverse relationship with socioeconomic status, with people in higher socioeconomic groups eating more fruit and vegetables than those in lower socioeconomic groups.

A central theme of government policy since the 1980s has been that individuals need to take responsibility for their own health and adopt more healthy behaviours, thus reducing the burden of care on the state. Every English public health White Paper (DH, 1998, 2004, 2010) has focused on the responsibility of individuals to make healthier choices. By contrast, the socioeconomic and environmental determinants of individual health-related behaviours have been relatively neglected. In relation to food choices, there has been increased attention to the role of social and environmental influences and a recognition of the 'obesogenic environment' (Foresight, 2007). This is consistent with an ecological model of food consumption, in which behaviour is said to be influenced by the interaction of individual, social and physical environmental variables. For example, incomes in the poorest households have failed to rise in proportion to food costs, and the increased numbers of supermarkets at the expense of local shops has given rise to food deserts in many poor neighbourhoods (see www.poverty.ac.uk/tags/food-poverty).

The English national strategy on obesity, *Healthy Weight, Healthy Lives* (DH, 2008), identified a focus on the early prevention of weight problems to avoid the 'conveyor belt' effect into adulthood, with the focus on children part of government's 'duty of care' to minors. Reducing the consumption of foods that are high in fat, sugar and salt and increasing the consumption of healthier food such as fruit and vegetables, as well as getting people to take physical exercise as a normal part of their day, were also seen as priorities.

Education is often seen as the key to enabling people to change their health-related behaviours. The assumption is that if people are informed about the link between their behaviour and health, they will act in a rational manner and make efforts to change. There have been many reports and campaigns highlighting the negative impact of a poor diet on health (WHO, 2013). However, it is clear that providing such information is, by itself, insufficient to change behaviour. Health promoters recognize that education is only part of the story and tend to adopt a broader view. People's behaviour is based on attitudes, beliefs and cultural and social norms as much as it is based on knowledge. To change behaviour, mindsets and social norms also have to be targeted and changed. This may be achieved in different ways, ranging from social marketing and mass-media campaigns aimed at changing attitudes, such as 5 A Day (www.nhs.uk/livewell/5aday/Pages/5ADAYhome.aspx), to policy-making aimed at changing the environment in which choices and decisions are made, for example banning the advertising of junk food targeted at children or a 'fat tax' on junk food. Health promotion encompasses the whole spectrum of activity and health promoters may be involved in educational campaigns, designing media messages and campaigns, campaigning for organizational change, or political lobbying for policy change. Health promoters have been active in setting up weight loss programmes, food co-ops and food gardens, healthy school meals and the banning of vending machines, and launching mass-media campaigns.

There is no single way to promote healthy eating or tackle obesity. Most interventions are multicomponent, including education and environmental change. For example, a review of healthy eating programmes for teenagers (www.eppi.ioe.ac.uk) detected at least some positive effects on healthy eating but noted that little evidence is available from the UK. The review synthesized evidence from studies of young people's views and found clear views on healthy eating. Barriers to healthy eating included the cost and poor availability of healthy foods and the association of these foods with adults/parents. In contrast, 'fast foods' were widely available, tastier, and associated with pleasure, friendship and being able to exercise choice.

The above account of health promotion approaches to the promotion of healthy eating demonstrates the variety of strategies and the range of disciplines and knowledge underpinning them. It follows that health promoters therefore have to be skilled in various different techniques and approaches. Tackling healthy eating is not the province of any one professional group – be it dieticians, teachers or medical staff. A key requirement, then, is the ability to work successfully with others – to communicate effectively with others, gain support from different key players, and facilitate effective partnership working. To do this successfully requires, in turn, an understanding and recognition of the contribution of the various academic disciplines in which different practitioners are rooted.

Health studies and employability

An additional challenge to interdisciplinary study and practice is that professional identity makes it hard to view and understand the concept of health in new or different ways (Duncan, 2007). Different practitioners and professionals are allied to particular disciplines. For example, sociology underpins social work practice, whereas biology underpins medical practice. Professions are defined in part by their disciplinary knowledge and expertise. The traditional consensual functionalist definition of a 'profession' is of an occupation possessing desirable traits including a body of theoretical knowledge (Parsons, 1954). Critical perspectives on professions retain disciplinary expertise as part of the definition of a professional. For example, Larson (1977) uses the term 'professional project' to refer to members of an occupation working collectively to improve their status and economic position. A key plank in this enterprise is the professional claim to knowledge, ratified through training and registration. Different professions use training and registration to create their own boundaries, reinforcing disciplinary boundaries and thereby magnifying them.

In addition to professional barriers, there are also professional hierarchies. The three traditional professions (medicine, law and the clergy) tend to retain the highest status and position in society. Health is commonly interpreted as healthcare, and healthcare and service delivery have historically been 'owned' by medicine, medical practitioners and nurses. Medicine, informed by biology and science, has dominated the health arena. By contrast, social care, 'owned' by sociology and social workers, has been a relatively subservient aspect of health but is increasingly important and integrated with healthcare.

There are many benefits, academic and practical, to appreciating the concepts, methodologies and insights that different practitioners and professionals bring to bear on health-related issues. Many different practitioners focus on protecting, enhancing and promoting the health of their service users, each in their own unique way. For example, occupational therapists focus on service users regaining the skills and functions that enable independent living, whereas health visitors focus on parenting and the healthy development of children. Multiprofessional or interprofessional ways of working, where different professions work together across professional and organizational boundaries, is commonly cited as a goal for healthcare. The intention of such programmes is to increase mutual professional knowledge, promote teamwork, and encourage multiskilled professionals who can look beyond their particular specialism. Unfortunately, what is often cited as 'interprofessional education' is nothing more than shared learning in which professional groups, for example social workers, health visitors and mental health nurses, may learn together on common core programmes, specialist elements being presented separately for each professional group.

In practical terms, understanding the focus and approach of different practitioners enables and enhances multiprofessional working centred on service users' needs. The basic premise of this book is that working together across disciplinary and professional boundaries has a positive impact on health. Working in partnership with service users and other service providers means health needs can be identified and met in a more holistic and sustainable manner. By engaging in truly interdisciplinary perspectives and action, the health and wellbeing of people will be maximized.

This hierarchy of professions presents yet another barrier to interdisciplinary study and practice. However, in order to aspire towards the provision for service users of seamless care that spans medical and social services, it is important to appreciate the contributions that different professions and disciplines can make towards the promotion of health.

Although health studies has no direct link to a single profession and does not offer a training for a specific role, many students will go on to pursue a career in health and social care, some as frontline practitioners, some in an increasing range of 'lifestyle adviser' posts and some as managers. The value of a broad and fluid approach is recognized in the recent emergence of generic posts that cross specialist and professional boundaries, such as 'children's worker'. By studying health in an interdisciplinary way, through health studies, students who wish to embark on a related career will find themselves better equipped to work with other professionals, patients, managers and the general public. Acknowledging and understanding the diversity of perspectives on the concept of health is the first step in successful partnership working.

The QAA *Subject Benchmark Statement for Health Studies* (2007) includes the following employability skills that can be gained by studying health studies:

- The ability to analyse health and health issues, and health information and data that may be drawn from a wide range of disciplines

- The ability to synthesize coherent arguments from a range of contesting theories relating to health and health issues

- The ability to draw on the personal and lived experience of health and illness through the skill of reflection and to make links between individual experience of health and health issues and the wider structural elements relevant to health.

It is the goal of this book to provide a resource to enable students to attain these skills. Drawing on the contributions from a range of specialist practitioners and academics, this book presents a variety of perspectives and methodologies that address health issues.

Using this book

This book presents each discipline separately, showing what it can contribute to the understanding of 'health'. Each chapter is clearly signposted and structured for ease of reading and study. Key terms are highlighted in bold in the text and the complete Glossary of highlighted terms is at the end of the book. Interspersed in the text are interactive features:

- *Questions* for discussion, reading and exploration as a learning task

- *Thinking about* to enable the reader to use their experience to understand and apply concepts

- *Examples* to illustrate concepts or methodologies or explore contemporary issues

- *Connections* make links to other chapters, flagging up shared concepts or methodologies.

The complex health issue of food, health and obesity is addressed by each discipline in a case study at the end of the chapter. This discussion of a common issue throughout the book suggests that one level of explanation or single field of knowledge is inadequate and encourages the reader towards a more holistic interpretation. By comparing the different disciplines' approaches and strategies to issues regarding food, nutrition and obesity, it is hoped that the reader will appreciate the value of interdisciplinary and multiprofessional ways of working.

We hope this book will provide a tool to encourage students to explore the meaning and promotion of health across different academic disciplines and professions, and thereby contribute to the promotion of health and wellbeing.

References

Ben-Shlomo, Y., Mishra, G. and Kuh, D. (2014) *A Handbook of Epidemiology*. New York: Springer.

Conrad, P. and Jacobson, H.T. (2003) Enhancing biology? Cosmetic surgery and breast augmentation, in S. Williams, L. Birke and G. Bendelow (eds) *Debating Bilology: Sociological Reflections on Health, Medicine, and Society*. London: Routledge, pp. 223–35.

DH (Department of Health) (1998) *Saving Lives: Our Healthier Nation*, Cm 4386. London: TSO. Available at www.gov.uk/government/uploads/system/uploads/attachment_data/file/265576/4386.pdf (accessed 16/3/2014).

DH (2004) *Choosing Health: Making Healthy Choices Easier*, Cm 6374. London: TSO. Available at http://webarchive.nationalarchives.gov.uk/+/dh.gov.uk/en/publicationsandstatistics/publications/publicationspolicyandguidance/dh_4094550 (accessed 16/3/2014).

DH (2008) *Healthy Weight, Healthy Lives*. London: DH. Available at http://webarchive.nationalarchives.gov.uk/20100407220245/http:/www.dh.gov.uk/prod_consum_dh/groups/dh_digitalassets/documents/digitalasset/dh_084024.pdf (accessed 16/3/2014).

DH (2010) *Healthy Lives, Healthy People*, Cm 7985. London: TSO.

Duncan, P. (2007) *Critical Perspectives on Health*. Basingstoke: Palgrave Macmillan.

Foresight (2007) *Tackling Obesities: Future Choices*. Project report. London: Government Office for Science/DH. Available at www.gov.uk/government/uploads/system/uploads/attachment_data/file/287937/07-1184x-tackling-obesities-future-choices-report.pdf (accessed 16/3/2014).

Gard, M. and Wright, J. (2005) *The Obesity Epidemic: Science, Morality and Ideology*. London: Routledge.

Lang, T. and Heasman, M. (2004) *Food Wars: The Global Battle for Minds, Mouths and Markets*. London: Earthscan.

Larson, M. (1977) *The Rise of Professionalism: A Sociological Analysis*. San Francisco: University of California Press.

McKeown, T. (1976) *The Role of Medicine: Dream, Mirage or Nemesis*. Oxford: Nuffield Provincial Hospitals Trust.

Parsons, T. (1954) The professions and social structure, in T. Parsons, *Essays in Sociological Theory*. Glencoe, IL: Free Press, pp. 34–49.

QAA (Quality Assurance Agency for Higher Education) (2007) *Subject Benchmark Statement for Health Studies*. Gloucester: QAA.

Sontag, S. (1989) *AIDS and its Metaphors*. London: Penguin.

WHO (World Health Organization) (1946) *Preamble of the Constitution of the World Health Organization*. Geneva: WHO.

WHO (1984) *Annex 1: A Discussion Document on the Concept and Principles of Health Promotion*. Copenhagen: WHO Regional Office for Europe.

WHO (2013) *Obesity and Overweight*. Fact sheet No 311. Available at www.who.int/mediacentre/factsheets/fs311/en/index.html (accessed 7/11/2013).

S.H. CEDAR

Human biology and health

Overview   23

Introduction   23

Part 1 The contribution of biology to health studies   24
Cell theory   25
Homeostasis   29
Genes and genetics   30
Ill health and disease   33

Part 2 Theoretical and research approaches   36
Induction   38
Deduction   38
Proof and falsification   39
Experimentation   40
Techniques   41

Case study Biological explanations for obesity   43
Summary   46
Questions for further discussion   47
Further reading and resources   47
References   47

Learning outcomes

This chapter will enable readers to:

- Gain an appreciation of the scope of human biology, the framework of homeostasis and health, and the use of biology to examine ill health and disease
- Be aware of the scientific methods used by biologists, bioscientists and biomedical scientists
- Understand how biology can contribute to the analysis of physical aspects of human health

Overview

Natural sciences seek to explain the natural world, while social sciences seek to explain human societies, culture and belief. This book is largely made up of social science disciplines, but because its focus is health, the natural sciences and, in particular, biology, offer a fundamental perspective. Natural science limits what it investigates to the natural phenomena in the universe. It does not investigate human feelings, morals or beliefs as cultural phenomena. Biology contributes to the study of health by providing knowledge of the body's functions and how these are interlinked. These issues are illustrated later in the chapter using a biological analysis of food, nutrition and obesity. Human biology concerns how the body functions in terms of its cells, tissues and body systems. This chapter will briefly explain some biological theories such as the function of cells in all organisms; how each body system contributes to the maintenance of a constant internal environment (homeostasis) for its cells; and gene theory. Most importantly, biology is a science and **science** is an experimental, evidence-based pursuit. The discipline of science dates back about 2,500 years to ancient Greece (Wolpert, 2000). It is derived from the Greek *episteme*, which distinguishes science as knowing not only that something is so, an act of experience, but also why it is so, an act of the 'knowledge of first causes', as Aristotle would say in his *Metaphysics* (Finley, 1963). It uses scientific methods variously described as induction, deduction, falsification and hypothetico-deduction. This chapter will explain the principles and processes of the scientific method.

Introduction

Biology is the science of life (from the Greek words *bios*, life, and *logos*, reasoned account). It is the study of living organisms, what they are made of and how they function, how they interact with each other and with the environment, the effect they have on the environment and the environment has on them. In biology, humans are seen as just one type of organism, one species or race. Species are defined as of one kind when they can breed together and have viable offspring. As all humans can do this, all humans, biologically, are one species or race. In this chapter, while biology applies to all living organisms, it is the human species, *Homo sapiens*, that interests students of health.

Biology is the study of living organisms and their environment. It can be divided into subcategories, such as human biology, immunology, genetics, anatomy and physiology. Anatomy is the study of the structure of organisms, what they look like, their form. It is used in evolutionary biology to see similarities and differences between species and in medicine to see normal, healthy forms from abnormal ones. It can also be used to look at the structures of organs within a body, such as the structure of the heart, lungs or blood vessels. Physiology, meaning the study (*logos*) of nature or origin, is the study of the living processes within an organism, such as breathing, moving, eating, eliminating, growing, reproducing and dying. In fact, these processes are often used as the activities of daily living, which are used to access the ability of a person to maintain an independent, healthy, age-appropriate lifestyle (Cedar, 2012). It includes how the entire organism as well as organs, cells and molecules maintain the system. These physiological processes are carried out by anatomical structures and thus there is a link between the form of an organ and its function. Biology encompasses anatomy and physiology, as well as the subdivisions mentioned previously, and will be used here as the generic study in which human biology and health sit.

Science can be divided into 'pure' (also called 'basic') and 'applied'. Pure or basic science is the description, explanation and understanding of phenomena and this understanding can be applied to many areas. From this, you can understand that science intends to be universal, applicable everywhere. Applied science is the application of pure or basic scientific principles to meet a specific, recognized need, for example biomedical science applies scientific principles and methods to human illness in the hope of treating a disease. In addition to all the specialized applied fields within biology, many applications of biology such as medicine involve many additional specialized subdisciplines. The remit of biology, however, is not to cure human disease, but to understand how living organisms work, their physiology and what life is. Science aims to be politically neutral, objective and reproducible. It also, like philosophy from which it derives, aims to be universal in its findings rather than culturally particular. However, the application of science by society for dangerous or deadly ends, such as the development of the nuclear bomb or indeed genetic engineering, cannot be ignored.

Because the physiology of health relies on biological underpinnings, students of health studies will need to understand the biology and its associated academic disciplines if they want to work later in nutrition or sports or exercise science.

Part 1 The contribution of biology to health studies

example 1.1

Application of biology to contemporary health issues

- To understand the functions of the body
- How the body adapts to its environment such as cold or lack of energy
- The resiliency factors that buffer individuals from changes in their environment

- How health shapes the individual life course and vice versa
- The manifestations of disease and its pathogenesis
- How genetic understanding can improve fertility and protection against disease

Biology is a scientific discipline that contributes to our understanding of the bodily processes and functions that keep us alive in various states of health. The case study example of obesity illustrates how a biological framework can identify the cause of a health problem and contribute to its management or cure. Similarly, a knowledge of the molecular composition of foods and their biochemical behaviour enables effective nutrition for the needs of the person. The distinction between the biological science and its medical application is therefore an important one. Biology studies how a body functions; it is not of itself clinical. Biology informs medicine but has a separate identity. Medicine without an underlying understanding of biology would rely on belief and myth rather than scientific evidence. This chapter demonstrates the use of a biological framework in the analysis of physical and chemical aspects of health. Biology is interested in the normal, functioning organism, but it is often when an organism is not functioning that new ways of seeing how it normally functions are revealed. When an organism is not functioning normally, it is said to be diseased or in ill health and the cause can be investigated. Through this, causes such as infections, traumas, genetics, degenerative diseases and cancers have been discovered.

? What examples are there of biological knowledge contributing to human health?

The biological model shows that health is due to physiological processes in the body and ill health is also due to physiological processes in the body and those biological processes have a chemical (matter and energy) basis. Humans are made of matter and spend a lot of time extracting energy from food; for example, calories are a measure of how much energy some matter, called food, contains. Thus, biology studies the interactions between the internal environment of the body and the external environment in which the body, the organism, lives. It also studies what the body is made from and how that works. All living organisms including humans (but excluding viruses) are made up of cells. Cells are microscopic (can only be seen with a microscope) and can combine to make multicellular tissues, organs and organisms such as humans.

Cell theory

Cells are the smallest functioning unit within which life can be carried out; they are like little chemical factories. Some organisms are composed of just one microscopic cell and are said to be 'unicellular'. Humans are composed of billions of cells and are thus 'multicellular'. Cells arise from other cells through growth in size, doubling of the genetic material within the cell, and division of this genetic material between the two new cells. This form of growth is called 'binary fission', where one cell divides into two. In multicellular organisms, every cell in the organism's body is produced from a single cell in a fertilized egg, which then produces progeny cells by binary fission. These then go on to do the same. Humans are composed of about 10^{13} cells (ten trillion cells), each derived from previous cells by this method. All the cells in the embryo and fetus are thus derived from the fertilized egg cell by binary fission using nutrients from outside the fetus to fuel its growth. Figure 1.1 shows a typical animal cell.

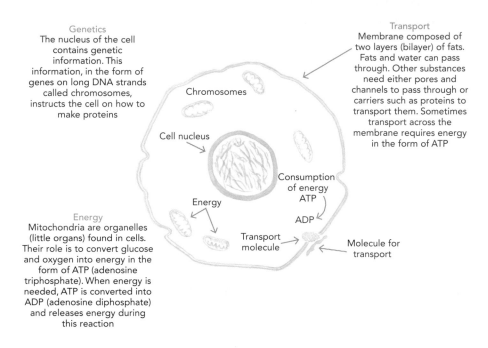

Genetics
The nucleus of the cell contains genetic information. This information, in the form of genes on long DNA strands called chromosomes, instructs the cell on how to make proteins

Transport
Membrane composed of two layers (bilayer) of fats. Fats and water can pass through. Other substances need either pores and channels to pass through or carriers such as proteins to transport them. Sometimes transport across the membrane requires energy in the form of ATP

Chromosomes

Cell nucleus

Consumption of energy ATP

Energy

ADP

Energy
Mitochondria are organelles (little organs) found in cells. Their role is to convert glucose and oxygen into energy in the form of ATP (adenosine triphosphate). When energy is needed, ATP is converted into ADP (adenosine diphosphate) and releases energy during this reaction

Transport molecule

Molecule for transport

Figure 1.1 **A typical animal cell**

Within each cell are little organs, organelles, which carry out the physiological function of the cell. There are organelles, such as the nucleus, that carry the genetic material we inherited from both our parents, which we copy into each cell in our body. The genes carry the information on how to make proteins. In the cytoplasm are ribosomes where the proteins, which consist of long chains of amino acids, are assembled. Also in the cytoplasm are mitochondria, known as the powerhouse of the cell. Mitochondria are organelles that convert foods into energy.

The main source of food for this is sugar, such as glucose, which is brought to every cell in the body from the digestive tract due to the digestion of sugar-containing foods such as carbohydrates. The sugar in the cell reacts with oxygen brought to the cells from the air in the lungs. Both the sugar from the gastrointestinal (GI) tract and the oxygen from the lungs are transported to every cell in the body by the blood. Once in the cell, the sugar and oxygen react in the mitochondria. From this reaction, energy is released as adenosine triphosphate (ATP). This energy is used to fuel all the reactions of the body, such as contracting muscles, including the muscles of the heart that pump the blood and the muscles that open the lungs to allow air to enter, actively transporting substances across cell membranes, producing hormones, and generating resting potentials in the nervous system that allow us to think. Thus, mitochondria are the energy producers of the cell and the body, vital organelles that allow us to function.

Mitochondria have their own genetic material separate from that of the cell, the nuclear genetic material. Errors in mitochondrial genetic material (mtDNA) can have serious consequences on metabolism. This genetic material is inherited maternally and copied into every cell of the body during growth of the embryo and during regeneration of tissue to replace worn-out or damaged tissue. This DNA is susceptible to damage by reactive oxygen species (e.g. free radicals) but has many mechanisms to protect itself.

Tissues are groups of structurally and functionally similar cells. Tissues can be solid such as skin, or liquid such as blood. From the post-embryonic stages onwards, tissues are categorized into four types:

- *Nervous tissue*, comprising
  - the cells that conduct electrical potentials (neurons)
  - the support cells (glia)

- *Muscle tissue*, comprising
  - the skeletal, voluntary muscle we use in locomotion
  - the smooth, involuntary muscle that moves our internal organs, such as the waves of contraction (peristalsis) that move food through the GI tract
  - cardiac muscle that pumps blood into the blood vessels for transport around the body

- *Connective tissue*, comprising many cells types, including
  - bone, cartilage and tendons, as part of the skeleton
  - blood cells and liquid plasma
  - fibroblasts and their secretions, such as collagen and elastin
  - adipose fat tissue
  - dermal layers

- *Epithelial tissue*, comprising
  - epidermis and endodermis, lining outer surfaces such as skin and inner surfaces such as blood vessels and kidney tubules.

Much of biology is interested in how all these different types of tissue arise during development from the fertilized egg cell. Thus, development is not only a case of proliferation of many cells to form the human body, but different types of cells, through a process called 'differentiation'. Biology is also interested in how cell numbers and differences are maintained during homeostasis and health, discussed below.

Organs are specialized structures composed of tissues that carry out certain functions. The heart, for example, is an organ that pumps blood, whereas the stomach is an organ that breaks down food. Organs can work together in systems such as digestion to carry out particular functions involved in sustaining the life of the organism by maintaining optimal conditions for cells, of which the organism and its organs and tissues are composed. A multicellular organism, such as a human, carries out the functions necessary to keep itself alive, as illustrated in Figure 1.2.

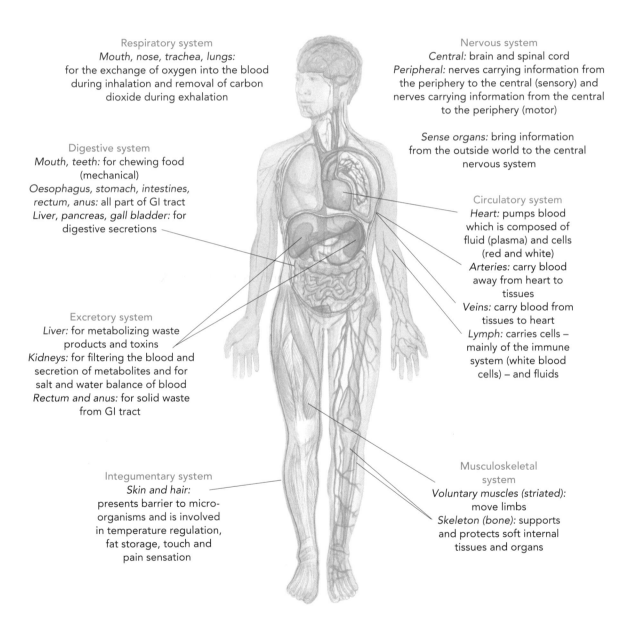

Respiratory system
Mouth, nose, trachea, lungs:
for the exchange of oxygen into the blood during inhalation and removal of carbon dioxide during exhalation

Digestive system
Mouth, teeth: for chewing food (mechanical)
Oesophagus, stomach, intestines, rectum, anus: all part of GI tract
Liver, pancreas, gall bladder: for digestive secretions

Excretory system
Liver: for metabolizing waste products and toxins
Kidneys: for filtering the blood and secretion of metabolites and for salt and water balance of blood
Rectum and anus: for solid waste from GI tract

Integumentary system
Skin and hair: presents barrier to micro-organisms and is involved in temperature regulation, fat storage, touch and pain sensation

Nervous system
Central: brain and spinal cord
Peripheral: nerves carrying information from the periphery to the central (sensory) and nerves carrying information from the central to the periphery (motor)

Sense organs: bring information from the outside world to the central nervous system

Circulatory system
Heart: pumps blood which is composed of fluid (plasma) and cells (red and white)
Arteries: carry blood away from heart to tissues
Veins: carry blood from tissues to heart
Lymph: carries cells – mainly of the immune system (white blood cells) – and fluids

Musculoskeletal system
Voluntary muscles (striated): move limbs
Skeleton (bone): supports and protects soft internal tissues and organs

Figure 1.2 Organs and body systems

thinking about Think about a disease or condition you have read about where a physiological process is said to be involved, for example weight management using low glycaemic index (GI) foods. How could an understanding of digestion be helpful in assessing the role of GI foods?

The introductory chapter highlights how genetics raises many important issues for health in fields such as population-based genetic screening and antenatal care. The ethical and legal issues regarding human embryo research are discussed in Chapter 12. See www.hfea.gov.uk (the Human Fertilisation and Embryology Authority website) for further up-to-date details regarding this issue.   connections

Homeostasis

The external environment varies all the time. Sometimes it is daylight and sometimes night. Sometimes it is hot and sometimes cold. Sometimes it rains and sometimes it is dry. Sometimes there are tornados and earthquakes and sometimes there are floods and volcanic eruptions. Living organisms, however, are composed of cells and cells like a fairly constant environment. Living organisms cannot control the external environment, but they can control their own internal environment. A central concept in biology is the maintenance of a stable internal environment known as **homeostasis**. The body is a hugely complex anatomical structure consisting of cells, tissues and organs that work together to carry out the physiological functions necessary to keep itself alive. All cells, whether from plants, bacteria, frogs or humans, have some common properties and need to carry out certain functions to maintain themselves – to keep themselves alive. In order to carry out these functions, cells must maintain themselves within strict and quite narrow ranges. Humans have cells that function only within a temperature range around 37°C and strict oxygen/carbon dioxide limits. Other cells, such as those of aquatic organisms or plants, have different ranges, but they still need to be kept within their optimal limits for the cell to survive and flourish. When conditions veer outside these limits, life is threatened, and the cell, the organ or the whole organism may die. Knowing what these limits are is part of the subject of biology and health.

The mechanisms enabling a cell to stay within its optimal range are part of a system called homeostasis. In 1865, Claude Bernard first observed that:

It is the constancy of the internal environment which is the condition of free and independent life. All vital mechanisms, however varied they may be, have only one object, that of preserving constant the conditions of life in the internal environment. (Bernard, [1865] 1957)

Bernard's concept remains the framework within which biology and biomedical science operates. Cells are bathed by interstitial fluid, which is their internal environment. This fluid provides nutrients and oxygen to sustain the life of each cell. Waste products from the cell's metabolism are added to the internal environment before being removed to the blood and then disposed of in various ways. If the nutrient and oxygen supply are compromised and waste products accumulate, the cells would clearly die.

The biological model of health, therefore, is one where we maintain ourselves homeostatically, taking in what we require, making new cells and proteins as needed and excreting waste products as appropriate. Sometimes our internal environment is challenged. For example, if we tear our skin, we can heal it ourselves. We may at first bleed, leaking liquids from our body. We may get an infection in the area from bacteria or viruses that enter at the wound site, but we have the immune system that detects and disables outside organisms. We will go through a process of stopping the bleeding, haemostasis, making a scar over the wound to seal it up before making new skin. The paradigm is essentially simple: if something happens to change the internal environment, physiological pathways are in place to reduce the extent of the change and return to the status quo.

connections	Chapter 2 describes how the concept of balance for health has been understood historically.

Genes and genetics

Each cell contains genetic information within its nucleus. This information is specific to itself, the individual and the species from which it comes, in our case human. While our genomes, our entire genetic content, may differ from one person to another, 98% of human **genes** are shared by our nearest biological relatives, the apes.

The function of genes is to instruct our cells how to assemble individual amino acids into long polymers called **proteins**, akin to joining letters together to make words. Our genes, of which we have about 30,000, contain information on how to synthesize all the proteins that humans need, each gene containing the instructions for how to make a particular protein (a particular word). Nearly all the functions of our bodies are carried out by proteins. For example, there are a variety of proteins, such as:

- Enzyme proteins that help convert chemicals from one form to another form, which can be used in the body

- Neurotransmitter proteins that convey information in the brain and nervous system

- Transport proteins that carry insoluble material around the body, for example haemoglobin is a transport protein for oxygen.

Proteins can be found in the food we eat – you are what you eat. When we eat, proteins contained in the food are broken down into their individual amino acids and then reassembled into other proteins needed to carry out various body functions. Excess amino acids are further broken down and eliminated in urine. Genes tell our body how to put together amino acids to build proteins. Each cell in the body can synthesize its own proteins to keep itself alive as an independent entity because it has the instruction manual, the genetic material, which is contained in the cell nucleus telling the cell how to do so. The cell can thus generate and maintain itself; it is an independent entity and exists in a community of cells. Organisms are also able to pass on this genetic information from generation to generation via reproduction. If a gene is defective or mutated, it cannot build a particular protein so the function that protein carries out is no longer performed. This is turn can alter the function of a tissue and lead to disease or ill health.

In the twentieth century, genetic material was shown to be made of a chemical called deoxyribose nucleic acid (DNA), long polymers of nucleotide bases, held in place by a deoxyribose sugar. The structure of DNA was shown to be a double helix (Watson and Crick, 1953) and its replication was elucidated. As each cell has to copy (double) its genetic content and then divide it between two daughter cells, the growth of cells started to be understood in molecular detail. This understanding of basic biological mechanisms has had a great impact on our understanding of cancer.

example 1.2

Chromosomal and genetic disorders

While we can inherit many genetic disorders, some disorders are due to chromosomes. Chromosomes are the packaging devices of genes. As we have so many genes, they are held on long chromosomes. Humans have 23 pairs of chromosomes (46 in total). One of each pair is donated from the mother, the other from the father. Of these chromosomes, 22 pairs are called 'autosomal' (of the body) chromosomes, while there is one pair that has two distinct versions, the sex chromosomes, X and Y. Some disorders are caused by chromosomal abnormalities. The chromosome numbers, the karyotype, are usually written as 46XY. Abnormal chromosome numbers will thus differ from this. Examples include Down syndrome (extra chromosome 21), Turner syndrome, lacking one sex chromosome (45X0) and Klinefelter's syndrome (a male with two X chromosomes – 47XXY).

Some disorders are caused by the inheritance of defective genes from the parents. In this case, the genetic disorder is known as a 'hereditary disease'. This can often happen unexpectedly when two healthy carriers, each having one copy of a defective recessive gene, reproduce and pass on both defective copies to their offspring. It can also happen when the defective gene is dominant.

A genetic, recessive disease can result in a serious metabolic problem. For example, most of us have a protein with the ability to digest a particular amino acid called phenylalanine. If we cannot break down phenylalanine, it accumulates to toxic levels in our bodies. The resulting disease is called phenylketonurea (PKU). PKU in early development has a deleterious effect on the nervous system. All newborn babies in the UK are tested for the ability to digest phenylalanine (the Hicks test). In the future, biologists hope genetic therapy will replace faulty genes with effective genes that produce the functioning protein.

The human genome project has now plotted the precise sequence of genetic codes in human cells, both nuclear and mitochondrial. It is hoped that this will allow the development of new knowledge on the causes and mechanisms of disease. A relatively simple DNA test can immediately predict whether or not someone will develop cystic fibrosis, for example. But the most common chronic diseases – cancer, diabetes, heart disease, stroke and dementia – are far more complex. Genes do influence their risks, but the inherited component is more in the nature of an increased risk rather than a direct cause as genes act in the environment of the other genes and their products, proteins, in the body and the body interacts with the external environment. Lifestyle factors such as diet and smoking habits, and the environment in which we live and work are also involved.

'Gene therapy' is the term used to describe correcting potentially deleterious genes. While we can now screen and detect many genes, we have not been able to replace them in adults. It would be possible to do so in embryos, but the genetic manipulation of human embryos is not permitted. The ability to carry out routine genetic screening has wider implications that could affect the lives of apparently healthy people. The presence of specific genes may result in individuals having difficulty obtaining life insurance, for example, and some employers (particularly in the US) require potential employees to undergo genetic screening for particular diseases. There are moves to regulate the use of this scientific information by the insurance industry and for changes to employment and anti-discrimination law.

The challenge for molecular biologists following the sequencing of the genome will be to find out what kinds of proteins are encoded in the DNA and, more importantly, what they do in living cells. A new name, 'proteomics', has been coined to cover this field of study, which, it is anticipated, will be technically much more challenging than the sequencing of genetic codes in DNA.

Additionally, the field of epigenetics is showing that genes become reprogrammed during development. This will impact on whether a gene is *expressed*, meaning whether it is translated from the genetic code of DNA into a protein or whether it remains silent and unexpressed in a cell. Obviously, expressing the wrong genes at the wrong time could have deleterious effects in health, such as cancer. Epigenetics and stem cell research are leading new ways of looking at how we develop and maintain our physiologies and thus what goes wrong in ill health.

A limitation to the application of genetic knowledge to health is that most diseases are multifactorial, having many factors such as genes, development and lifestyle. Multifactorial effects can be thought of as similar to continuous characteristics; due to their complexity, they are difficult to assess and it is then hard to ascribe a single gene to a disease. For example, cancers such as breast cancers have been shown to have a linkage to a particular variant of a gene called BRCA 1 or BRCA 2. However, possession of that version of a gene (allele) does not mean that you will get breast cancer, it increases your risk, but so do obesity and other factors (Calderon-Margalit and Paltiel, 2004).

example 1.3

UK Biobank

Biobanks contain blood or cell samples from large numbers of people. Genetic information from each sample is linked to the individual's medical history and lifestyle data. By following their health long term, researchers can work out why some people develop a particular disease while others do not. UK Biobank started in 2006 and will assess and take samples from 500,000 participants aged 40–69 at the start of the study, and then follow their health over subsequent decades. With their informed consent, participants will complete a detailed lifestyle questionnaire, be interviewed about their medical history, have several standard physical measurements (such as blood pressure, body size and lung function), and will donate blood and urine samples. Information about participants' health will then be obtained, with their permission, from medical and other health-related records. As long-term follow-up continues, medical researchers will be able to compare the lifestyle, genes and other factors of participants who develop some particular disease with those participants who do not. For common conditions, such as heart disease and diabetes, this will be possible within 5–10 years (http://genome.wellcome.ac.uk).

Ill health and disease

Diseases are brought about in various ways, the causes of which are the subject of many scientific and medical disciplines. Coronary heart disease, for example, is said to be linked to family history and specific risk factors such as the blood lipid level. The study of biology helps to explain the normal workings of the body and what goes wrong to cause disease. It therefore has a major impact on health and medicine.

Body systems such as the transport, digestive, respiratory and excretory systems are all involved in maintaining the life of the organism. If they do not operate correctly, the internal environment will not be kept under the optimal condition for the body cells and their chemicals to survive. The biological model of ill health is when we do not function homeostatically and are no longer capable of being independent. When the body cannot repair itself and maintain homeostasis (either alone, or assisted with drugs or technological interventions), death ensues.

All living organisms die. Humans die of one of four main causes:

- *Traumas* such as burns or car accidents remove more tissue than we can replace and challenge our homeostasis so far that we cannot recuperate

- *Infections* by microorganisms such as bacteria or viruses destroy tissue and create toxic levels of chemicals or foreign cells in our bodies

- *Degenerative diseases* caused by ageing or lack of vital nutrients (malnutrition) or water, where more cells are lost or energy expended than can be replaced or repaired

- *Cancerous growths* where more cells are made than are needed, thus replacing functioning tissue.

The biomedical model of health and all models of health attempt to increase the health of the individual as well as delay the inevitable, death. This process is carried out by interventions, including the use of chemical compounds called medication (both conventional and alternative), surgery, vaccinations and various manipulations such as physiotherapy. All clinical interventions are an attempt to restore homeostasis and delay death.

In the biomedical model of health, the root cause of an **illness** is sought. Patients present with symptoms (self-reported feelings such as pains that are either dull or sharp, prolonged or acute nausea, diarrhoea, dizziness and so on) and signs (measurable changes such as increased or decreased temperature) that tell them they are unwell. From these, the diagnosis starts to be made as to what is causing these symptoms and signs. Objective and verifiable clinical facts largely based on demonstrable physical changes in the body's structure or function thus form the basis of the doctor's diagnosis. These changes are measured and then compared with a range of normal physiological values. In medicine, disease implies an abnormality of structure or function, the need for correction and the idea that abnormalities are undesirable. Tests may then be run to see if there has been an infection or blockage in blood vessels or altered heart rates, for example. From these tests, a diagnosis may finally be made as to what is causing the problem. Each disease entity has particular characteristics that identify it. Once this has been assessed, a treatment can be instigated. If, for example, one has diarrhoea, it may be due to food poisoning, that is, food infected with microbial organisms. A stool sample may be taken and analysed to see what bacteria, virus or fungi are causing the problem and a drug given to help kill the particular infectious agent. In the meantime, knowing about the GI tract where the food is digested, the clinician will recommend taking in more fluid to avoid the dehydration caused by losing water in loose stools – the large colon (also called large intestine or large bowel) is responsible for the absorption of water from the faeces before defecation. Knowing the basic biology and applying it in medicine allows for diagnosis and treatment.

connections	The biological perspective emphasizes the natural state but in Chapters 4 and 7 a social constructionist view is described, which sees illness, health and disease as all relative concepts, differently experienced. Chapter 7 describes these by reference to culture.

The understanding of health and disease in medicine thus follows a process of:

- Initial diagnosis based on signs and symptoms

- Tests to identify cause, for example X-ray or ultrasound, microbiological tests for infection

- Diagnosis

- Treatment based on interventions known to have a beneficial effect on the condition.

The advantage of a medical model of health is that it is **pathogenic** – it seeks out the cause of a disease. This approach is sometimes called **reductionist**, in that it seeks to explain the experience of ill health in terms of the material functioning of the body, assuming that there is a single cause of a disease and that is what needs eradicating or treating. A biologist would say it is merely seeking the proximal (at close proximity) or ultimate cause of a disease, while a sociologist might look to the environment, whether physical, economic or social, to find the cause of ill health, a distal (at a distance) cause.

> The introductory chapter discusses a holistic approach to studying health and Chapter 5 discusses the social determinants of health.   **connections**

The concept of **holism** is that there is not one cause for disease. Disease is caused by many factors (multifactorial) and their interrelationship. The ill individual must be treated as a whole person with a specific identity, socioeconomic status, history and personality. For example, in an infectious disorder, a reductionist approach would be that a virus has invaded the body and caused an illness. A holistic view might look at lifestyle, beliefs and socioeconomic class as potential causes of the disease. For example, in the early 1980s when AIDS was first reported, the main risk factors found in epidemiological studies highlighted a risk between Kaposi's sarcoma (a type of cancer) with promiscuity, drug use or homosexuality (Marmor et al., 1982). While this may raise alarms, it did in fact point to areas of research suggesting that the cause of the increase in this cancer, usually seen in 70-year-olds and now suddenly seen in younger people, may be transmissible, particularly in blood. By 1985, the scientific research had shown that AIDS had a reductionist cause; it is caused by a virus (HIV) and if the virus attacks humans (some viruses attack other species), then it can attack all humans (Goedart and Gallo, 1985). Knowing that it is a virus allows possible treatments to be sought that eradicate the virus.

The reductionist model is the founding principle in the field of epidemiology. John Snow, one of the founders of epidemiology and the study of diseases in populations, discovered that the cause of an outbreak of cholera in London was due to a contaminated water supply. Later, the germ theory of Louis Pasteur was able to show that microorganisms such as bacteria can cause these pathogenic diseases. Without the work of John Snow, the cause of the disease would have been attributed to various factors and lifestyles as occurred in the attempts to ascertain the cause of AIDS.

> Chapter 3 discusses epidemiology and the contribution of John Snow.   **connections**

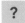 What are the strengths and limitations of the biomedical approach to studying health?

| connections | Chapter 2 shows how religious beliefs have played a major part in understandings of health and disease and the emergence of the biomedical approach to studying health. |

Reducing a disease to its root cause can liberate us from attributions involving blame. On the other hand, an illness has wider socioeconomic and environmental determinants and while reductionism looks at what caused the illness, it may not address the other factors or behaviours that led to the illness.

Part 2 Theoretical and research approaches

example 1.4

Examples of research in biological sciences

- Molecular biology and the study of gene structure and function
- Evolutionary ecology and behaviour, for example the development of immunity and the infections
- Biodiversity and ecology
- Molecular oncology and the development of metastasis
- Microbiology and the emergence and transmission of pathogenic bacteria
- Pharmacology and the development of drugs
- Toxicology and the effects of pollution
- Neurobiology and the organization of the cells of the nervous system and the failure of the circuits that process information in dementias, Parkinson's and motor neurone disease

example 1.5

Stem cells and regenerative medicine

Stem cell research is an area of basic biology and also an area of applied biology of biomedical interest. The work on stem cells in human biology results from work on the biology of stem cells in other species. In the 1960s and 70s, James Till and Ernest McCulloch (Becker et al., 1963) described the ground-breaking work on rescuing mice irradiated with potentially lethal doses by the reintroduction of donor bone marrow cells,

which formed colonies in the recipient that contained all the types of cells of the blood. These colony-forming cells are now called 'stem cells'.

In the 1970 and 80s, the eminent scientist John Gurdon worked with eggs from *Xenopus laevis*, a type of frog. These eggs are laid and fertilized externally and are rather large, lending themselves to manipulation. His work included transferring a nucleus with genetic information (DNA) from an adult cell into an egg that had had its nucleus removed. The egg developed into a normal tadpole and frog. This is how, many years later, Dolly the sheep was made by the scientist Ian Wilmut in 1997.

Transferring nuclei into eggs is a form of **cloning**. There are two types of nuclear cloning – therapeutic and reproductive. Both rely on the transfer of a nucleus from a somatic cell into a recipient cell – somatic nuclear cell transfer. Therapeutic cloning into an egg cell may yield embryonic stem cells for use in medical research and the development of stem cell therapies. Reproductive cloning aims to make a fully developed replica of the organism being cloned by implanting the altered egg cell into a uterus and allowing it to grow into an independent organism. It is not allowed for human reproduction.

Stem cells produce all the types of cells of the body during early development, the embryonic stem cells (ESC), while the adult or somatic stem cells (SSC) replace and maintain cell numbers in the adult (Cedar et al., 2006). The area of interest for stem cell researchers is how one type of cell, the stem cell, can make many types of functional end cells such as red blood cells, kidney cells and pancreatic cells. This process, as mentioned above, is called 'differentiation'. From a biomedical point of view, stem cell research (pure biology) has an impact on regenerative medicine (applied biology), an area of medicine hoping to replace worn-out or damaged cells as found in disease, trauma and ageing, for example replacing non-functioning or absent ß (beta) pancreatic cells in type 1 diabetes with laboratory grown ß cells. Stem cell research also has an impact on the mechanism of cancer cell growth, which may be a form of growth of aberrant stem cells. Given the shortage of donor organs for transplants, ESC may provide a pool of regenerative tissue, where cells can be grown by tissue engineering. ESC may be isolated from early embryos without cloning, but with the destruction of the embryo. Thus, there are major ethical issues surrounding obtaining stem cells from human embryos (Cedar, 2006). Stem cells have been grown from normal differentiated connective tissue cells called 'fibroblasts', and then 'undifferentiated' back to a more primitive stem cell state (Takahashi and Yamanaka, 2006; Takahashi et al., 2007). This process results in what is called 'induced pluripotent stem cells'. The science and technology is gradually advancing, fuelling hope to be able to address regenerative disorders and the degenerative disorders of ageing, such as Alzheimer's and heart disease.

Biology is a scientific discipline, science often being typified as a rational means of acquiring knowledge through the observation of physical phenomena. This is not the complete picture, as science is an experimental discipline where tests are carried out to try to ascertain the cause of phenomena. While one can say the cause of something is Z, to prove it in science, one must carry out an **experiment**. In experiments, all other possible causes are removed or held constant and Z is tested either by removing Z or adding Z. The result is whether the phenomena still occurs. Scientific methods are rigorous and systematic. Scientific truths are thus an attempt to be objective, that is, independent of any particular researcher's beliefs or views (Chalmers, 1983). Its methods attempt, as far as possible, to reduce the influence of bias when testing a **hypothesis** or **theory**.

Scientists are interested in how events happen, that is, the cause of an event, and investigate this using an experiment. Science has been described as empirical, but this is incorrect as empiricism relies on experience and denies causation. One of the principles in science is that our own senses are limited. We see a small fraction of the electromagnetic spectrum, for example, and we call it 'visible light'. But there are signals our senses cannot detect. So, relying solely on one's senses, empirically, is limiting in trying to understand the whole nature of the universe. Science is thus not empirical (Okasha, 2002). Scientists use a number of logical ways to think about a problem and account for observable events. These logical ways include induction and deduction.

connections	Chapter 3 considers the nature of the scientific method in relation to the study of patterns of disease in populations.

Induction

Induction is the process of recording a large number of observations over a wide range of conditions until a universal statement or law can be induced that applies to all the individual observations. For example, the endocrine glands regulate a number of functions of the body. Using the inductive approach, observations by many scientists showed that the underfunctioning of an endocrine gland caused a deficiency syndrome. Such observations were made on people with diseases such as diabetes mellitus, which results from a deficiency of the hormone insulin, produced by the pancreas gland. Symptoms such as loss of weight, hunger, thirst and the production of a large amount of sugar in urine were observed. The experimental removal of the pancreas from animals also resulted in the deficiency state. Induction therefore identified the universal law that the underfunctioning of an endocrine gland causes a deficiency syndrome. This then has uses and can be applied to many situations, avoiding having to start from scratch each time an event, diabetes mellitus for example, occurs.

Deduction

The description of science as entirely inductive misses out the mental processes of theorizing. Science often progresses via suggesting an explanation or scientific theory, an 'informed guess' on how something might work, which lends itself to testing. **Deduction** is essentially logical reasoning. Deduction in science allows predictions to be made from its laws and theories as a way of testing them.

Using the example of endocrine glands, the universal statement is so far rather vague – an underfunctioning gland causes disruption in the body. This could apply to any gland or indeed organ. A criterion for endocrine glands, however, is that they secrete chemicals called 'hormones' into the blood, the hormones acting on tissues distant from the gland itself. Logically, then, if the gland is an endocrine gland, injecting extracts of the gland into the blood will reverse the deficiency syndrome. Here, one has gone from a general law to deduce, or predict, a logical event that should follow from this law.

Scurvy was a disease suffered particularly by sailors in the seventeenth and eighteenth centuries when they were at sea for a long period of time, which eventually became linked to a lack of vitamin C. Americans may still describe British people as 'Limeys', a reference to the sailors who carried fresh fruit, particularly lemons and limes, on voyages, because these fruits contain vitamin C. Contemporary explanations for scurvy might look to a lack of access to fresh fruit, a lack of education on nutrition, the relatively high cost of fresh fruit or possibly cultural reasons for not eating fresh fruit. All these indirect reasons do not deny that the cause is lack of vitamin C, a scientific finding. The cure is known only because of scientific investigations into normal physiology and biochemistry. Therefore biology, albeit not a medical science, still has a direct impact on our health.

example 1.6

Inductive reasoning and the example of eugenics

Eugenics is a term coined in 1883 by Francis Galton, who defined it as 'the science of improvement of the human race germ plasm through better breeding'. Galton thought that if characteristics were inherited, it would be possible to improve the 'stock' of the population through selective breeding. Galton knew that the poor were less healthy than the rich and decided that the way to improve the health of the nation was to let only healthy (and rich) people breed. Galton made the mistake of conflating poverty with health and coincidence for causation. He falsely inferred that the poor health of poor people was inherited, or in their genes. He decided, therefore, that to avoid having unhealthy people in the population, the poor and unhealthy should be encouraged not to breed. This is a piece of logical induction based on a false hypothesis. Galton's motives in improving the health of the nation, a public health initiative, may have been good, but his understanding of the cause of ill health was unsound.

Proof and falsification

How do we know when a law or theory is true or proven? Induction and deduction have their place, but can it ever be said that enough observations have been made to prove a law, or that enough predictions based on that law have been tested? Scientists are not naive observers – they make sense of observations through pre-existing theory, building on previous scientific information.

Falsification, as propounded by Karl Popper in the 1950s, acknowledged that scientists have some preconceptions about how phenomena happen. Popper also argued that is never possible to prove that something is true. The next observation might disprove the theory. Popper (1959) suggested that good science starts with a hypothetical explanation that is falsifiable – **the null hypothesis.**

Logically, deductions can be made from the hypothesis, and these can be tested. If the hypothesis does not stand up to testing, it is rejected; if it does, the hypothesis is not rejected, instead it is subjected to even more rigorous testing. This description of science, the hypothetico-deductive method, is still accepted today. This process builds evidence supporting a hypothesis, but at the same time acknowledges the hypothesis is not an absolute truth, but a conditional truth. Science is therefore evidence based and its findings are in a constant state of flux, unlike absolute beliefs or morals that are held to be fixed and inviolable.

Kuhn (1962) suggested that science progresses by a series of revolutions. A number of contrary findings may challenge the existing explanatory framework. This leads to an alternative paradigm or framework being proposed that explains existing incompatible findings. A **paradigm shift** then occurs, whereby scientists adopt a new explanatory system. Einstein's law of relativity is an example of a paradigm shift from Newtonian physics.

Experimentation

The relationship between cause and effect is tested by experiment. Science is a systematic discipline involving the recording of observations made under carefully controlled conditions. The observations are a way of testing an idea. The observations can be caused by altering phenomena experimentally and seeing the outcome. The results of scientific research are publicized and opened up for testing, that is, the same piece of work could be repeated by another person and identical results obtained. The equipment used must be accurate and reliably measure whatever data are being recorded. The methods are clearly described in papers so that they can be repeated by others.

The unravelling of a biological pathway usually requires some intervention or interference whereby the changes can be noted and inferences drawn; for example, if it is suspected that a gland in one part of the body controls another by hormones, the removal of that gland will result in physiological changes in the effector. If the hypothesis is that one part of the body controls another by nerves, cutting or inactivating the nerves will prevent the control system working and there will be clear differences between the observations recorded in the control (uncut) group and in the experimental (cut) group.

The important point to experimentation is, however, that if an experiment disproves a hypothesis, then the hypothesis is incorrect and a new one must be proposed. Hypotheses that are consistently confirmed can be considered acceptable 'theories' or 'laws' of nature. A key aspect of the **scientific method** is that, regardless of how many times a theory has been confirmed or rejected, it is always subject to the addition of new data. This explains why science continually finds new explanations to understand the universe and is not about protecting the status quo. It also explains why many subjects of interest cannot be 'scientifically' investigated because no rigorous experiment can be undertaken where just one variable is tested. When observing phenomenon, explanations for the observed effect need to be tested before causation can be established. Just because two things happen together doesn't mean that one causes the other. To establish this means controlling for various influences that may contribute to the relationships between things. Biology, as a natural science, is able to test for causality by undertaking a controlled experiment.

Chapter 3 further defines the concepts of causation and association. The nature and process of 'social' experiments in randomized controlled trials is also discussed in Chapter 3.   **connections**

example 1.7

Clinical interventions: the double-blind trial

The double-blind clinical trial is a piece of applied science. It seeks to understand *whether* something works, not *how* something works. In a double-blind test, patients are selected who all have the same clinical problem. They are then divided into two groups and one is given the trial intervention, for example a new medicine, and the other group is given a 'placebo' – an intervention that looks like the trial intervention, but which has no active ingredient. This is a blind trial as the patients do not know which group they are in so that their expectations of a drug's efficacy cannot mask their reactions to the drug. The trial is made double blind by not letting the clinical staff administering and

measuring the trial intervention know whether their group is being given the trial drug or intervention or the placebo. This is to avoid staff influencing patients' responses. If an intervention is to be deemed effective, it must work better than the placebo.

The placebo effect is a well-known phenomenon, whereby people given a neutral or ineffective intervention may still get better and heal themselves. This could be due to psychological or self-healing factors. Some of those on the trial may have got better without any medical intervention through their own homeostatic mechanisms. All medicines and surgical interventions are thus tested in clinical, double-blind trials. Although it is impossible to control all variables in patients, these trials provide the best evidence we can gather.

Techniques

The systematic collection of measurements, often in a controlled setting such as a laboratory, is what distinguishes science. The measurements often require instruments and the development of science has been closely tied to their invention and development.

In vitro (literally 'in glass') studies are those undertaken outside the body. It is possible to keep organs alive outside the body by providing them with fluid that mimics interstitial fluid, the internal environment. It is clearly easier to manipulate the organ concerned and observe and measure its responses when it is separated from the rest of the body. Techniques developed in studying cells have, for example, resulted in the possibility of in vitro fertilization and the subsequent birth of babies to couples who are unable to conceive and bear children naturally.

Techniques can be subdivided into invasive and non-invasive, in other words, in terms of whether or not they involve introducing substances into the body. Arterial blood pressure can be measured invasively by inserting a cannula into an artery and connecting it up to a pressure-measuring machine. Alternatively, the sphygmomanometer measures blood pressure non-invasively.

Clinical observations of patients with congenital deficits or hyperfunction, particularly in the field of endocrinology, have led to information on the actions of hormones. An overactive gland exaggerates the normal effects of the hormone(s) secreted. For example, patients with an overactive thyroid gland show symptoms of a raised metabolic rate, including weight loss, feeling hot and an increased pulse rate. The actions of the thyroid hormones are thereby revealed. Conversely, an underactive thyroid results in symptoms of a reduced metabolic rate, such as mental and physical lethargy, and a tendency to put on weight, feel cold and have a slow pulse. Such non-invasive observations preceded the experimental manipulations of endocrine glands. Following observational studies, the hormones from the gland were isolated and purified, the hormone structure was identified and in some cases synthesized.

As all ill health and disease has an underlying biological cause, biological research has been central to health. For instance, if someone is suffering from malnutrition, a lack of the correct nutrients, biological research can investigate which nutrients are missing. This may involve taking blood and urine samples and the use of food diaries to investigate which nutrients are missing. Clinical investigations usually require testing patients' tissue or fluids. These are linked to the patient's vital signs, their respiratory, heart or blood gas levels; for example:

- Type 1 diabetes: urine samples will be taken to see if glucose is present (glucose should not be present in normal urine)

- AIDS: blood will be taken to confirm the presence of the HIV virus

- Meningitis: cerebrospinal fluid is taken from the meninges of the spinal cord to test for the presence of bacteria or virus causing the disease

- Myocardial infarction: the electrical conduction by nerve cells, the blood flow in vessels and the anatomical integrity of the heart will be investigated.

All clinical investigations involve testing biological components. Either anatomical features will be investigated to ascertain if any damage has occurred and follow up on wound healing and whether the anatomical integrity has been restored (e.g. after fracturing a bone) or physiological processes will be monitored (e.g. in diabetes, the utilization and elimination of glucose will be investigated).

Imaging techniques introduced in the 1970s have enabled studies of internal organs to be undertaken for research and clinical investigation. The techniques or 'scans' include:

- *computed tomography (CT):* CT scans use rotating X-rays projected through the body to produce a series of images that are combined by computer to produce a 'slice' through the body.

- *magnetic resonance imaging (MRI):* uses magnetic fields and radio waves to energize hydrogen atoms in the body. Three-dimensional colour images are produced of tissues (soft and hard), comparative metabolic activity and blood flow.

- *positron emission tomography (PET):* PET scans are taken following the injection of a radioactive molecule such as glucose into the bloodstream. The more active a tissue is, the more glucose it takes up, the fate of the radioactivity being analysed by the computer, which produces a colour map reflecting different levels of metabolic activity. By such means, particular areas of the brain can be 'seen' to be associated with specific functions: the occipital lobes are, for example, more active when the eyes are open, whereas the hippocampus is active in memory tasks.

case study biological explanations for obesity

Food, nutrition and obesity are all subjects studied in biology and have biological explanations. A biological framework can be used to understand the causes of the symptoms of obesity as well as assisting the identification of which particular mechanism or function is impaired and causing the obesity. Once the causal mechanisms are understood and identified, attempts may be made to manage, control or remove the causes of obesity.

To grow, replace worn-out cells, maintain our internal environment, and have energy to carry out all our physiological activities, we need to ingest appropriate chemical matter from the external environment (Cedar, 2012). What we ingest we call 'food'. This food is composed of chemical matter. Food is nutritious if it allows all the activities we need for homeostasis and growth and it contains nutrients, a subset of chemical matter that maintains us, as opposed to the chemicals that do not or are harmful if we ingest them.

The food that is habitually eaten or ingested by organisms to provide nutrition is part of their 'normal' diet. Food contains a variety of nutrients that are absorbed by organisms and used for energy, growth and repair. Humans need to eat food containing six kinds of nutrients in order to maintain healthy bodies:

- Carbohydrates: for energy
- Fats: for energy
- Proteins: for growth and replacement
- Vitamins: as antioxidants and coenzymes in metabolic reactions
- Minerals: for osmotic balance, nerve conduction and muscle contraction
- Water: for osmotic balance, maintenance of normal blood pressure, metabolic activity, transport and diffusion of chemicals around the body.

Energy (calories) comes from food such as carbohydrates and fats, which can be converted by the cell into a chemical called adenosine triphosphate (ATP) to do work. When energy is needed, for example during physical exercise, the ATP that has been formed from sugar is converted into adenosine diphosphate (ADP), releasing energy for other reactions during this process. Sugars are then metabolized to reform the ATP from ADP.

Fats are macromolecules composed of long chains of fatty acids. Fat, or adipose tissue, is used to store energy, provide insulation and protect the organs. Fat contains more calories, and thus more potential energy, than carbohydrates and sugars. When necessary, fat can be converted into energy. When food containing more calories than are used is consumed, the excess is stored as fat. If an individual is habitually eating more than their body uses, and is storing a large amount of excess fat, this condition is known as 'obesity'.

There are three different ways of calculating obesity:

1. The *body mass index* (BMI) is a person's weight in kilograms divided by the square of height in metres. A person with a BMI of above 30 is considered to be obese.
2. The *waist-to-hip ratio* assesses how much body weight is carried around the stomach, known as 'central adiposity'. Increased central adiposity is a risk factor for the development of type 2 diabetes (Folsom et al., 1993; Simpson et al., 2007; Zhang et al., 2007), and is associated with coronary vascular disease (Yusuf et al., 2004).
3. The *percentage of body weight that is body fat*. Men with over 25% body weight as fat and women with over 30% body weight as fat are considered to be obese. The best means of measuring body fat is underwater weighing, but skinfold testing (to measure the subcutaneous fat layer) and bioelectrical impedance analysis may also be used. All these measures require specialist facilities and personnel, so are not as readily accessible as BMI or waist-to-hip ratios. There are different types of fat in the body and it is fat surrounding organs and inside blood vessels that is thought to be the more dangerous than fat under the skin, although fat under skin is indicative of the fat in organs and blood vessels.

There are many biological explanations for obesity but the root cause is believed to be the consumption of more calories as food than are being converted and used as energy to do work. In other words, there is more input than output.

The identification of the obesity gene in 1994 triggered a growth of research into the genetic determinants of body weight. Whether there is a genetic propensity towards fatness has long fascinated scientists (Leibel et al., 1990). Those who have argued for a genetic explanation point to the genes that affect calorie consumption and feelings of hunger and satiation. Genes produce proteins and there is evidence that some peptides (small proteins) produced by the stomach and GI tract may affect calorie intake. The discovery of leptin (see Freidman and Halaas, 1998) triggered research into the many hormonal mechanisms implicated in appetite control, food intake, storage patterns of adipose tissue and the development of insulin resistance (Flier, 2004). Ghrelin, another peptide, increases during fasting and is reduced in response to a meal. Ghrelin and leptin are thought to be complementary in their influence on appetite, with ghrelin affecting short-term appetite and leptin affecting long-term appetite. Low fat stores trigger a reduction in levels of leptin, which stimulates food-seeking behaviour. Insulin and leptin hormones are secreted in proportion to the amount of adipose tissue (fat) in the body, stimulating receptors in the brain to reduce food intake. If the genes involved in the production of these peptides, insulin or hormones are functioning abnormally, or are absent, normal feelings of satiety would be affected, which could cause habitual overeating, resulting in obesity. A small percentage of obese people are leptin deficient, and many more obese people are leptin resistant.

The mediators mentioned above affect appetite by acting on the hypothalamus, the part of the brain that processes signals related to metabolic state and energy storage. One theory is that one region of the hypothalamus, the lateral hypothalamus, affects feelings of hunger, while another region, the ventromedial hypothalamus, affects feelings of satiety; however, this theory has been challenged by more recent research (Flier, 2004). An analysis of trials on the link between leptin and obesity showed no link between the gene and obesity (Paracchini et al., 2005).

Isolating any individual gene(s) responsible for obesity has proved elusive until recently. However, in 2007, the results were published from a large study originally set up to identify susceptibility to type 2 diabetes (Frayling et al., 2007). People with type 2 diabetes were more likely to have a particular variant of the fat mass and obesity-associated gene, known simply as FTO, which was also shown to be linked to increased body weight. FTO comes in two varieties, and everyone inherits two copies of the gene. The variant making people fatter differed from the other version of the FTO gene by a single mutation in the DNA sequence: 16% of people have two copies of the high-risk variant, 50% have one high-risk and one low-risk, and 34% of people have two low-risk variants

The study found that people with two copies of the particular 'fat gene' variant had a 70% higher risk of obesity than those with two copies of the other variant and weighed 3 kg more. In each case, the extra weight was entirely accounted for by more body fat, not greater muscle or extra height. The 50% of subjects who inherited one copy of each FTO variant had a 30% higher risk of obesity.

These findings must be treated with caution: FTO will not be the only gene that influences obesity, and inheriting a particular variant will not necessarily make anyone fat. Again, correlation does not prove causation. Except in rare cases, such as Prader-Willi syndrome, obesity is not caused directly by genes but it may explain how people with apparently similar lifestyles differ in their propensity to put on weight.

An even more contentious theory is that obesity may be 'caught'. Exposure to adenovirus 36, commonly associated with coughs and colds, can induce stem cells from fat tissue to become fat cells (Dhurandhar et al., 2000; Vangipuram et al., 2004). In laboratory experiments, mice and chickens infected with the virus put on much more fat than uninfected animals. The same virus is more prevalent among overweight people, a strong indication that it may also cause obesity in humans.

Recent work by Everard et al. (2013) has revealed changes in the flora or the gut where bacteria reside. In the large colon, there are many commensal bacteria aiding digestion and vitamin K production. One such bacteria, *Akkermansia muciniphila,* may be at a slightly higher concentration in normal mice compared to obese mice. This bacteria is involved in the digestion of mucins and these findings may have similar results in humans, the idea being that increasing certain normal flora of the gut may reduce obesity. These bacteria may have been reduced previously due to diet, other infections or even antibiotics taken after illness as medicine or found in foods as part of the farming process.

Biology also offers insights into how food production can impact on health. Science discovered some of the hormones that increase growth rates, and they have been used in food production. However, these hormones may also affect the consumer of the food. Genetically modified foods tend not to need the addition of so many external chemical additives. Eating foreign genes should not be a problem as every cell has genes in it and all vegetables, fruits and meats (including fish, which are animals too) are composed of cells containing genes. We are always eating 'foreign' genes and digesting them into their component parts, nucleotides,

LIBRARY, UNIVERSITY OF CHESTER

which we can reuse in our own bodies. Thus, they are nutrients.

With the exception of infectious diseases, no other chronic disease has increased so rapidly as obesity (see Chapter 3). Notwithstanding these emerging genetic and contagion explanations, the primary biological explanation is the imbalance between calories consumed and calories expended, with the excess of calories ingested being turned into fat. Lifestyle factors such as changes in diet and exercise patterns are the most likely candidates as causal factors for the rise in obesity levels. The availability of processed food from a variety of different countries may be one factor, while reduced physical activity due to sedentary work and leisure patterns may be another. In America, reliance on energy-dense, fast-food meals tripled and calorie intake quadrupled between 1977 and 1995 (Lin et al., 1999). Genetic explanations or contagion theories that explain perceptions of hunger or satiety or fat deposition may, in the future, offer the possibility of screening or treatment, but, in the meantime, lifestyle and environmental changes offer the only realistic way of tackling obesity.

Summary

- For most people, health is associated first and foremost with a physical state of being. Having knowledge of biological frameworks, pathways and mechanisms contributes to our understanding of this physical state of being

- The scientific discipline of biology helps us to uncover universal mechanisms that regulate the body (homeostasis)

- People's interpretation of bodily symptoms and states is highly varied and is related to many other non-physical factors, such as social factors and cultural beliefs. Biology provides a means of arriving at a common baseline understanding of what is occurring inside the human body by means of rigorous scientific methods

- Biology contributes in many ways to human health. Once processes have been understood, effective interventions may be proposed and refined. Biology is, however, distinct from medicine, its investigations and research being neither limited nor dictated by medicine

- Understanding biological concepts, frameworks and research methods enables us to discover the complexity and self-regulating nature of the human body. This in turn assists us in understanding what is happening in altered states of health, whether caused by assaults from the external world, for example infection or an extremely hostile environment, or internal errors in regulation, for example genetic conditions such as haemophilia. Understanding physical states of being is a crucial aspect of the wider task of understanding human health

- Clinical interventions seek to restore the normal, physiological processes and homeostasis of the body. Without understanding the biology of these processes, clinical interventions would not be effective

Questions for further discussion

1. Is homeostasis the same as health?
2. Are genes the primary determinants of disease?
3. What is obesity? What are its causes?
4. Will genetically modified foods reduce the extraneous chemicals in our diet?

Further reading and resources

Cedar, S.H. (2012) *Biology for Health: Applying the Activities of Daily Living*. Basingstoke: Palgrave Macmillan.
Written for students in all areas of health. A new, clear and innovative way of explaining the biology of health by focusing on the activities of daily living that are used as indicators of healthy lives.

Chalmers, A.F. (1999) *What is this Thing Called Science?* (3rd edn). Buckingham: Open University Press.
Highly readable excursion into the nature of scientific research, gently exploding many of the myths about the nature of science.

Davey, B. (2001) The nature of scientific research: biomedical research methods, in K. McConway and B. Davey (eds) *Studying Health and Disease* (2nd edn). Buckingham: Open University Press.
Useful summary of the main issues in general scientific and biological research relating to health in particular.

Wolpert, L. (2000) *The Unnatural Nature of Science*. London: Faber & Faber.
Witty and entertaining book on the origin of science and what science is, intended for the general reader.

www.wellcome.ac.uk
Wellcome Trust contains details of the human genome project.

www.hfea.gov.uk
The Human Fertilisation and Embryo Authority is an excellent site to see the debates on stem cell research.

References

Becker, A.J., McCulloch, E.A. and Till, J.E. (1963) 'Cytological demonstration of the clonal nature of spleen colonies derived from transplanted mouse marrow cells'. *Nature* 197: 452–4.

Bernard, C. ([1865] 1957) *An Introduction to the Study of Experimental Medicine*. Mineola, NY: Dover.

Calderon-Margalit, R. and Paltiel, O. (2004) 'Prevention of breast cancer in women who carry BRCA1 or BRCA2 mutations: a critical review of the literature'. *International Journal of Cancer* 112(3): 357–64.

Cedar, S.H. (2006) 'Stem cell and related therapies: nurses and midwives representing all parties'. *Nursing Ethics* 13(3): 292–303.

Cedar, S.H. (2012) *Biology for Health: Applying the Activities of Daily Living.* Basingstoke: Palgrave Macmillan.

Cedar, S.H., Cooke, J.A., Luo, Z. et al. (2006) 'From eggs to embryonic stem cells: biopolitics and therapeutic potentials'. *Reproductive Biomedicine* 13(5): 725–31.

Chalmers, A.F. (1983) *What is this Thing Called Science?* Buckingham: Open University Press.

Dhurandhar, N.V., Israel, B.A., Kolesar, J.M. et al. (2000) 'Increased adiposity in animals due to a human virus'. *International Journal of Obesity and Related Metabolic Disorders* 24(8): 989–96.

Everard, A., Belzer, C., Geurts, L. et al. (2013) 'Cross-talk between *Akkermansia muciniphila* and intestinal epithelium controls diet-induced obesity'. *PLoS* 110(22): 9066–71.

Finley, M.I. (1963) *The Ancient Greeks*. Harmondsworth: Penguin.

Flier, J. (2004) 'Obesity wars: molecular progress confronts an expanding epidemic'. *Cell* 116(2): 337–50.

Folsom, A.R., Kaye, S.A., Sellers, T.A. et al. (1993) 'Body fat distribution and 5-year risk of death in older women'. *Journal of the American Medical Association* 269(4): 483–7.

Frayling, T.M., Timpson, N.J., Weedon, M.N. et al. (2007) 'A common variant in the FTO gene is associated with body mass index and predisposes to childhood and adult obesity'. *Science* 316(5826): 889–94.

Friedman, J.M. and Halaas, J.L. (1998) 'Leptin and the regulation of body weight in mammals'. *Nature* 395(6704): 763–70.

Goedert, J.J. and Gallo, R.C. (1985) 'Epidemiological evidence that HTLV-III is the AIDS agent'. *European Journal of Epidemiology* 1(3): 155–9.

Kuhn, T. (1962) *The Structure of Scientific Revolutions*. Chicago: University of Chicago Press.

Leibel, R.L., Bahary, N. and Friedman, J.M. (1990) 'Genetic variation and nutrition in obesity: approaches to the molecular genetics of obesity'. *World Review of Nutrition and Dietetics* 63(1): 90–101.

Lin, B.H., Guthrie, J. and Frazao, E. (1999) Nutrient contribution of food away from home, in E. Frazao (ed.) *America's Eating Habits: Changes and Consequences*. Washington DC: US Department of Agriculture, Economic Research Service, pp. 213–39.

Marmor, M., Friedman-Kein, A.E., Laubenstein, L. et al. (1982) 'Risk factors for Kaposi's sarcoma in homosexual men'. *Lancet* 1(8281): 1083–7.

Okasha, S. (2002) *Philosophy of Science: A Very Short Introduction*. Oxford: Oxford University Press.

Paracchini, V., Pedotti, P. and Taioli, E. (2005) 'Genetics of leptin and obesity: a HuGE review'. *American Journal of Epidemiology* 162(2): 101–14.

Popper, K. (1959) *The Logic of Scientific Discovery*. London: Hutchinson.

Simpson, J.A., MacInnis, R.J., Peeters, A. et al. (2007) 'A comparison of adiposity measures as predictors of all-cause mortality: the Melbourne collaborative cohort study'. *Obesity* 15: 994–1003.

Takahashi, K. and Yamanaka, S. (2006) 'Induction of pluripotent stem cells from mouse embryonic and adult fibroblast cultures by defined factors'. *Cell* 126(4): 663–76.

Takahashi, K., Tanabe, K., Ohnuki, M. et al. (2007) 'Induction of pluripotent stem cells from adult human fibroblasts by defined factors'. *Cell* 131(5): 861–72.

Vangipuram, S.D., Sheele, J., Atkinson, R.L. et al. (2004) 'A human adenovirus enhances preadipocyte differentiation'. *Obesity Research* 12(5): 770–7.

Watson, J.D. and Crick, F.H.C. (1953) 'A structure for deoxyribose nucleic acid'. *Nature* 171: 737–8.

Wolpert, L. (2000) *The Unnatural Nature of Science*. London: Faber & Faber.

Yusuf, S., Hawken, S., Ounpuu, S. et al. (2004) 'Effect of potentially modifiable risk factors associated with myocardial infarction in 52 countries (the INTERHEART study): case-control study'. *Lancet* 364(9438): 937–5.

Zhang, X. Shu, X.-O., Gong, Y. et al. (2007) 'Abdominal adiposity and mortality in Chinese women'. *Archives of Internal Medicine* 167(9): 886–92.

LOUISE HILL CURTH

History and health

Overview	51
Introduction	51
Part 1 The contribution of history to health studies	53
Developments in concepts of health and disease: six non-naturals	59
Developments in medicine and healthcare	63
Part 2 Theoretical and research approaches	66
The development of the discipline	66
The historical method: using sources, oral history	68
Case study Food safety and bread in Victorian England	70
Summary	72
Questions for further discussion	72
Further reading and resources	72
References	73

Learning outcomes

This chapter will enable readers to:

- Understand what it is meant by history and how it can be applied to health
- Gain an overview of the discipline and development of the history of health and illness, including its theoretical and methodological approaches
- Reflect on the insights that history can give to our understandings of health, illness and healthcare

Overview

'History' is a broad discipline that focuses on the study of the past. This can include how individuals and groups of humans or animals behaved and interacted, as well as the ways in which politics, religion or economics affected past societies and cultures. Studies can also concentrate on a vast range of locations or periods of time, from the ancient world into the present day. The study of the history of health and illness is a relatively new subdiscipline, which examines questions such as the ways in which individuals, communities and societies have defined, experienced and responded to health issues over time. It is also increasingly linked to the concept of 'one medicine' or 'one health', which recognizes the inseparable links between humans and animals.

Part 1 will examine the ways in which people in the past understood concepts such as 'health', the evolution of ideas, institutions and language, and how they related to contemporary social, scientific and cultural factors. Part 2 provides an examination of theoretical and research approaches used by historians, interspersed with short examples taken from historical sources ranging from the seventeenth century to the present day.

Introduction

? How might the study of history provide insights into understanding modern ideas on health?

In the eyes of many people, the discipline of history is about memorizing dates, names and events that happened long ago. Although this can be a component of historical study, history does, in fact, focus on much more than that. As Duffin (2010, p. 7) has noted, it allows people 'to ponder how things came to be in the past … and challenges them to explain how things that we currently think are so wrong were seen as "right" in the past'. History is also a highly interdisciplinary field, closely linked to many of the topics covered in this book, including cultural studies, epidemiology, ethics, social policy and sociology. However, unlike many other disciplines, history can also provide 'a dimension of longitudinal meaning over time' (Black and MacRaild, 2000, p. 3).

There are various names for the subdiscipline of the history of health and illness, with the most common being 'medical history'. As this chapter discusses later, the topics and the ways in which they are examined have changed and continue to change. At one time, the discipline of medical history referred to the study of 'great doctors' and 'great medical discoveries'. Over the past few decades, however, it has increasingly come to focus on the ways in which our predecessors understood ideas of health and illness and how the societies in which they lived chose to deal with related issues. Accounts of the history of medicine often focus on individuals such as Edward Jenner and Louis Pasteur and their contributions to understanding immunology and vaccination, or

Florence Nightingale's role in the development of nursing as a profession. But the history of medicine and health is much more than a focus on a small group of doctors and scientists making great discoveries. It explores the development of healthcare and medicine, seeking to understand the factors contributing to change, such as technological developments, religion or war. History also studies how health and disease affected society – the way people lived, what they ate and drank, how they organized their private and public hygiene and healthcare, and how they coped, physically as well as spiritually, with pain, illness and death.

The first part of this chapter looks at how people in the past defined health and disease and how these ideas were constructed and contextualized. It will also illustrate how ideas about the mind and body, the environment, natural and supernatural causation and morality influenced these choices. The chapter goes on to look at the ways in which healthcare was organized, from the role of healers to the organization or institutionalization of medicine, the status practitioners enjoyed in society, and the ways in which medical authority and competence were established and maintained.

As in all areas of academic study, there are many different ways in which key terms can be defined. One of the main unifying factors behind medical history studies is the need to understand and agree on definitions for 'health' and/or 'illness', which have changed dramatically over time. There is a large body of contemporary literature that discusses what human health means today in Western Europe. However, the most commonly used definition is still that coined by the World Health Organization in 1946. This states that health is 'a state of complete physical, mental and social well-being, not merely the absence of disease or infirmity' (WHO, 1946). The most striking part of this statement is the suggestion that a 'complete' state of mental and social wellbeing could ever actually exist. Other components are also problematic, such as what wellbeing means, and it fails to acknowledge patterns of social inequality. One accepted interpretation of 'being healthy' relates to the ability to carry out various 'social roles'.

connections	Chapter 5 examines the link between health and social life in greater detail.

The contemporary idea that health is the opposite of disease is firmly linked to the medical model of biomedicine, which is predominant in Western Europe and the Americas. Biomedicine's major focus is on various types of external pathogens that attack living creatures. Since this is centred on the idea of bacteria and viruses, it follows that a body that has been invaded by disease entities would no longer be in a state of wellbeing. In order to treat what is a pathological process or deviation from a biological norm, the modern medical profession relies mainly on technological interventions (Boyd, 2000).

connections	Chapter 1 explores the contribution of biology to the study of health and disease.

Furthermore, our medicalized healthcare system attempts to generalize causes of disease, how they will affect living creatures and how they can be treated. In many ways, this has turned the 'art of healing' into what might be called 'merely repair work' (Kang, 2004, p. 81). Although there has recently been a growing interest in social and/or psychological factors, for most health professionals the emphasis is still on finding new drugs or treatments to eradicate the effects of the attacking pathogens.

Part 1 The contribution of history to health studies

example 2.1

The application of history to the study of contemporary health issues

- How the modern idea of a 'healthy lifestyle' originated
- How medicines and healthcare systems

have developed over time and shaped contemporary experience
- How hospitals and other medical institutions have evolved
- The growing popularity of complementary and alternative medicine

Every society and culture has its own ways of defining what health and illness mean and how they can be dealt with. The predominant model in Western Europe is that of **biomedicine**, which rests on the idea of pathogens attacking the body. This is an ontological model, which views disease as a real, independent entity, and suggests that it is the bacteria or virus that is being treated, not the individual. These generic diseases 'cause' a pathological state that will produce the same effects and can therefore be treated in a similar way in all patients. Once the cause is identified, treatment can begin and, in theory, lead to comparable outcomes (Bates, 2000).

Chapter 1 explores the biological definitions of disease in relation to pathology and deviation from the norm. Chapter 3 explores how epidemiology studies patterns of disease.   **connections**

One of the major problems with this model is that the emphasis on pathogens attacking the body fails to acknowledge the mental, social and cultural factors that might also be involved. This is one of the main reasons for the growth in the West of complementary and alternative medical systems. There are many different types throughout the world, of which herbal, homeopathic and naturopathic medicines are just a few examples. In other parts of the world, there are many other medical belief models. Traditional Chinese medicine, for example, is based on the concept that disease results from disruption in the flow of qi and/or an imbalance in the forces of yin and yang. Four of the

most commonly used treatments for rectifying this imbalance are herbs, meditation, massage and acupuncture. In India, the traditional system of Ayurveda
aims to integrate the body, mind and spirit to prevent and treat disease. As
with traditional Chinese medicine, this model includes the use of herbs and
massage, as well as yoga.

The study of medical history shows that the Western biomedical focus
is diametrically opposed to the ways in which previous generations thought
about health and illness. In the past, the main focus was on health, in terms of
creating a healthy body and maintaining it through a healthy lifestyle. As the
following examples show, the ways in which health-related terminology has
changed over time helps to provide insights into the past.

> **?** Historians argue over whether specific events lead to revolutions in thought.
> Can you think of any examples where there has been a radical shift in ways
> of thinking about disease?

Historically, the meaning of the word 'disease' was very different, in that it
focused on the holistic nature of health, which included the state and feelings of
the patient. The mid-eighteenth-century definition of disease, for example, was
'the state of a living body wherein it is prevented from the exercise of any of its
functions' (Allen, 1765). A hundred years before that, the word 'distemper' was
used in place of disease, meaning any excess of heat or cold in the body of man.
By the nineteenth century and the discovery of microorganisms, there began a
new way of thinking about the individual as a cause agent in disease.

The term 'health' is difficult to define because it can be a subjective and/or
an objective phenomenon. It is also a term that differs according to people and
their society, culture and the time in which they live. Many definitions emphasize elements such as adaptability and coping. Kovacs (1989, p. 261) suggested
that health is a 'physical or mental state ... which is capable of adapting to
the natural and social-environmental surroundings of the individual with the
appropriate advantage or disadvantage ratio for the body and spirit'. In the
mid-eighteenth century, the surprisingly similar definition was 'a proper dispo-
sition of the several parts to perform their respective functions, without any
impediment or sensation of pain' (Anon, 1765). The unifying theme in these
definitions seems to be that of being able to function in society to an appropriate degree. This would be influenced, and therefore differ, according to the
place and time under study. Daily requirements in pre-modern, or developing
society, for example, might include being healthy enough to carry out strenuous agricultural labour. This is dramatically different from the demands made
on the human body in most modern white-collar jobs.

Being healthy enough to carry out work tasks or leisure activities varies
across social, ethnic and age groups, by gender and over time. In some segments
of modern British society, it is generally not considered to be morally or ethi-
cally wrong to stay home from work if someone feels unwell. However, before
the advent of paid sick days in the early twentieth century, most workers

would have had economic and moral reasons for not staying home unless they were acutely ill. The concept of retirement would also have been unfamiliar to people in the past, who considered themselves healthy enough to continue working as long as they were physically able. For the elderly, the threat of ending up in the poor house was partially removed by Lloyd George's introduction of pensions in 1908, followed by the National Insurance Act 1911 (Boyer, 2009).

Chapter 9 examines the development of the welfare state in the UK.   **connections**

There have also been major changes over time in the types of medically related institutions and the conditions they cater for. For example, early 'mental asylums' were radically different from modern Western institutions. The ways in which mental disorders were defined, labelled and diagnosed have also changed dramatically over time. In medieval and early modern Europe, madness was generally linked to the body being possessed by evil spirits or the devil. The term 'devil's bath', for example, referred to such spirits causing physical disorders as well as terrifying dreams and attacks of 'raving' (Clark, 1997). Until the mid-nineteenth century, the two main forms of lunacy were either melancholia or mania. Thomas Sydenham distinguished hysteria from madness and argued that the most common symptoms of hysteria were pains in the back (Sloan, 1996). Eccentric or other types of deviant behaviour that might be categorized today as mental illness were accepted or tolerated in seventeenth- and eighteenth-century society.

? How does the study of history help to understand the complexity of psychiatry as a specialty?

In the past, religious beliefs played a major role in helping people understand and come to terms with their state of health. Whether one was healthy or ill was linked to whether God (or Gods) wished to bless or punish an individual. Furthermore, illness could be used to punish individuals, communities or even nations through epidemics or other natural disasters. In order to stay healthy people had to try to live a good life free of sin (Thomas, 1991).

A popular literary device in the sixteenth and seventeenth centuries was to use the analogy of a body being a fortress under perpetual threat by enemies. This was likely to have been a familiar idea to readers accustomed to Christian imagery of the body protecting the soul from the devil. Furthermore, comparing the body to a fort constantly under attack was something that most people would have been able to empathize with in an age of recurring social upheavals, political conflicts and wars. In 1681, Richard Saunders argued that:

> tis simple reason ... to keep out an enemy, then to let him in, and afterwards to beat him out, so doubtless if men in the Government of their health would use Reason more, they would use the Physician less.

thinking about Does the analogy of health under attack still make sense in Britain today?

The idea that mental disorders were a sickness, rather than a form of heavenly punishment, meant that they could, in theory, be treated medically. These were considered organic complaints that could be treated by 'nerve doctors' or a system of hydrotherapy. Such views were strongly supported by William Battie, the founding medical officer of St Luke's Hospital in London. In his *Treatise on Madness* written in 1758, Battie also argued that mad people should not be shut up in prisons along with criminals, but should be placed in special asylums. Earlier asylums banned visitors and advocated a range of treatments including sedative opiates or brandy to stimulate patients suffering from melancholy (Shorter, 1997).

The numbers of people placed in such institutions rose dramatically between the beginning and end of the nineteenth century. The famous psychiatrist Henry Maudsley, who has a London hospital named after him, saw insanity as a form of regression back to our animal nature, a sort of backwards evolution. He argued that rather than the mind being an intangible or 'incorporeal essence', it was simply a part of the body and that 'the manifestations of mind take place through the nervous system' and should, therefore, be treated by medical means (Maudsley, 1871, p. 12).

In reality, the rapidly increasing number of asylums and their correspondingly larger number of patients meant that they were often little more than a way of keeping undesirables out of public sight. By the early twentieth century, the poor treatment of English mentally ill patients had gone so far that in 1918 'a third of the asylum population died in the space of twelve months' (Scull, 1977, p. 13). The death of such large numbers of institutionalized people was thought to have been due to poor nutrition. It seems likely that substandard living conditions would also have had a major impact on morbidity and mortality rates.

The importance of a good health regimen or what we would now call a 'healthy lifestyle' has been recognized since ancient times. The principles behind this can be traced back to the *Hippocratic Corpus*, a body of around 60 texts on health and illness. Although there is some uncertainty about individual authors, they are thought to have been written in the fourth century BC by followers of Hippocrates, who is often referred to as the 'father of medicine'. Although a vast range of topics were covered in these texts, the most important component for health was considered to be that of food and drink (Schiefsky, 2005).

The *Hippocratic Corpus* also introduced the idea that disease was caused by different types of imbalances of the four humours within the body. Although these humours were always in flux, the aim was to keep them as balanced as possible. As every living creature was thought to have a unique humoural combination, this was a complicated undertaking that required detailed medical knowledge and an in-depth understanding of the individual in question. Figure 2.1 illustrates the four humours of black bile, blood, yellow bile and phlegm and their related qualities. It was thought that all bodies had a predominance of one humour, depending on a variety of factors, ranging from the time they were born to the place where they first saw light. Each of the humours was linked to the four primary elements of earth, air, fire and water, which were further tied to the four material qualities of heat, dryness, coldness and wetness, and the four seasons of the year. Autumn, for example, was thought to be cold and dry, as was the humour called black bile. This meant that if black bile was the predominant humour in a person's body, they would have a cold and dry constitution and therefore be susceptible to hot and wet diseases (Wear, 2000).

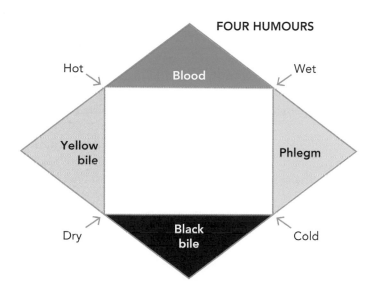

Figure 2.1 **The humoural theory**

The relationship between health and the four humours was further refined by Galen of Pergamum (*c.* 131–200 AD). As a prominent physician and prolific writer, Galen is credited with rationalizing Hippocratic ideas on diagnosis and prognosis (French, 2003). Unlike biomedicine, Hippo-Galenic or Galenic medicine focused on health and the holistic nature that underlies it (Porter, 2002). Humouralism rested on the idea that 'disease was an integral part of the self … [and] the world of God and nature', rather than on our modern view that disease can be viewed in isolation as a 'generic entity'. In other words, the emphasis was on the individual and their experiences rather than on some external 'attacker'. A state of health could be defined as when the four humours within the body were 'in their natural state, or while they balance one another in quality, quantity and mixture' (LeClerc, 1699, pp. 195–6). Such a functionalist description did not suggest that a perfect state of wellbeing was possible. It also acknowledged that being healthy could mean different things, as humans and animals were thought to have their own unique constitution or complexion.

Galen's theory about the 'non-naturals' was that these were one of the three basic types of phenomena whose mixture would define whether an individual was healthy or diseased. They comprised:

- 'thynges naturall': included the four elements of earth, air, fire and water, which manifested themselves as the four humours.

- 'thynges not naturall': these had the power to alter one's humoural balance, thereby destroying the desired state of health. According to Galenic thought, there were six non-naturals – 'ayre', 'meate and drinke', 'slepe and watch', 'mevying and rest', 'emptynesse and replettion' and 'affectations of the minde'.

- 'thynges ageynst nature': these are the 'contra-naturals', which literally meant against the naturals. They consisted of pathological conditions made up of 'syckenesse, cause of syckenesse and accidents whiche foloweth syckenesse' (Niebyl, 1971, pp. 486–92; Sotres, 1998, p. 291).

Although little could be done to alter the naturals or the contra-naturals, it was believed that the non-naturals could be manipulated in order to protect the health of individuals. It was generally accepted that the most effective way to do this was by following a daily health regime based on living by 'Rule and wholesome Precepts', which would result in a stronger body and mind (Maynwaring, 1669). The earliest and best-known medieval treatise on the topic was the *Regimen sanitatis salernitannum* (*Salernitan Regime of Health*). Commonly credited to Arnald of Villanova (1240–1311), it was composed of verses that discussed the relationship between health and the Galenic non-naturals. The poem was associated with the tenth- and eleventh-century medical school of Salerno, a city that played a major role in the revival of classical medicine in the Christian West. Legend has it that its medical school based its teachings on the writings of Hippocrates, said to have been brought to Salerno by a Latin, a Jew, an Arab and a Greek. Regardless of whether this was merely an apocryphal story, it was presumably meant to suggest that the regimen was universally supported by members of the medical profession. The *Salernitan Regime of Health* became so popular that it appeared in at least 240 versions in Latin and multiple editions in English and other European languages over the following centuries (Porter, 1996).

Interestingly, the basic rules involved in this are almost identical to modern recommendations on living a healthy lifestyle. Although there is much debate as to the exact definition of the term, it is generally accepted that it has to do with making 'good' choices about diet, exercise and lifestyle. Prevailing attitudes about what these actually consist of illustrate both change and continuity with those in the past. In common with advice in the past, this includes an emphasis on food and drink, as well as the other traditional 'non-naturals' of sleep, exercise and avoiding stress. Some of the differences can be attributed to changing variables such as limited income or restrictions linked to ethnicity or age.

Developments in concepts of health and disease: six non-naturals

Air

Although concern about the quality of the air we breathe often seems to be a modern issue, it actually dates back to Hippocratic writers who believed that air was the most powerful of all things, linked not only to human and animal life, but also to the transmission of disease (Longrigg, 1998). What we now refer to as 'air pollution' is said to emanate from a number of sources, including industry, agriculture, services, households, solid waste management, and road, air and sea transport. With the exception of air transport, all these factors also featured in the creation of polluted air or miasma. Toxic air could also be created through the work of butchers, tanners or farm workers, as well as from human or animal excrement. Battlefields full of rotting bodies were thought to exude dangerous fumes, as would swamps and muddy areas or stagnant water (Corbin, 1996).

The growing industrialization of England in the latter part of the eighteenth century created new forms of air pollution in the inner cities in which factories were located. This, along with the lack of a sanitation for the urban poor, was thought to be the reason for outbreaks of highly contagious fevers in Manchester, Liverpool, Stockport, Newcastle, Leeds and London in the 1790s. They were also linked to the growing concern about public health and the subsequent involvement of paternal social reformers such as William Wilberforce (1759–1833) and Jeremy Bentham (1748–1832) (Bynum, 1996).

Chapter 3 describes John Snow's early epidemiological work in documenting the spread of cholera in London during the 1850s.

connections

Motion and rest

There are obvious parallels between the perceived importance of exercise in early modern and twenty-first-century England. However, for many centuries, writers of popular medical texts included homilies such as 'Exercise is best, For him that in old Age would live at rest' or 'for the man that is in health, exercise is the only medicine' (Neve, 1671; Trigge, 1681). There were two main types of exercise, the first consisting of vigorous physical movements, generally related to one's work or daily duties, that would result in deeper and/ or quicker breathing. The second included activities undertaken consciously, during one's leisure time, for the purpose of being healthy (Arcangeli, 2003).

Exercise, when taken in moderation, was considered to be a vital part of a good health regime. According to contemporary theory, exercise increases the heat of the body, keeps muscles limber, allows the body to sweat (thereby removing harmful humours) and improves transpiration (Arcangeli, 2003). To modern ears, however, some of the socially acceptable forms of exercise in early modern England were not likely to provide such results.

In early modern England, social forces exerted a great deal of pressure on contemporary ideas of appropriate physical activities. These might be determined by variables such as age, gender, socioeconomic class and ethnicity, as well as by prevailing politics. The types of acceptable exercise were heavily influenced by social and cultural considerations and also varied according to one's gender or constitution. While men could partake of a range of strenuous activities, it was generally recommended that women take up gardening instead (Laurence, 1996). Walking was also seen to be an excellent form of exercise for men and women, particularly if it was done in the countryside. Activities such as hunting, leaping or swimming, however, were generally portrayed as only being suitable for male members of the gentry or nobility (Peachem, 1622). Football was a popular sport for men lower down the social scale, as were a number of other games that involved running (Underdown, 1995).

Religion was another factor that had a major impact on what types of exercise were considered appropriate and when they were allowed to take place. The 'Declaration of Sports' issued by the Crown in 1618 and 1633 proclaimed that sports were only permissible after evening prayer was over. This meant that for most people, Sundays and church festivals were the only leisure time when they were allowed to enjoy such exercise. Many Puritans believed that the entire day should be committed to religious rejoicing and the praising of God, and that even watching others play on the Sabbath was a sin (Malcolmson, 1973).

Sleep and waking

Modern studies suggest that men and women who sleep fewer than seven to eight hours at a time have a higher mortality rate than their better rested contemporaries (Heslop et al., 2002). Insufficient sleep is also known to affect mental functions such as concentration as well as general mental wellbeing (Gale and Martyn, 1998). Early modern English writers reached similar conclusions, based on a collection of ancient texts on hygiene or the nature of what might now be called 'healthy lifestyles'. According to Nicholas Culpeper (1657, p. 129), the time spent sleeping would 'comfort nature much, refresheth the memory, cheers the spirits, quickens the senses'.

Diet

Dietetics has been called one of the most ancient branches of the therapeutic art, despite the fact that our modern definition is somewhat different from that of the past. In the early modern period, 'dietetics' encompassed a range of considerations, from the humoural qualities of different types of food and drink to the most appropriate times for consumption. The text *On Ancient Medicine*, part of the *Hippocratic Corpus*, suggests that 'in the beginning', humans and beasts were able to be nourished and grow by eating fruits, brush and grass but they then began to seek more differentiated forms of nourishment. The types of food and drink that this referred to changed dramatically over the centuries in response to socioeconomic and cultural factors.

During the medieval and early modern period, diet was considered 'the mother of diseases' because it was the most often consumed and longest internalized component of the non-naturals (Pelling, 1998). As such, it was thought to lead the way to a variety of illnesses, from gout to death. Such beliefs were based on centuries of empirical evidence of seeing the consequences of overeating and drinking.

> The case study in Chapter 3 shows how overconsumption of food and drink and a sedentary lifestyle are associated with obesity and subsequently high rates of mortality and morbidity, based on evidence from clinical studies.   **connections**

The components of what constitutes healthy eating are linked to a range of popular, scientific and political discourses and their corresponding implications for shaping individual and public behaviour (Guptil et al., 2013). Nutritional medicine, just one aspect of twenty-first-century healthcare, focuses on the use of specific nutritional factors in conjunction with the elimination of toxic and/or allergenic materials from the daily diet (Fulder, 1996). Although the terminology differed somewhat in the seventeenth century, the principle was almost exactly the same. People were advised to eat a varied diet, with the proviso that the type and quantity of food to be ingested depended on each person's gender, age and constitution.

Evacuation and retention

It was widely accepted that good health was linked to the periodic removal of excessive humours. This was done by regularly purging the system as a preventive measure. The modern definition of purging refers to emptying the bowels, perhaps through the assistance of colonic irrigation. However, in the medieval and early modern period, this was only one of many different methods used to remove unwanted materials from the body.

There were a number of different ways in which to purge offensive matter from almost every natural or artificial bodily orifice. Generally, they began with phlebotomy, or bloodletting, which comes from the Greek words *phleps* (vein) and *tome* (incision). Vomiting, 'neesing' (sneezing) and 'gargarismes' (gargles) were three popular methods for clearing the upper body. A more general, overall method was causing the body to sweat.

connections   Chapter 1 discusses how science now understands the physiological pathways that regulate processes such as sweating.

What might be called 'sexual evacuation' was also considered to be an important part of a good health regime. In moderation, and at the correct times of the year, sexual intercourse was an important part of good health. In broad humoural terms, females were 'cold and wet' and males were 'hot and dry'. It therefore followed that married women needed to have regular intercourse in order to avoid humoural imbalances. Galenic theory held that if 'natural seed' was kept too long within the body, it would turn into poison. So, for married men, too, regulated and moderate sexual emissions played a major part in the preservation of health. On the other hand, too much sex would weaken the seed and could result in stunted or deformed offspring (Stone, 1979; Crawford, 1994).

According to contemporary stereotypes, abstinence or even moderation would be almost impossible for many married men. The reason and the blame for this lay with their wives, who were cursed with voracious sexuality that could make them physically demanding whatever the season. Such behaviour could adversely affect their men, as too much sex was thought to weaken their seed and therefore their general health (Crawford, 1994; Fletcher, 1995). The physical reason for this had to do with Galenic theory, whereby men were thought to be hotter and drier than women. In some cases, women's urge to obtain sperm to counteract their colder and wetter complexions could spiral out of control (Weisner, 1998). Sexually transmitted diseases, such as 'the French pox' (now called syphilis), were another possible consequence of uncontrolled sex, then as now.

Passions and emotions

A final, but important component of a healthy lifestyle involved keeping a rein on one's emotional state. Judging by the vast number of texts on the subject, there was a great deal of interest in learning how to avoid or suppress excessive feelings of pride, anger, envy, malice, sorrow and fear. Such themes are still evident today, in the academic press and the multitude of popular self-help books and articles printed in the mass media. Some studies suggest that such negative emotions increase mortality rates following a myocardial infarction, or even play a role in the onset of coronary disease (Kubzansky and Kawachi, 2000).

?   Why is an understanding of past concepts of health and illness important?

Since all societies experience disease and illness, it follows that they also develop various practices to deal with them. Inherent in this framework would be people playing the role of carers or healers, whether on a formal or informal basis. It would also include the use of some types of medicinal ingredients, whether organic or inorganic substances. The study of medical history helps to provide insights into contemporary beliefs and practices, which in turn provide a greater understanding of how our current ideas have developed. In addition, the study of health and illness in the past can help to enhance current understandings of theoretical and cultural beliefs and practices and their ethical basis.

Developments in medicine and healthcare

Since ideas about what constitutes health and illness are linked to the society and culture in which they take place, it is understandable that they will change over time. While biomedicine is the dominant model in the West today, it should not be used to judge or denigrate earlier belief systems. The historical bonds between human and animal health still exist under the heading of 'one medicine'. This term refers to the inextricable interconnection between humans, animals and their social and ecological environment. Schillhorn van Veen (1998) has argued that Western Europe had 'one medicine' until the Industrial Revolution. Thirty years ago, Schwabe (1984, p. 30) emphatically stated that there has never been a 'difference of paradigm between human and veterinary medicine'. This concept is even more popular today, although it is increasingly being referred to as 'one health' rather than 'one medicine' (Zinsstag et al., 2011, pp. 148–56).

A great deal of our modern knowledge base can be traced back to much earlier times. As already mentioned, the theory of the four humours is attributed to the work of Hippocrates and Galen. Although the medieval period is no longer referred to as the 'Dark Ages', there is still a stereotype that there were few changes in medical knowledge between the sixth and fourteenth centuries AD. In fact, there is evidence that contemporary medical practice was influenced by ancient Greek writings and writings from the Byzantine Empire. This was also the period when medicine began to be taught at what would become great universities on the Continent and in England, such as Padua, Bologna, Paris, Montpelier and Oxford (Nutton, 1996). The early modern period of medicine continued to be based mainly on ancient Greek ideas, including continuance of the practice of bloodletting based on the four humours, and religious ideas still held sway. However, the growth of 'new science' in the late seventeenth century began to have an effect on beliefs and practices, and the influence of the Church declined.

example 2.2

The body as a machine: the contribution of dissection and anatomy

The ideas of Thomas Sydenham (1624–89) led to a great advance in the treatment of patients. He recognized the importance of detailed observation, record-keeping and the influence of the environment on the health of the patient. During the eighteenth century, through a series of painstaking dissections, William Harvey was able to demonstrate that the body contains only a single supply of blood and the heart is a muscle pumping it round a circuit. Research into general anatomy and physiology led to new 'mechanistic' theories, whereby the body was seen to be comparable to a machine. The development of the microscope enabled organisms to be studied. The study of microbes, or microbiology, and the increased knowledge of pathogenic microbes led to the development of new medicines to tackle infectious diseases. By the late eighteenth century, the use of infected matter from smallpox victims was being used as a preventive measure in parts of Europe. However, the practice of inoculation is credited to Edward Jenner, an English country doctor who injected patients with cowpox to protect them against smallpox.

? Which factors had the greatest influence on the development of modern medicine?

It is misleading to suggest that changes in medicine occurred in a linear chronological fashion. All historical change is a consequence of many developments:

- the pressures of the economy and need for trade

- urbanization, war and nationalism

- developments in education and its institutions

- religious beliefs and the relative importance of religious institutions

- scientific and technological developments.

example 2.3

Changes in the management of infectious diseases

From the fourteenth to seventeenth centuries, bubonic plague killed millions of people across Europe. From 1347 to 1352, 25 million people died. One-third to one-half of the European population was wiped out. Until the late eighteenth century, outbreaks were dealt with by emergency measures and regulations dealing with disposal of the dead and rubbish. Venice established a system of epidemic control by setting up special hospitals to house the sick and their contacts, burning a dead person's clothes and restricting travel. Humans were seen as the vectors of disease and so a person required a clean bill of health before they could enter the city.

From the mid-nineteenth century, changes in surgery can be attributed to improved surgical instruments from manufacturing industry, and the discovery of anaesthetics such as ether, chloroform and cocaine allowed surgeons to take more time over operations. During the Industrial Revolution, means of communication such as the telegraph and railways also meant scientists and doctors were able to communicate with each other and contributed to the development of ideas.

There have been many institutional and structural changes in how healthcare for humans has been organized and administered over the centuries. European hospitals, for example, date back over 1,000 years. Their purpose, however, has changed dramatically since the Middle Ages. Unlike modern hospitals, medieval ones did not provide a range of specialized medical services, but were more similar to what are now called 'hospices'. In fifteenth- and sixteenth-century London, there were up to 30 hospitals, which served a range of purposes. St Bartholomew, for example, treated the sick, while St Thomas was for poor elderly people. Bridewell was a hospital for 'the idle poor', while 'lunatics' were placed in Bethlem, more commonly known as 'Bedlam' (Slack, 1997, p. 236). Over time, these evolved into centres for patients who required rest and fairly simple treatments, while excluding those with infectious diseases.

There were also many changes over the centuries in how such institutions were funded. In eighteenth-century Europe, many voluntary hospitals were endowed with properties or funded by the church or state. In England, however, they were supported mainly through charitable contributions, subscriptions, fundraising events or collection boxes (Berry, 1997). Since its foundation in 1948, the majority of British hospitals and healthcare have been provided by the state- (that is, tax-) funded NHS. This has been joined by a rapidly growing private sector offering biomedical and alternative therapies, as well as services offered by voluntary or charitable organizations (Rivett, 1998).

There are also a number of state-funded healthcare systems in Continental Europe. Italy, for example, has the similarly named 'Servizio Sanitario Nazionale'. The principle of free at the point of use healthcare was also first introduced in Italy in 1948, although it took several decades before it came to fruition (Turati, 2013). Russia also provides nationalized clinics, although their chronic underfunding and understaffing has led to many people being forced to pay for private services (Nazarova, 2009).

Despite the similarities between many modern health systems in European countries, there are also differences linked to varying sociocultural ideas. Some of these are linked to issues of decentralization. For example, the division of Germany after the Second World War resulted in different types of healthcare in the new countries of East and West Germany. In addition to differences in funding and technology, these included a greater acceptance of complementary medicine in the West. After the fall of the Berlin Wall in 1989, however, the reunified country was said to have returned to its 'common medical heritage' (Payer, 1996, p. xii). Today, Germany has a system based on public and private services. Unless a person is covered by private health insurance, this involves mandatory participation in a statutory insurance scheme.

Chapter 9 discusses how an analysis of comparative welfare systems can contribute to understanding the factors influencing social policy.

connections

Part 2 Theoretical and research approaches

example 2.4

Examples of historical health research

- Medical beliefs and practices in the past
- The institutionalization of medicine and medical care

- Preventive and 'preservative' medicine
- The growth of 'one medicine' or 'one health'
- The development of mental healthcare and changing ideas on mental illness

The development of the discipline

History, as with all the other disciplines described in this book, has its own approach to researching and explaining its core questions. Thucydides (*c.* 460–400 BC) is credited with having begun the scientific approach to history in his work *The History of the Peloponnesian War*. In his historical method, Thucydides emphasized chronology, a neutral point of view, and that the human world was the result of the actions of human beings, not divine intervention. In the twentieth century, historians focused less on epic narratives, which often tended to glorify the nation or individuals, and more on realistic chronologies.

As de Blécourt and Usborne (1999, p. 283) pointed out, different times produce different types of historians. One hundred years ago the field of medical history was dominated by men whose main interest was in the history of 'great doctors' and the (supposedly) unilinear path of scientific, medical progress. These men were not academics but 'physician[s], trained in the research method of history' (Sigerist, 1951, p. 15). This was part of the Whiggish school of history, which argues that the past consists of a 'noble ... crusade marching into the present' (Duffin, 2010, p. 446). In medical history, this resulted in viewing the past as a time of 'ignorance, superstition and suffering', which moved in a single path towards modern, 'scientific' medicine (Lindemann, 1999, p. 278).

Fortunately, the tendency to negate earlier medical practices and practitioners is no longer the norm. Medical history is now a greatly expanded discipline encompassing a range of subjects in humanities and social sciences. In fact, according to one historian, the entire field 'is expanding at break-neck speed' (Burnham, 2007, p. 1). This has resulted in a variety of new ways of looking at issues of health and illness, with many historians now focusing almost entirely on the close link between illness, society and healing (Wilson, 1993).

The latter part of the twentieth century saw the burgeoning of a new type of social history with highly segmented subdisciplines. Each of these has developed its own sources, methods, topics, problems and concerns. Taken literally, the term 'social history' refers to the history of societies, or social structures, processes and trends. In this respect, its focus and thinking is closely linked to the sociological paradigm of social constructionism, which suggests that knowledge is not an independent reality, but is linked to social relations and, therefore, subject to change. The focus of social history has shifted away from looking at how organizations such as charities and governmental bodies dealt with social problems, such as poverty or ignorance, in the 1970s. This was followed by an examination of everyday life, in the home and the workplace. A third stage focuses more on particular groups, such as the working class or women (Tosh, 2002). Although the main current interest is on patients' points of view, many medical historians work in other areas, depending on their own academic background and interests.

Karl Marx's interpretation of history, generally referred to as 'the materialist conception of history' or 'historical materialism', stresses the important relationship between economic production, social institutions and the everyday life of people (Green and Troupe, 1999). Critics have argued that Marxism attempted to 'reduce all of history to material causes ... overlooking the influence of ideas, personalities and emotions' (Appleby et al., 1994, p. 80).

Marxist studies on the history of health-related issues would be likely to focus on issues of political and economic power operating within a capitalist society. Studies of the early modern period, for example, would have looked at the role the bourgeoisie played in contemporary healthcare provision (Elton, 2002). In the modern period, such studies might look at the way in which the NHS mirrors society's class structure through control over health institutions, stratification of health workers, and limited occupational mobility (Waitzkin, 1978).

One example of the use of Marxist theory can be found in a study of mental illness and the evolution of mental health policy. As a Marxist historian, Scull disagreed with the commonly held view that the growth of mental asylums in the nineteenth century was linked to growing urbanization and industrialization. Instead, he argued that their phenomenal rise was related to 'the emergence of segregative control mechanisms and the growth of an ever more highly rationalized capitalist order' (Scull, 1977, p. 221). A more recent example of this theory would be that poor mental health is linked to increasing working hours, compromised safety at work, lower job satisfaction, and insecurity (Larkin, 2011).

example 2.5

Foucault and history

Michel Foucault (1926–84) was a French philosopher and historian who believed that the body could be seen as an object and instrument of political power. His writings, which first appeared in the 1960s, emphasized the types of power biomedical practitioners and the state held over their patients. This included the ability to relabel or 'medicalize' various types of conditions that had not formerly been seen as medical problems, such as pregnancy (Waddington, 2011).

Discipline and Punish (1977), one of

Foucault's most famous works, focused on Western penal systems. Based on French sources, Foucault gives a series of eighteenth-century examples of disciplinary regimes, including army barracks, schools and hospitals. Foucault shows how, in such institutions, the keeping of records on individual cases and examinations, for example parades in the army, tests in schools and consultants' rounds in a hospital, helped control the subjects and made each one's progress visible.

The historical method: using sources, oral history

History is studied through the assessment and interpretation of **evidence** and thus entails using primary sources. In general, there are two main types of source material used by historians:

1. *Primary* material is that written or compiled by people living in the time period under study. This might include handwritten letters, journals or other accounts, printed pamphlets or books, newspapers or journals. If the subjects of interest are still alive, primary material might also include taped or transcribed interview notes.

2. *Secondary* sources can date from any time after the period under study. They can include commentaries on earlier events, government reports or statistics, official documents, newspapers, journals or television or radio programmes.

Examples of primary sources include the texts on healthy living printed in the sixteenth and seventeenth centuries.

example 2.6

Almanacs as a historical source

Almanacs are one of the oldest known forms of literature, dating back to the manuscript texts on lunar and planetary motion from the third century BC (Parker, 1975). By the Middle Ages, the genre had grown into a highly popular annual means of using astrological calculations to predict events for the coming year. The first printed almanac was published by Johannes Gutenberg in 1448, eight years before his famous Bible. By the 1470s, large numbers of almanacs were being printed in various European countries (Capp, 1979). The first domestically printed edition appeared in England in 1537, and quickly become what one historian has called a 'scientific bestseller' (Jones, 1999; Simons, 2001).

Printed in their hundreds of thousands every year, these cheap, annual publications targeted and were read by a wide cross-section of the public, making them the first true form of British mass media. The main purpose of almanacs was to disseminate information about the movements of the stars and planets and their subsequent effects on all living things. However, most included a range of other interesting, useful and/or entertaining topics, including a great deal of information on popular beliefs and practices (Hill Curth, 2007).

Although some authors provided more medical material than others, all advice was divided into preventive and remedial treatments for humans, and often for animals as well. The major emphasis was on preserving a state of health by following a good health regimen, based on the Galenic non-naturals. If someone was unlucky enough to fall ill, almanacs also provided advice on remedial treatments or medicines that could be prepared either at home or by an apothecary. By the latter part of the seventeenth century, this material was joined by a growing number of advertisements for what might be called 'self-help' books, as well as medical services and implements such as trusses or fake eyeballs. In addition, the advertisements illustrate the early growth of ready-made, prepackaged and branded proprietary medicines (Hill Curth, 2002).

Another example of primary material are letters, which became widely used as a means of communication as literacy levels increased in the late nineteenth century. During periods of war, the letters from soldiers and others provide insight into wartime conditions and their impact on health. For example, during the Boer War there was movement of nurses both to and from South Africa from many parts of the world. This was part of the greater movement of nurses during the colonial expansion. This created a mixing of ideas and experiences termed the 'nursing diaspora' (Rafferty, 2005; http://boerwarnurses.com).

Oral history is seen as mainly a methodological approach, but it could be argued that the growing number of theories on memory and subjectivity takes it further than that. Green and Troupe (1999, p. 130) have argued that oral history is a product of the 1960s and was developed in order to reach otherwise 'marginalized or neglected social groups such as women or ethnic minorities'. Since that time, however, the approach has tended to focus on the 'subjective and collective meaning embedded in the narrative'.

Oral history is an ideal methodology for academics interested in the health beliefs and practices of subjects who are still living. For example, in 2005, the Department of Health began an oral history project to document the experiences and commitment of those from the Caribbean who helped set the foundations for today's NHS between 1948 and 1969. The growth of new forms of mass communication, such as the internet, has also made it possible for the results of such studies to be disseminated to a vast audience. In 2005, the Wellcome Trust set up a website to disseminate the results of an oral history project, which involved the stories of 100 people diagnosed with diabetes between 1927 and 1997 (www.diabetes-stories.com).

case study food safety and bread in Victorian England

Until 1875, there were few effective controls on the content or quality of food and drink on sale to the public. Now far more additives are present in foods than ever before, but their use is, by and large, monitored and controlled. Food safety remains a major public concern and, in recent years, the UK has seen concerns over salmonella in eggs and bovine spongiform encephalopathy (BSE) in beef. Analyses of these crises have tended to focus on the processes of large-scale food production and the ways in which health risks are communicated to the public. This case study examines the role of bread as a staple part of the diet of Victorian England.

The production, distribution and cost of bread as a staple food have been matters of great social and economic importance for many years. In 1815, for example, the Corn Laws raised the duty on imported wheat, which led to increased prices and subsequent riots in many cities. This case study will examine the development of a new way of making bread in mid-Victorian London. This was a period when most urban dwellers were suffering from poor nutrition, polluted air and water supplies, overcrowded living conditions, and the ravages of infectious diseases (Hardy, 1988). Since most Londoners did not have the facilities, or time, to make their own bread, many were forced to buy highly adulterated loaves produced in underground bakeries by 'sickly, perspiring men who worked round the clock' (Baker, 1858, p. 4). Karl Marx (cited in Kimber, 2005) noted the problems of poor bread in the first volume of *Capital*, commenting:

> Englishmen, with their good command of the Bible, knew well enough that man, unless by elective grace a capitalist, or a landlord, or the holder of a sinecure, is destined to eat his bread in the sweat of his brow. But they did not know that he had to eat daily in his bread a certain

quantity of human perspiration mixed with the discharge of abscesses, cobwebs, dead cockroaches and putrid German yeast, not to mention alum, sand and other agreeable mineral ingredients.

Marx noted the testimony to the 1855 parliamentary committee that, because of adulterations, 'the poor men who lived on two pounds of bread a day did not take in one fourth of that amount of nutrition'.

There were two main reasons why food and drink were adulterated. The first was to make products more attractive to customers, for example adding chalk to milk to increase its whiteness, or dyeing used tea leaves to render them brown again. The second reason was to increase bulk; for example, in bread-making, a range of potentially dangerous additives were added to increase bulk and produce a more attractive loaf. According to a study carried out in 1855, bread could be adulterated with mashed potatoes, alum and sometimes, although rarely, with sulfites of copper (House of Commons, 1856).

The public outcry about food safety became so great that, in 1869, Hansard reports Lord Eustace Cecil calling upon Her Majesty's government to 'give their earliest attention to the widespread and most reprehensible practice of using false weights and measures and of adulterating food, drink and drugs'. The first Food Adulteration Act was passed in 1860, followed by a revised Adulteration of Foods Act in 1872. The Sale of Food and Drugs Act was passed in 1875, which required local authorities to appoint public analysts as well as providing workable measures against adulteration (French and Phillips, 2000).

In addition to concerns about adulteration, there were concerns with the way in which commercial bread was manufactured. The majority of London bakeries were situated underground, with the 'conveniences' situated in one corner opposite the dough troughs in the other, and open drains running the length of the room. 'Sulphurous fumes' from the furnace mixed with flour dust and moisture from the bread rendered the air almost impossible to breathe (*British Baker, Confectioner and Purveyor*, March 1894, p. 589). Instead of skilled bakers, owners hired sweated labourers with poor personal hygiene who worked round the clock in overheated filthy conditions. These men suffered a range of health problems, from heat exhaustion to pneumonia, heart failure, chest and lung damage from the flour dust, and uncomfortable rashes on their hands, known as 'baker's itch'. A study in 1848 found that, of 111 bakers examined by Dr Guy, none were in 'robust health' (Petersen, 1995).

Traditionally, bread has been made by hand out of a mixture of flour, water, salt and yeast. In addition to worries about the workers who were handling commercial dough, there were also concerns about the effects that bread prepared with yeast could have on health. This was due to a prevailing idea in mid Victorian London that 'fermented bread has a tendency to ferment a second time in the stomach, and thus bring on acidity and other inconveniences' (Dodd, 1856, pp. 203–4). The contemporary discovery that carbon dioxide could be used instead of yeast gave rise to a new type of bread developed by Dr John Dauglish in the late 1850s. His products were referred to as 'aerated' bread, after the carbonated water he used as a raising agent instead of yeast. The product was also free of any adulterants and was produced almost entirely by machinery.

This new bread proved so popular that Dauglish was able to find investors to help build the Aerated Bread Company (ABC). One of the major reasons for the young firm's success was undoubtedly that they played on public concerns about food safety by developing a bread that would now be referred to as a 'health food'. The ABC advertised heavily in the daily newspapers, promising readers that their bread was 'untouched by hand in its entire manufacture'. Furthermore, it was not only 'most valuable' for 'sustaining the health of children' but it would even 'give great relief to persons suffering from acidity of the stomach, flatulence, heartburn and loss of appetite' (*Daily News*, 1886). Aerated bread was 'tried dietetically' at Guy's Hospital and by numerous London physicians who were willing to vouch for its health value (Lobb, 1860). The growing popularity of aerated bread during this period suggests either that consumers believed its consumption aided their health, or it actually did so.

Although the ABC began simply as a manufacturer of bread, it soon developed into an outfit with multiple retailing outlets. As the size of its distribution network increased, so did its product line. ABC swiftly moved from simple white loaves into other types of baked goods. Within the first decade or so of its existence, it developed a new form of catering for light refreshments to provide additional outlets for its products. The company continued to grow through a mixture of good business practices, as well as adopting novel concepts and technologies. By the end of the century, an article in *The Master Baker* (1899) lauded the ABC as being 'the leading company, notwithstanding the ever-increasing competition of its younger, and perhaps more enterprising rivals'. The ABC is an example of an organization that developed in response to the increasing demand for variety and volume of cheap, unadulterated bread. As the original company prospectus stated:

> Wherever the aerated bread has been introduced it has obtained favour with the Public and support from the Medical Profession, by its perfect cleanliness and purity, and wholesome and nutritious qualities; and it must, when supplied in quantity, supersede the use of fermented bread. (Aerated Bread Company Prospectus, 1862)

Summary

- Views on what constitutes a state of health and/or illness are dependent on society and culture, as well as the time period in which they take place
- Medical history is an interdisciplinary subject heavily influenced by social sciences and humanities
- While medical history was once concerned only with 'great doctors' and 'great discoveries', it now focuses on the ways in which people understood and experienced states of health and illness

Questions for further discussion

1. Why do ideas about what constitutes 'health' differ over time?

2. What arguments would you use to justify including a historical perspective in health studies?

3. What kinds of methods can be used to disseminate information about health and healthcare to the public?

4. What accounts for the dominance of the biomedical model in the twentieth century?

5. What influence can or should history have on the development of policy in relation to healthcare?

Further reading and resources

Burnham, J. (2007) *What is Medical History?* London: Polity.
Provides an excellent overview to many different facets of medical history, including discussions of the changing roles of healers and patients and how concepts and types of diseases have changed over time.

Duffin, J. (2010) *History of Medicine: A Scandalously Short Introduction* (2nd edn). Toronto: University of Toronto Press.
Good starting point for those with little or no knowledge of this topic, offering an introduction to a number of areas for further study.

Porter, R. (1999) *The Greatest Benefit to Mankind: A Medical History of Humanity*. London: Fontana.
Written by one of the foremost medical historians of the late twentieth century, this is one of his most comprehensive and important works on the history of medicine.

Webster, C. (ed.) (2001) *Caring for Health: History and Diversity*. Buckingham: Open University Press.
Excellent compilation of essays, providing an analytical overview of the historical development of Western models of health between the sixteenth and late twentieth centuries.

There are some journals and websites with a specific focus on history and health or medicine, for example *Journal of the History of Medicine and Allied Sciences*, *Medical History*, and *Social History of Medicine*. Websites include:

- www.nimr.mrc.ac.uk British Official Publications
- www.nlm.nih.gov US National Library of Medicine
- www.nlm.nih.gov/hmd National Institute for the History of Medicine
- www.wellcome.ac.uk Wellcome Trust

The Wellcome Trust is a global charity that includes a study of the history of medicine at www.wellcome.ac.uk/About-us/Publications/Wellcome-History, and also funds an exhibition at the London Science Museum at www.sciencemuseum.org.uk/broughttolife. aspx?gclid=COykp8Hss8ECFSj3wgod0bsAtA.

References

Allen, J. (1765) *A Complete English Dictionary*. London.

Appleby, J., Hunt, L. and Jacob, J. (1994) *Telling the Truth about History*. London: W.W. Norton.

Arcangeli, A. (2003) *Recreation in the Renaissance: Attitudes toward Leisure and Pastimes in European Culture, c.1425–1675*. Basingstoke: Palgrave Macmillan.

Baker, A. (1858) An Address to Master and Journeymen Bakers Dedicated to the General Board of Health and the Medical Profession. London.

Bates, D.G. (2000) 'Why not call modern medicine alternative?' *Perspectives in Biology and Medicine* 43(4): 502–18.

Battie, W. (1758) *Treatise on Madness*. London: Whiston and White.

Berry, A. (1997) 'Balancing the books: funding provincial hospitals in 18th century England'. *Accounting, Business and Financial History* 7(1): 1–30.

Black, J. and MacRaild, D.M. (2000) *Studying History*. Basingstoke: Palgrave – now Palgrave Macmillan.

Boyd, K.M. (2000) 'Disease, illness, sickness, health, healing and wholeness: exploring some elusive concepts'. *Medical Humanities* 26(1): 9–17.

Boyer, G.R. (2009) Insecurity, safety nets and self-help in Victorian and Edwardian Britain, in D. Ellis, F. Lewis and K. Sokoloff (eds) *Human Capital and Institutions: A Long-run View*. Cambridge: Cambridge University Press, pp. 46–90.

Burnham, J. (2007) *What is Medical History?* London: Polity.

Bynum, W.F. (1999) *Science and the Practice of Medicine in the Nineteenth Century*. Cambridge: Cambridge University Press.

Capp, B. (1979) *Astrology and the Popular Press: English Almanacs, 1500–1800*. London: Cornell University Press.

Clark, S. (1997) Demons and disease: the disenchantment of the sick (1500–1700), in M. Gijswijt-Hofstra, H. Marland and H. de Waardt (eds) *Illness and Healing Alternatives in Western Europe*. New York: Routledge, pp. 38–59.

Corbin, A. (1996) *The Foul and the Fragrant: Odour and the Social Imagination*. London: Papermac.

Crawford, P. (1994) Sexual knowledge in England 1500–1750, in R. Porter (ed.) *Sexual Knowledge, Sexual Science: The History of Attitudes to Sexuality*. Cambridge: Cambridge University Press, pp. 82–107.

Culpeper, N. (1657) *Galen's Art of Physick*. London: Peter Cole.

De Blécourt, W. and Usborne, C. (1999) 'Situating alternative medicine in the modern period'. *Medical History*, 43(3): 376–92.

Dodd, G. (1856) *The Food of London*. London: Longman, Brown, Green and Longmans.

Duffin, J. (2010) *History of Medicine: A Scandalously Short Introduction* (2nd edn). Toronto: University of Toronto Press.

Elton, G.R. (2002) *The Practice of History* (2nd edn). Oxford: Blackwell.

Fletcher, A. (1995) *Gender, Sex and Subordination in England 1500–1800*. London: Yale University Press.

Foucault, M. (1977) *Discipline and Punish: The Birth of the Prison*. London: Allen Lane.

French, M. and Phillips, J. (2000) *Cheated not Poisoned? Food Regulation in the United Kingdom 1875–1938*. Manchester: Manchester University Press.

French, R. (2003) *Medicine before Science: The Business of Medicine from the Middle Ages to the Enlightenment*. Cambridge: Cambridge University Press.

Fulder, S. (1996) *The Handbook of Alternative and Complementary Medicine*. London: Vermillion.

Gale, C. and Martyn, C. (1998) 'Larks and owls and health, wealth and wisdom'. *British Medical Journal* 317(7174): 1675–7.

Green, A. and Troupe, K. (1999) *The Houses of History: A Critical Reader in Twentieth-century History and Theory*. Manchester: Manchester University Press.

Guptil, A., Copelton, D. and Lucal, B. (2013) *Food and Society: Principles and Paradoxes*. Cambridge: Polity.

Hansard (1869) False Weights and Measures and Adulteration: Observations. HC Deb 05 vol 194 cc718-36. Available at http://hansard.millbanksystems.com/commons/1869/mar/05/false-weights-and-measures-and (accessed 7/10/2014).

Hardy, A. (1988) 'Diagnosis, death, and diet: the case of London, 1750–1909'. *Journal of Interdisciplinary History* 18(3): 387–401.

Heslop, P., Smith, G.D., Metcalfe, C. et al. (2002) 'Sleep duration and mortality: the effect of short or long sleep duration on cardiovascular and all-cause mortality in working men and women'. *Sleep Medicine* 3: 305–14.

Hill Curth, L. (2002) 'The commercialisation of medicine in the popular press: English almanacs 1640–1700'. *The Seventeenth Century* 17: 48–69.

Hill Curth, L. (2007) *English Almanacs, Astrology and Popular Medicine 1550–1700*. Manchester: Manchester University Press.

House of Commons (1856) *Report from the Select Committee on Adulteration of Food*. London: HMSO.

Jones, S.D. (2004) 'Mapping a zoonotic disease: Anglo-American efforts to control bovine tuberculosis before World War I'. *Osiris* 19: 133–48.

Kang, S. (2004) Cultural assumptions of medical theory and practice, in M. Evans, P. Louhiala and R. Puustinen (eds) *Philosophy for Medicine: Applications in A Clinical Context*. Oxford: Oxford University Press, pp. 65–83.

Kimber, C. (2005) 'Marx and Engels on food adulteration'. *Socialist Worker* 2 April, 1945.

Kovacs, J. (1989) 'Concepts of health and disease'. *Journal of Medicine and Philosophy* 14(3): 261–7.

Kubzansky, L. and I. Kawachi (2000) 'Going to the heart of the matter: Do negative emotions cause coronary heart disease?' *Journal of Psychosomatic Research* 48: 323–37.

Larkin, M. (2011) *Social Aspects of Health, Illness and Healthcare*. Maidenhead: Open University Press.

Laurence, A. (1996) *Women in England 1500–1760*. London: Phoenix.

LeClerc, D. (1699) *The History of Physick, or an Account of the Rise and Progress of the Art*. London: D. Brown.

Lindemann, M. (1999) *Medicine and Society in Early Modern England*. Cambridge: Cambridge University Press.

Lobb, H.W. (1860) *Hygiene of Bread*. London.

Longrigg, J. (1998) *Greek Medicine from the Heroic to the Hellenistic Age: A Source Book*. New York: Routledge.

Malcolmson, R. (1973) Popular recreations before the eighteenth-century, in R. Malcolmson (ed.) *Popular Recreations in English Society 1700 1850*. Cambridge: Cambridge University Press, pp. 5–15.

Maudsley, H. (1871) *Body and Mind*. New York: D. Appleton.

Maynwaring, E. (1669) *Vita sana and longa: the Preservation of Health and Prolongation of Life*. London: JD.

Nazarova, I. (2009) Access to health care and self care, in N. Manning (ed.) *Health and Health Care in the New Russia*. Farnham: Ashgate, pp. 173–200.

Neve, R. (1671) *Merlinus Verax, or, An Almanac*. London.

Niebyl, P.H. (1971) 'The non-naturals'. *Bulletin of the History of Medicine* 45: 486–92.

Nutton, B. (1996) The rise of medicine, in R. Porter (ed.) *Cambridge Illustrated History of Medicine*. Cambridge: Cambridge University Press, pp. 52–81.

Parker, D. (1975) *Familiar to All: William Lilly and Astrology in the Seventeenth Century*. London: Cape.

Payer, L. (1996) *Medicine and Culture*. New York: Henry Holt.

Peacham, H. (1622) *The Complete Gentleman: The Truth of our Times, and The Art of Living in London*. London.

Pelling, M. (1998) Attitudes to diet in early modern England, in M. Pelling *The Common Lot: Sickness, Medical Occupations and the Urban Poor in Early Modern England*. London: Longman, pp. 38–63.

Petersen, C. (1995) *Bread and the British Economy c. 1770–1870*. Aldershot: Ashgate.

Porter, R. (1993) Man, animals and medicine at the time of the founding of the Royal Veterinary College, in A.R. Mitchell (ed.) *History of the Healing Professions*, 3. Wallingford: CAB International, pp. 19–30.

Porter, R. (1996) Medical science, in R. Porter (ed.) *The Cambridge Illustrated History of Medicine*. Cambridge: Cambridge University Press, pp. 154–202.

Porter, R. (2002) *Blood and Guts: A Short History of Medicine*. London: Penguin.

Rafferty, A.M. (2005) 'The seductions of history and the nursing diaspora'. *Health and History* 7(2): 2–16.

Rivett, G. (1998) *From Cradle to Grave: The First 50 Years of the NHS*. London: King's Fund.

Saunders, R. (1681) *Apollo Anglicanus*. London.

Schiefsky, M. (2005) *Hippocrates on Ancient Medicine*. Leiden: Brill.

Schillhorn van Veen, T.W. (1998) 'One medicine: the dynamic relationship between animal and human medicine in history and at present'. *Agriculture and Human Values* 15: 116.

Schwabe, C. (1984) *Veterinary Medicine and Human Health*. Baltimore: Johns Hopkins University Press.

Scull, A. (1977) 'Madness and segregative control: the rise of the insane asylum'. *Social Problems* 24(3): 337–51.

Shorter, E. (1997) *A History of Psychiatry*. London: Wiley.

Sigerist, H. (1951) *A History of Medicine,* vol. I. Oxford: Oxford University Press.

Simons, R.C. (2001) ABCs, almanacs, ballads, chapbooks, popular piety and textbooks, in J. Barnard and D.F. McKenzie (eds) *The Cambridge History of the Book in Britain*, vol. 4. Cambridge: Cambridge University Press, pp. 504–14.

Slack, P. (1997) *Hospitals, Workhouses and the Relief of the Poor in Early Modern*. London: Routledge.

Sloan, A.W. (1996) *English Medicine in the Seventeenth Century*. Durham: Durham Academic Press.

Sotres, P.G. (1998) The regimens of health, in M. Grmk (ed.) *Western Medical Thought from Antiquity to the Middle Ages*. Cambridge, MA: Harvard University Press, pp. 291–319.

Stone, L. (1979) *The Family, Sex and Marriage in England 1500–1800*. Cambridge: Cambridge University Press.

Thomas, K. (1991) *Religion and the Decline of Magic*. London: Penguin.

Tosh, J. (2002) *The Pursuit of History* (3rd edn). London: Longman.

Trigge, T. (1681) *Calendarium Astrologicum*. London.

Turati, G. (2013) The Italian Servizio Sanitario Nazionale: a renewing tale of lost promises, in J. Costa-Font and S. Greer (eds) *Federalism and Decentralization in European Health and Social Care*. Basingstoke: Palgrave Macmillan, pp. 47–120.

Underdown, D. (1995) Regional cultures? Local variations in popular culture in the early modern period, in T. Harris (ed.) *Popular Culture in England, c.1500–1850*. Basingstoke: Macmillan – now Palgrave Macmillan.

Waddington, K. (2011) *An Introduction to the Social History of Medicine*. Basingstoke: Palgrave Macmillan.

Waitzkin, H. (1978) 'A Marxist view of medical care'. *Annals of Internal Medicine* 2: 264–78.

Wear, A. (2000) *Knowledge and Practice in English Medicine 1550–1680*. Cambridge: Cambridge University Press.

Weisner, M. (1998) *Women and Gender in Early Modern England*. Cambridge: Cambridge University Press.

WHO (World Health Organization) (1946) *Preamble of the Constitution of the World Health Organization*. Geneva: WHO.

Wilson, A. (1993) A critical portrait of social history, in A. Wilson (ed.) *Rethinking Social History: English Society 1570–1920*. Manchester: Manchester University Press, pp. 1–25.

Zinsstag, J., Schelling, E., Waltner-Toewsm, D. and Tanner, M. (2011) 'From one medicine to one health and systemic approaches to health and wellbeing'. *Preventative Veterinary Medicine* 101(3/4): 148–56.

NICOLA CRICHTON and ANNE MULHALL

Epidemiology and health

Overview   79

Introduction   79

Part 1 The contribution of epidemiology to health studies   80
The emergence of the evidence-based healthcare movement   83
The link between ill health and socioeconomic conditions   85
Concepts of health and disease in medical epidemiology   87
Social epidemiology   89

Part 2 Theoretical and research approaches   91
The natural history of disease   92
Identifying risk   93
Classifying disease   93
Diagnosing and treating disease   94
Surveillance and the planning and evaluation of health services   94
The methodologies used by epidemiology   96

Case study Trends in obesity   104
Summary   108
Questions for further discussion   108
Further reading and resources   108
References   109

Learning outcomes

This chapter will enable readers to:

- Define different epidemiological approaches and be aware of their importance to healthcare
- Understand where epidemiology stands in relation to other disciplines in healthcare
- Describe the different research designs used by epidemiology
- Gain an appreciation of the concepts of health and sickness as they are used in epidemiology

Overview

Epidemiology is the study of how diseases are distributed among different groups of people and the factors that affect this distribution. Accurately recording who in a defined population contracts a disease (the disease rate) also makes it possible to explore factors that might affect disease acquisition. Disease patterns are traditionally studied in relation to time, place and person. For example: Does the disease occur during particular seasons? In certain geographical locations? Age groups? Do those who become sick differ in their lifestyle habits from those who remain healthy? In this way, epidemiology tries to predict conditions (risk factors) that might lead to disease, and thus to identify strategies that might be used to prevent its occurrence. Moreover, once someone has contracted a disease, epidemiology can help to identify prognostic factors, which indicate how quickly or severely the disease may progress. The natural history of diseases (how they develop and progress over time) is thus central to epidemiology. Since it is concerned with rates, epidemiology focuses on populations of people rather than single individuals.

Part 1 explores the approach of epidemiology to healthcare problems and how health and disease are conceptualized in epidemiology. Part 2 describes how epidemiological data are collected and analysed. The chapter concludes with a case study discussing how epidemiology studies public health issues such as obesity by analysing its distribution and seeking to explain its causes.

Introduction

Epidemiology – derived from the Greek *epi* (upon), *demos* (people), *logos* (science) – is the science of how often and why diseases occur in different groups of people. It is concerned with the who, what, where, when and how of disease causation (Valanis, 1999). This focus on health and disease in human populations, as opposed to individuals, is central to epidemiological theory and the research methodologies that it uses. Epidemiologists are concerned with the experience of groups, the differences between groups and whether chance might have affected these differences or whether they provide clues to the **aetiology** or cause of disease.

Four questions drive the discipline:

- Who becomes sick or is most likely to be affected by a disease or condition?

- Why do particular people become sick?

- When are people most likely to be affected?

- How effective are the available treatments and preventive strategies?

In many ways, epidemiologists are like detectives trying to understand if a disease occurs at particular times, in particular groups and what might be the reasons for this. The focus of epidemiology has traditionally been a concern with disease. The study of the distribution of disease (mortality and morbidity) – descriptive epidemiology – has been central to public health strategy. It identifies and quantifies ill health problems in communities, whether nations or smaller groups within nations, and assesses the scope for prevention. The assessment of population health is not, however, straightforward. A wide range of data is available to illustrate different aspects of a population's health – the illnesses and diseases experienced, how many people are born and die, and the lifestyles and health behaviours of the population. This chapter argues that, as health is not easily defined, a broader view of epidemiology is needed that uses methodologies incorporating lay perceptions and perspectives. In identifying health problems, a social epidemiology focuses not just on biomedical causes but also on socioeconomic factors.

Part 1 The contribution of epidemiology to health studies

---

example 3.1

The application of epidemiology to contemporary health issues

- Population or community health assessment, for example the monitoring of reports of communicable diseases in the community
- Determinants of a disease or condition, for example whether a particular dietary component such as alcohol influences the risk of developing cancer

- Evaluation of the effectiveness and impact of an intervention, for example cholesterol awareness programme through quasi-experimental study design
- Analysis of historical trends and current data to project future public health need
- Clinical trials randomizing communities into different strategies for risk reduction

---

For hundreds of years, certainly long before the founding of the discipline, people have been trying to make sense of why disease occurs at certain times, in certain places and in certain people. Some early commentators suggested that supernatural events caused sickness, whereas others, such as Hippocrates, related disease to lifestyle and environmental conditions. Although the cause of disease was often historically unknown, links between certain conditions (perhaps something to do with the climate or geography) and the occurrence of disease were made.

example 3.2

John Snow and the Broad Street pump

During the early nineteenth century, severe cholera epidemics threatened London, and John Snow, a doctor, became interested in the cause and transmission of the condition. In 1849, he published *On the Mode of Communication of Cholera*, suggesting that cholera is a contagious disease caused by a poison in the vomit and stools of cholera patients. He believed that the main means of transmission was water contaminated with this poison. This differed from the commonly held theory that diseases were transmitted by inhaling vapours or miasmas.

In 1854, 500 people died in the Soho area of London. By plotting the geographical location of each case, shown in Figure 3.1, Snow deduced that the deaths occurred in people living close to a water pump in Broad Street, yet a workhouse with 535 inmates close to the pump had had only four fatalities. On investigation, Snow found that the workhouse had its own water pump and had not used water from the Broad Street pump. Snow made sure that the handle of the pump was removed, and from then on the number of new cases declined. Although the epidemic was probably self-limiting, this showed the importance of mapping mortality.

Snow later provided further convincing evidence to support his theory and clarified the mode of transmission of cholera. Carefully documenting the incidence among subscribers to the city's two water companies, he showed that the disease occurred much more frequently in the customers of one of them, which took its water from the lower Thames where it had become contaminated with London sewage.

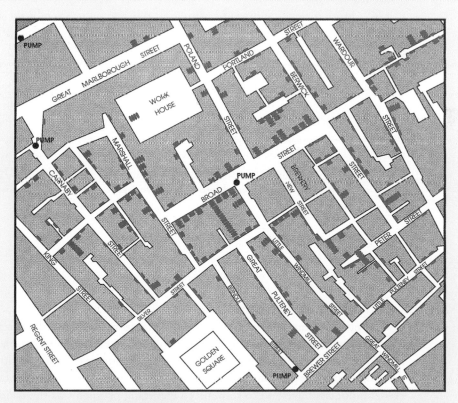

Figure 3.1 **Snow's map of Soho**

connections	Chapter 6 uses a different type of mapping to show the cholera cases during the 1854 epidemic in London.

Much early epidemiological work centred on identifying the causes of infectious diseases and involved the initiation, in the mid-nineteenth century, of a public health movement based on the work of sanitary inspectors and engineers. Although the public health movement recognized the link between environmental conditions and health, the motives of reformers such as Edwin Chadwick (1800–90) were not so much to improve the conditions of the poor but to maintain economic and moral stability. With the acceptance of the germ theory of disease (rather than the theory of miasma, 'bad air', which was previously dominant), the therapeutic era of public health began. This focused more on treatment than on prevention. The foundation of the NHS and the professionalization of medicine further contributed to the emphasis on therapeutic medicine.

connections	Chapter 2 examines early understandings of health and disease and developments in scientific understanding.

In the 1970s, however, this perspective was challenged by McKeown's (1976) observations that immunization and therapy had shown little effect on mortality compared with socioeconomic factors. The modern view of disease causation relies on multifactorial explanations. There may be a particular agent of disease (for example a microorganism or a dietary substance such as fat); however, a complex of social factors may lead people to behave in particular ways, and these behaviours (for example smoking or a lack of exercise) contribute to disease. These behaviours are a response to the conditions in which people are born, grow, live, work and age. It is now recognized that these circumstances are shaped by the distribution of money, power and resources at global, national and local levels (see the World Health Organization's inquiries into the social determinants of health at www.who.int/social_determinants/en).

connections	Evidence of the inverse relationship between health and socioeconomic status is discussed in Chapter 5, and Chapter 6 highlights the influence of the natural, built and social environments on health.

Although epidemiology and public health have always played a part in health service planning, their role has waxed and waned according to prevailing health problems, the ways in which society perceives those problems and the subsequent government policy devised to counteract them. In addition to recognizing the importance of socioeconomic factors in the genesis of disease, epidemiologists have had to respond to changing problems as the incidence of infectious disease has (at least in the Western world) declined. The simplistic one agent/one disease model had to be abandoned as epidemiology struggled with more complex problems, such as heart disease and cancer that have no obvious single cause, as well as mental and physical illnesses.

Epidemiology has gained increasing importance as a result of:

- the need to collect data to plan services and ascertain the quality of services

- the emergence of the evidence-based healthcare movement and the desire for evidence-based health policy

- the acknowledgement that ill health is linked to socioeconomic factors and the continuing focus on tackling health inequalities.

The emergence of new infectious disease threats, such as HIV/AIDS, MRSA (methicillin resistant Staphylococcus aureus, an antibiotic-resistant infection commonly found in hospitals), SARS (severe acute respiratory syndrome), A/H5N1 ('bird flu') and Ebola, have kept the surveillance role of epidemiology in the news headlines. *The World Health Report 2007: A Safer Future: Global Public Health Security in the Twenty-first Century* calls for global cooperation in surveillance to control outbreaks (WHO, 2007). The emergence of major threats to life expectancy in high- and low-income countries from the lifestyles we adopt adds a new focus to the epidemiological work on more complex health problems such as cancer and heart disease (WHO, 2002).

Common to many healthcare systems in high-income countries has been an increasing emphasis on the provision of a service to consumers and a demand for quality care that was cost-effective. As part of strategic planning, health and local authorities have instituted mechanisms to determine the need for health services in their local community and the extent to which that need was being met. Epidemiology and demography (the study of population size, density, growth and distribution) provide the tools to collect the 'hard' data that are used to plan services and ascertain quality. All health and local authorities now collect large data sets of demographic, fertility, mortality and morbidity trends, which can be used to identify geographic variations and local patterns. (See, for example, the use of such data to tackle public health issues at the Association of Public Health Observatories at www.apho.org.uk and the Office for National Statistics at www.statistics.gov.uk.)

The emergence of the evidence-based healthcare movement

Over the past 30 years, a strong movement towards the use of more evidence in healthcare has been promoted by governments and the professions. For example, the National Institute for Heath and Care Excellence (NICE: www.nice.org.uk) was created in 1999 as an independent organization responsible for producing national (England and Wales) guidance on treatments and public health that was evidence based. It is argued that if healthcare professionals based more of their decisions on evidence, the quality of care could be standardized and improved, in some instances also saving costs. Thus, there is a drive towards increasing clinical effectiveness. For many, such evidence takes the form of research, such as surveys and clinical trials, which produces quantitative data. Many of these designs have a foundation in epidemiology.

The rise of **evidence-based practice** in healthcare was strongly influenced by a group of clinicians who advocated the principles of clinical epidemiology (Sackett et al., 2004; Fletcher and Fletcher, 2013). In their interactions with clients, most healthcare professionals go through a process of gathering information about, for example, physical and psychological symptoms, the results of investigations, social circumstances, cultural histories and so on. In medicine, such information is required to answer certain questions, such as: Is this person sick? Do I need to do further tests? What is the optimal treatment for this condition? The answers to these questions form the basis of the subsequent action taken by the doctor. Clinical epidemiology aims to provide a scientific basis for this decision-making process.

thinking about One of the consequences of the evidence movement is the increased availability of information for the public. How able do you feel to evaluate treatment choices when you are unwell?

connections   Chapter 11 explores the economic basis for healthcare decisions, and Chapter 12 discusses the ethical dilemmas posed by such decision-making.

example 3.3

Screening for prostate cancer

The question of whether men should be routinely offered a **screening** test for prostate cancer provides an example of where the science of epidemiology can be applied at the level of individual patient encounters.

There are few advantages in instituting a screening procedure for a condition for which no treatment exists, or in which early treatment is no better than late treatment. From a socioeconomic viewpoint, it is reasonable to screen only for conditions that have a relatively high incidence and cause a considerable burden of suffering, although any one individual may take a different view on this. The acceptability of screening tests and the potential of reaching those at most risk is also important. It is well known that those who take up screening for cervical cancer are, in

fact, those least at risk of this disease. Finally, it is important to establish the trustworthiness of any screening test.

Substantial increases in the incidence of prostate cancer have been reported in many countries over the past 30 years. This apparent rise may be due to increased detection and/or increasing numbers at risk (older men) due to the ageing population. However, there is also controversy over the accuracy of the screening procedure, which consists of a blood test, a rectal examination and an ultrasound scan. (See www.cancerresearchuk.org/about-cancer/type/prostate-cancer for some of the main arguments.)

In deciding whether a test is trustworthy and suitable for use, doctors must consider the following question: How often does the test produce a false-positive result (when a person would be wrongly classified as having the disease) or a false-negative result (when a person would be wrongly classified as being disease free)? Diagnostic tests are discussed later in the chapter.

There is also an ethical problem of identifying individuals as 'diseased' when in fact their condition causes few problems. Screening for prostate cancer may identify individuals with early disease that may remain unsymptomatic and untroubling. Such individuals may even die 'with' the disease rather than 'of' the disease (Mettlin et al., 1991).

The UK National Screening Committee (www.screening.nhs.uk/uknsc) regularly reviews whether evidence supports the introduction of new screening, for example for ovarian cancer and osteoporosis.

? When the Scrutiny Committee of Birmingham City Council (2004) produced its report *Children's Nutrition: Obesity*, it found no hard data on the levels of childhood obesity in Birmingham:

> The committee ... believes that it is vital that local data on childhood obesity prevalence is collected and analysed, both to monitor the size of the problem and also to estimate the impact of actions to reduce obesity on population health. (p. 15)

How might such data be collected?

The link between ill health and socioeconomic conditions

The early history of epidemiology illustrates how it recognized the association between socioeconomic status and ill health, but with the rise of a powerful medical establishment, the public health function and preventive medicine were upstaged by an emphasis on therapeutics. More recently, the significance of social inequalities and poverty in the genesis of disease has been widely recognized even by governments (Marmot et al., 2010) and thus emphasized the central role of epidemiology. Social epidemiology goes beyond establishing that associations exist between static socioeconomic factors and ill health, to examining why they exist and how to begin to tackle these inequalities.

Traditionally, epidemiology has valued most highly the information interpreted within the scientific medical model. Lay and medical interpretations of risk differ and this may help explain why laypeople do not necessarily follow widely promoted public health messages such as those about smoking cessation. The recognition by public health professionals of lay epidemiology may be important in understanding and overcoming barriers to public health and in implementing health programmes, especially preventive programmes such as smoking cessation (Hunt and Emslie, 2001; Lawlor et al., 2003). People's understandings and explanations for their own health and illness and how information fits in with their beliefs and experiences have a role in the promotion of health.

Lay interpretation of risk is sometimes termed 'lay epidemiology' (Hunt and Emslie, 2001), which describes the processes through which health risks are understood and interpreted by laypeople (Allmark and Tod, 2006). Other authors have extended the scope of lay epidemiology to include lay information gathering, so lay epidemiology is the process whereby laypeople gather evidence and use experts in their midst to understand the epidemiology of diseases. It is a process often associated with political activism.

---

example 3.4

Lay interpretations of risk

Hunt et al. (2001) discuss lay constructions of a family history of heart disease and personal risk. They identify that medical or epidemiological and lay constructions of the factors contributing to a person having a 'family history' of heart disease acknowledge the importance of the number, age at death and biological relationship of the index person to affected relatives. However, there are also important differences in notions of what constitutes a 'premature' death, the fluidity and ambivalence that many people (particularly men from manual backgrounds) feel about whether or not they have a family history, and the distinction commonly drawn by people between having a family history and whether or not this puts them at increased personal risk.

The pursuit of epidemiological knowledge by laypeople is triggered by their dissatisfaction with the explanations provided by the conventional scientific community. It is often fuelled by environmental concerns, or the failure of government responses or public inquiries to satisfy ordinary people. Recent examples of lay epidemiology in action include recognition of Gulf War syndrome after a long struggle between Gulf War veterans and the scientific and military communities, PIP breast implants and the risk to health (Example 3.5), and the health risks from fracking (Finkel and Law, 2011).

---

example 3.5

Lay epidemiology and the health risks of Poly Implant Prostheses (PIP) breast implants

This case study illustrates the way in which the scientific evidence of ill health may differ from people's lived experience.

In March 2010, the French regulator for medical devices discovered that the manufacturer of PIP breast implants had been using industrial-grade silicone instead of medical-grade silicone in its breast implants. Between 2001 and 2009, about 94,000 implants (representing around 47,000 women) were sold in the UK alone, with about 95% being fitted privately. Following the French regulators discovery, the UK's Medicines and Healthcare products Regulatory Agency (MHRA) issued a medical device alert banning clinicians from using the PIP implants. The question remained whether the devices were a risk to health. Toxicology tests on samples of the filler material in France and the UK suggested there was no significant health risk for women who had received the implants. However, the women themselves thought otherwise and began the PIP Action Campaign (http://pipactioncampaign.org) and started compiling evidence from women about the health effects of leaking and ruptured PIP implants.

In December 2011, concerns over cancer risk and increasing reports of ruptures led the French government to recommend the removal of PIP implants. However, in the UK, the expert panel's interim report (Keogh, 2011) concluded there was no clear evidence at present that patients with PIP implants were at any greater risk of harm than those with other implants. The report emphasized the poor quality of data available and promised a further assessment in the near future. The final report (Keogh, 2012) acknowledged the evidence of the increased risk of rupture of PIP implants in comparison to other types of implant, but the policy recommendation was against routine removal. The report stated that the NHS would support removal of PIP implants if, following a clinical assessment, a woman with her doctor decided that it was right to do so. However, the NHS will only pay for replacement if the NHS did the original operation.

At the heart of the dispute lay the claim to validity of the different types of evidence that each party held. The lay epidemiologists of the PIP Action Campaign carefully collected data gleaned from people's experience, whereas the expert panel collected objective scientific evidence from toxicological studies, medical records and clinical measurements. Each party considered their evidence to be equally valid, but only one party (legitimized by the government and adherence to the principles of scientific epidemiology) was in a position to significantly influence the outcome of the event. In the UK, for many of the women affected, the dilemma remains of the risk to their health from a ruptured implant versus the risk to their self-confidence and mental health from being unable to pay for new implants – self-confidence being a common reason for seeking implants originally. For these people, health was not simply constructed through a narrative of biological dysfunction.

For a short summary of the assessment of the risks, see Spiegelhalter et al. (2012).

Concepts of health and disease in medical epidemiology

Before we can fully understand the contribution that epidemiology makes to healthcare, it is necessary to explore how concepts such as health, disease, normality and abnormality have traditionally been conceptualized. For many of those working in healthcare, epidemiology remains firmly associated with medicine and the methods of natural science. The following definition reflects this link with biology and physiology:

> the study of a disease or a physiological condition in human populations and of the factors which influence that distribution ... Thus epidemiology can be regarded as a sequence of reasoning concerned with biological inferences derived from observations of disease occurrence and related phenomena in human population groups. (Lilienfeld and Stolley, 1994, p. 4)

Epidemiology has, however, begun to expand to encompass other perspectives based on worldviews and theories drawn from other disciplines within the social sciences.

In medicine and epidemiology, health has been defined as the absence of disease. This is, however, quite a simplistic definition, and the World Health Organization (WHO, 1946) has specified that health is 'a state of complete physical, mental and social well-being, not merely the absence of disease and infirmity'. Even this definition has attracted criticism as commentators search for a broader, more positive concept of health (Seedhouse, 2002). The major problem with this definition is that disease or physiological status does not fully embrace the image of health held by most people. Many other factors – social, psychological, spiritual and environmental – are involved in perceptions of health. Hence, the term **quality of life** is often used to describe a person's health state.

Illness can be defined as a state of poor health, subjectively perceived, regardless of whether a person has a disease. A person may simply feel unwell. In medicine, disease means a diagnosable condition of abnormality. It can be used broadly to mean any condition that causes discomfort or dysfunction (**morbidity**) and/or death. A person with undetected high blood pressure who feels in good health would be diseased, but not ill.

connections   Chapter 1 outlines the biomedical definition of health as an organism's ability to efficiently respond to challenges (stressors) and effectively restore and sustain a state of balance, known as 'homeostasis'.

In its studies of populations, epidemiology is concerned with categorizing people into groups according to whether they are normal (that is, disease free) or abnormal (that is, diseased). Reference is usually made to particular physical and biochemical parameters, for example blood count, body weight, concentration of liver enzymes, absence of cellular changes and so on, in order to define normality. Each of these characteristics will have a normal range below or above which disease may be indicated.

thinking about Can you think of any tests or investigations you have undergone that used definitions of normality?

One example is the test for anaemia. If your haemoglobin level were found to be below 12 mg/100 ml, you would be recalled for further measurements and might be recommended an iron supplement. The recognition of normality and abnormality within epidemiology is often based on precise measurements of the type made in the biological and physical sciences. It is important that such measurements are *valid* (they measure what you think they are measuring) and *reliable* (repeated measurements coming up with the same result). Validity and reliability are much easier to measure when dealing with numerical data, which can be easily compared with a gold standard.

It is a short step, then, to see how, in this sort of system, phenomena that are readily measured and observed, for example serum cholesterol concentration, are attributed greater 'reality' than other phenomena such as nausea or wellbeing, which are more difficult to measure and for which normal ranges are less likely to have been defined (although scales have been developed to achieve this; see Bowling, 2004).

?   Why might it be difficult to identify and distinguish a 'normal' state?

Even when epidemiology and medicine confine themselves to using such objective, hard measures, difficulties may arise, for although in some cases there is a clear distinction between the values that are normal or abnormal in a population, more often than not the values for the diseased population overlap with those of the normal population, giving a 'grey' area. Difficulties then arise in trying to determine where the cut-off point between the two categories lies and thus the point above or below which disease may be defined. There may also be controversy between doctors over what the normal range should be. A good example here is that of blood pressure, for which, over the years, the 'normal range' has changed. Furthermore, the normal range may vary across different populations and different age ranges (see Fletcher and Fletcher, 2013).

By recognizing the differences and similarities between cases, epidemiologists are able to classify diseases. They have traditionally based such classifications of disease on the medical model. As we saw above, the medical diagnosis has become centred on science through the use of tests and technological procedures. The work of early scientists such as Louis Pasteur and Robert Koch suggested that each disease had a single, specific and objective cause, which, given the right treatment, could be selectively destroyed (as with the use of antibiotics to destroy infecting microorganisms). In the medical model, the classification of disease is based on demonstrable physical changes in the body's structure or function. If these deviate from the norm, the patient 'has' a disease.

Chapter 1 discusses the scientific model of disease causation.   **connections**

Each disease possesses certain recognizable characteristics that distinguish it from other diseases. Moreover, such diseases are considered to be universal in form and content, that is, they 'appear' in the same way in different people in different locations and at different times. Routine mortality statistics are based on this classification of the recorded cause of death. The WHO produces the *International Statistical Classification of Diseases and Health Related Problems* (ICD), which is used in most countries to classify and code mortality and morbidity.

Social epidemiology

Despite the apparently objective measures of disease, its assessment in a person is a social valuation, often with social consequences. Parsons (1951) put forward the theory that the sick role is a form of 'deviance' that is legitimized in the social world. People designated as 'sick' are exempted from normal activities and responsibility for their condition, but there is an expectation that the sick will acknowledge that the sick role is undesirable and seek help. The anthropologist Frankenberg (1980) suggests that the social environment or milieu is central to understanding what health and sickness are. He defines disease as a malfunction of structure or function, illness as a person's perception and experience of socially devalued states, and sickness as the social recognition of disease and illness.

What these sociological and anthropological perspectives have in common is their insistence that ill health is not just a malfunctioning of the physical body, but is instead closely affected by societal and cultural factors. In this respect, the views and ideas that laypeople have on how, when and why they become sick become important.

connections	Chapter 5 discusses the social construction of illness in detail, and Chapter 7 explores how health and illness are perceived differently in different cultures.

Since epidemiology is concerned with measuring the rate of health and ill health in populations and determining the reasons for it, it is clearly important that it takes full account of the different ways in which such concepts have been constructed.

> **?** If there are different perspectives on what constitutes health and sickness, how will this affect ideas of abnormality and disease?

The sociocultural view of abnormality suggests that although disease may be seen as a biological deviation, what is normal and abnormal is a social and moral judgement. Lewis (1993) contends that the diagnosis of abnormality is not confined to the medical domain but is a departure from some 'standard' of normality. He suggests that such standards are set by individuals and the society in which they exist. 'Normal' then becomes relative to circumstances and individuals – it is not a universal phenomenon that can be applied across all cultures and all occasions.

example 3.6

The social construction of illness

Schizophrenia provides an example of a socially constructed definition of mental illness. Statistics collected for a study in the Republic of Ireland showed that, on one day in 1971, 2% of males in Western Ireland were in a mental hospital. However, through an exploration of community definitions, it can be shown how abnormality and normality are 'constructed' by the community. Studies such as those of Scheper-Hughes (1978) and Dingwall (1992) show that quiet and eccentric individuals are tolerated, but those who violate the strong sanctions against expressions of sexuality, aggression and disrespectful subordination to parental or religious authority are perceived to be nonconformists and thus 'prime candidates for the mental hospital'. So, a large number of young bachelors had been labelled as 'mentally ill' and institutionalized.

The medical view is that nature produces diseases in constant and distinct ways. Diseases are not entities or things but a particular set of attributes characteristically shown by people who fall ill in this way. Diseases as such do not exist in nature but are produced by the conceptual schemes imposed on the natural world. Thus, some states of the body are valued and others are not, being deemed abnormal. Biological changes are undoubtedly a material fact, but the sociocultural viewpoint is that it is the significance of these changes that matters.

This part has illustrated how epidemiology has traditionally used medicine as the basis for its way of knowing about sickness and health – for building up its understanding of these concepts. The idea that diseases are entities defined through the methods and technologies of biology is, however, challenged by the sociocultural view. If epidemiology focuses only on the malfunctioning of the corporeal body, it is in danger of ignoring other aspects that are important in the generation of ill health. Moreover, it needs to take account of these other viewpoints in order to understand the considerable impact that the socioeconomic and physical environment have on people's health. Social epidemiology has been defined as the branch of epidemiology that studies the social distribution and social determinants of health and makes explicit their association with health and illness (Berkman and Kawachi, 2000; Krieger, 2001).

Part 2 Theoretical and research approaches

example 3.7

Examples of research in epidemiology

- Cancer prevention (see www.cancerresearch.uk), for example:
  - cigarettes with reduced yield of tar and nicotine do not reduce the risk of lung cancer
  - the association of obesity with increased death rates from at least ten cancer sites, including colon and post-menopausal breast cancer
  - the link between aspirin use and lower risk of colon cancer
- Research into particular conditions such as arthritis (see www.inflammation-repair.manchester.ac.uk/musculoskeletal/research/arc/), for example:
  - the co-morbidities associated with inflammatory musculoskeletal disorders and their impact on quality of life and mortality
  - the evolution from acute to chronic musculoskeletal pain
  - studies of bone health from childhood to very old age

- intervention studies to improve frailty, reduce pain and enhance quality of life
- Longitudinal studies to determine the factors influencing a phenomenon, for example:
  - the Twins Early Development Study (www.teds.ac.uk and www.twinsuk.ac.uk), which explores the influence of genes and environment on the aetiology of diseases
  - the Whitehall study of British civil servants and the factors that might contribute to their social gradient in death and disease (www.ucl.ac.uk/whitehallII/history)
  - the US Framingham Heart Study (www.framinghamheartstudy.org/about-fhs/history.php), which has explored the common factors or characteristics that contribute to cardiovascular disease since 1948
- Research into the impact on health of a new innovation, such as long-term mobile phone use (www.ukcosmos.org)

Epidemiology predominantly uses the conceptual framework of medicine to direct its activities, although other perspectives drawn from social science disciplines may also be illuminating. When it comes to looking at the practical ways in which epidemiology might contribute to healthcare, both these perspectives need to be considered. However, since epidemiologists have traditionally based their methods on medicine, rather more examples exist of activities within this sphere of influence.

Using medicine as its conceptual backdrop, epidemiology has been used in diverse ways (Valanis, 1999):

- determining the natural history of disease
- identifying risk
- classifying disease
- diagnosing and treating disease
- surveillance of health status
- planning health services
- evaluating health services.

The natural history of disease

In attempting to determine who, when and why certain people become sick, epidemiologists are interested in the entire natural progression of a disease, whereas many healthcare professionals, particularly those working in hospitals, are more focused on specific stages of the disease process, for example when the condition has been deemed serious enough by the patient to seek their advice. The natural history of a disease is generally described as the course it takes without medical intervention, whereas the clinical course is defined as that which evolves under medical treatment.

The natural history of a disease is useful in prognosis, which involves the prediction of events to come. In other words, it tells sufferers and their carers what they might expect in the future in terms of recovery, remission symptoms and their ability to 'carry on as normal' either now or at some time in the future.

Descriptions of the course of diseases reported in the literature may be susceptible to sampling bias. This is because such accounts are usually derived from specialist centres whose patients may not be representative of the whole spectrum of patients cared for in primary and secondary settings. Fletcher and Fletcher (2013) provide the example of multiple sclerosis to illustrate this. From the viewpoint of hospitals, multiple sclerosis must appear to be a lethal disease. A prognostic survey conducted in the community by Percy et al. (1971), however, demonstrated that 50% of diagnosed patients were alive 50 years after the onset – the same number as would have been expected to survive even if they did not have multiple sclerosis. Studies of the natural history of a disease must therefore take into account the full spectrum of people who might be afflicted.

thinking about Consider an illness you and someone you know have both had. Did your illness follow the same course? Did you have the same treatment?

Biological and physiological knowledge enables epidemiologists to understand more clearly how diseases are caused and thus hopefully how they might be prevented. Information concerning the early natural history of conditions is essential to the planning of timely interventions and the identification and treatment of high-risk groups.

Identifying risk

Risk refers to the likelihood that someone free of a condition but exposed to certain **risk factors** will subsequently acquire that condition. In today's society, we seem to be unable to escape from the idea of risk – the risk of toxic waste, climate change, infectious agents, bad driving, contaminated food, war, famine, our genetic inheritance.

For infectious diseases, it is quite simple to identify the relationship between the exposure to risk and an adverse outcome. However, in most chronic diseases, such as cancer and heart disease, the relationship between risk and disease is less clear. In these cases, it is difficult for clinicians to develop estimates of risk based on their own limited experience. An individual doctor will perhaps see neither the resulting outcome following an exposure nor enough patients to determine which of many possible risk factors are the most important. It is here that epidemiology, through its study of populations rather than individuals, can provide vital knowledge. With the use of case control and cohort studies (see below), risk and prognostic factors can be determined, which allows screening programmes and health promotion strategies aimed at changing risk behaviours to be established.

Classifying disease

Epidemiological data are used for the classification system, the ICD, which is central to modern Western medicine. The ICD was primarily disease oriented and a means of assigning the cause of death, but it now includes a wider range of health problems. The current version is ICD-10, which came into use in 1994 and is available online at www.who.int/classifications/icd/en. It encompasses infectious and parasitic diseases, diseases and their location in the body – malignant neoplasms (cancers), for example, being linked to sites such as the breast or pancreas – as well as a category on the factors influencing health status and contact with the health services. The 11th revision of ICD has begun and will continue until 2017.

? In what situations might the use of the ICD be limited?

Using the ICD can be problematic because:

- death certificates give no information about contributory behaviours such as smoking

- mental health problems are not identified because malfunctioning of the physical body is not present

- a wide range of factors, including environmental (e.g. housing), socioeconomic (e.g. poverty) or lifestyle (e.g. drinking), could contribute to the cause of death but these are not recorded on the ICD.

Diagnosing and treating disease

Diagnosing what is wrong with people is a central activity in medicine, often involving the application of diagnostic tests. The interpretation of these tests is quite difficult. Figure 3.2 illustrates some properties that clinicians may use to determine the usefulness of diagnostic tests. Test results may present four possible scenarios. Two are correct – a positive test in the presence of disease and a negative test in the absence of disease. Where tests mislead is when they present results that are false positive – a person is wrongly identified as having a disease – or false negative, a person is wrongly identified as being free of the disease. It would not be too serious if a false-positive test indicated that a patient had a urinary tract infection and should be treated with antibiotics. However, if a patient with breast cancer were given a false-negative result, the disease might progress beyond the stage amenable to treatment. In this latter case, we would want a test with high sensitivity that is unlikely to miss cases of disease. We would also, however, need a specific test since it would be traumatic if people without breast cancer were told that they had this disease and wasteful to treat people unnecessarily. Highly specific tests are unlikely to classify people without the disease as having it. New diagnostic tests should be compared with a gold standard (the best possible assessment of whether the condition is present or not, for example an expensive 'scan') to determine their appropriateness for use in different situations.

Surveillance and the planning and evaluation of health services

Surveillance and planning are interrelated. In epidemiology, surveillance involves the collection, analysis and interpretation of data about who is most at risk of contracting a disease, and where and when diseases are most frequently observed. Data on the incidence and prevalence of disease in a population are routinely collected, for example cancer registers, hospital episode statistics and general practice research databases.

Monitoring conditions in this way can alert health professionals to trends or unusual clusters of events. In many developed countries, infectious diseases

How accurate and reliable are diagnostic and screening tests? The 2 x 2 matrix below illustrates the relationship between the results of a diagnostic test and the actual presence of disease.

Disease

		Present	Absent	
Results of diagnostic test	Positive	True positive a	False positive b	a + b
	Negative	False negative c	True negative d	c + d
		a + c	b + d	a + b + c + d

Properties of the diagnostic test:

Sensitivity is the proportion of those with the disease who test positive

Sensitivity = $a/(a + c)$

Specificity is the proportion of those who do not have the disease who test negative

Specificity = $d/(b + d)$

Figure 3.2 **Screening tests**

must be notified to the appropriate authorities in order that outbreaks may be identified and confined. The surveillance of other conditions such as birth defects may identify possible causal agents. A knowledge of the distribution of disease in communities according to geographical location, age, ethnic origin, socioeconomic group and so on is obviously vital to the planning of healthcare services; epidemiology can provide the tools for such analyses.

The collection and analysis of data do not, however, occur in a social vacuum, and producing knowledge in a numerical form does not guarantee its objectivity. Statistics are collected and presented in different ways for all sorts of different reasons and to fit all kinds of different agendas. Whenever you are presented with health information data, some simple questions should be asked:

- Which population do the data represent?

- Is there any missing information?

- How have categories such as 'child' and 'elderly' been constructed, that is, how are they defined and by whom?

- Who collected the data and why?

- Do the data attempt to provide evidence to substantiate a particular viewpoint, for example the government's?

thinking about Can you think of an example in which data have been manipulated to present a particular picture, or where data may not be accurately recorded?

Despite Snow's epidemiological studies on the transmission of cholera, as late as 1885 the British authorities continued to insist that cholera was non-communicable, non-specific and endemic in Egypt; the government did not wish to accept that cholera originated in India because this would have disrupted Britain's substantial commercial and trade interests with that country. In Example 3.4 concerning the PIP breast implants, the expert panel found the data quality was poor and often not recorded in any systematic way or was not available. Attempts to create a registry of breast implants had failed due to women being unwilling to participate, a matter of regret when it came to trying to compile evidence of comparative risk of failure for different types of implant.

The methodologies used by epidemiology

Every discipline goes about its research in a particular way according to the paradigm within which its practitioners work. A paradigm is best understood as a worldview based on a set of values and assumptions that are shared by a particular group. Epidemiology has strong historical links with medicine, practitioners in both these disciplines tending to work within the natural science paradigm. The scientific paradigm is also often called the 'positivistic paradigm'.

The main tenets of this paradigm are as follows:

- Scientists believe that the social world and the physical world are physically real and objective and can therefore be known

- There are universal laws that predict and explain phenomena

- The data collected are usually quantitative.

connections   Chapter 1 demonstrates how the disciplines of biology, physiology and the study of the natural world are located in a scientific paradigm.

The assumptions that underpin the positivistic paradigm have certain consequences for research that is conducted through this perspective. Thus, natural scientists:

- seek cause-and-effect relationships

- attempt to generalize these relationships to populations other than the one under study

- ensure that researcher bias is carefully controlled

- reduce social situations down into smaller parts (perhaps two variables) for study.

Epidemiologists often use research designs that simply observe events as they happen in a population, rather than as they might happen in a controlled experiment. As a result, they are concerned with factors (other than the one under investigation) that might affect the outcome of the study or bias its results. **Bias** is the result of any process that causes observations to differ systematically from their true values. We consider three sources of bias:

- *Measurement bias:* Think of your bathroom scales: because they are not regularly calibrated, they might consistently tell you that you weigh three kilograms less than when you were weighed at the gym. This is a simple case of measurement bias.

- *Selection bias*: This may occur when subjects are recruited for a study. Many epidemiological studies compare the experiences or outcomes of two groups, one of which has been exposed to a risk factor and the other which has not. Since we are interested only in the effect of that risk factor, it is important that the two groups being compared do not differ in other significant ways that might affect the outcome. Selection bias occurs when the way in which subjects are selected distorts the outcome of the study. A study might, for example, be interested in finding out whether meditation reduces stress levels. A programme of meditation seminars is offered to the directors of a large City bank. The stress levels of those who undertake the programme is then compared with stress levels of those who chose not to attend. Selection bias is present if these two groups differ in other respects that may affect the degree to which they suffer stress. For example, those who volunteer for such programmes may be particularly health conscious and undertaking other strategies such as regular exercise, which might affect their stress level. In other words, the two groups are not comparable with respect to factors that might affect the outcome of the study.

- *Confounding bias:* This occurs when two factors are associated and the effect of one is confused with the effect of the other. An example is provided in a study of urinary tract infections in patients with catheters (Crow et al., 1986). When analysing the results of this study, it was found that females who were catheterized by doctors suffered fewer urinary tract infections than those catheterized by nurses. This might have led us to believe that nurses were less skilled at catheterization. However, the data also showed that doctors usually inserted catheters in the operating theatre and that women undergoing an operation were likely to receive antibiotics. These factors – the person doing the catheterization, the place of catheterization, and the receipt of antibiotics – were therefore confounding, and it was difficult to know which factor was responsible.

? What other factors might affect the results of a study?

Another factor that may affect the results of epidemiological studies is chance. Chance is random error. Unlike bias, which results in an observation being consistently above or below a value, chance is just as likely to deflect a measurement below as above its true reading. The probability of chance or random error accounting for the results of a study are estimated using statistics (the **p values** or probability values that you may have seen in research papers relate to this).

These two sources of error – bias and chance – are always carefully considered in the design and analysis of epidemiological studies.

Experimental studies

One of the principal aims of epidemiology is to identify cause-and-effect relationships, for example does asbestos cause small cell lung cancer?

A certain factor is sometimes the direct cause of a disease, and early epidemiologists who focused on infections certainly had considerable success in pinpointing their cause and thus controlling outbreaks. However, the focus of epidemiology is now firmly on chronic diseases. Most of these have multiple causes, and these causes, in turn, may have multiple effects. Heart disease, for example, has been seen in **association** with smoking, stress, obesity and high blood pressure, but smoking also causes chronic obstructive airways disease, bladder cancer and lung cancer. This intricate relationship between several factors, some known and some unknown, has been termed the 'web of causation'.

Bradford Hill (1897–1991), a British medical statistician, established certain criteria as a way of determining the causal link between a specific factor, such as cigarette smoking, and a disease, such as emphysema or lung cancer (Bradford Hill and Hill, 1991). Bradford Hill's criteria form the basis of modern epidemiological research and are outlined in Table 3.1. (See Bradford Hill and Hill, 1991, Ch. 28 for a detailed explanation and examples.)

The best way of establishing cause-and-effect relationships is through experimental research in which the investigator has a considerable degree of control over what is happening. In simple terms, in experimental studies, two groups of participants are assembled, one group receiving an intervention of some kind, perhaps a new drug treatment, the other group receiving nothing and acting as a control. In such studies, researchers have control over who is and who is not exposed to the intervention.

? Why might experimental studies be difficult to conduct with the public?

Human populations cannot always be easily studied in this way because of logistical or ethical problems. It would not, for example, be ethical to expose groups of people to potential risk factors for a disease. Nor is it feasible, over a period of time, to expose one group to a risk factor while ensuring another group, similar in all other respects, is not exposed to a risk factor. Much epide-

Table 3.1 **Cause-and-effect relationships**

Using the following criteria, it is possible to weigh up the evidence from a number of studies to decide whether a strong case exists for a particular factor being the cause of a disease, even when it has not been possible to undertake experimental studies. Consider the example of sun exposure as a cause of skin cancer.

1. Strength: the stronger the association, the more likely it is to be causative; that is, what is the risk of skin cancer in those exposed to the sun relative to those not exposed?

2. Plausibility: does it seem likely, according to what is known about the pathology and natural history of skin cancer, that sun exposure could be a causal factor?

3. Temporality: common sense would suggest that a cause needs to precede its hypothesized effect; that is, does exposure to the sun precede skin cancer?

4. Dose–response: if an increasing level of exposure leads to an increased incidence of disease, the case for cause and effect is strengthened; that is, are those who are most exposed to the sun, such as sunbathers or outdoor workers, more likely to get skin cancer?

5. Reversibility: if the removal of a risk factor reduces the incidence of disease, it may be its cause; that is, if sun exposure is reduced, through skin protection creams, covering up and not going out, as in Australia, does the incidence of skin cancer drop?

6. Consistency: if several studies all come up with the same answer, this provides strong evidence that the relationship is causal

miological research is conducted with naturally occurring populations, when it is not always possible to undertake experiments. It is important to assess the evidence from these other types of studies carefully.

Clinical trials used to test drugs are described in Chapter 1. **connections**

Two types of experimental study are used in epidemiology – clinical trials and preventive trials. In a clinical trial, the effect of a specific 'treatment' on people who already have a particular condition is studied. In this sense, 'treatments' may include not only drugs, but also equipment, for example different wound dressings, and 'procedures', such as different ways of organizing the A&E clinic). Preventive trials investigate the effect of a potential preventive measure in people who do not have the condition in question. A preventive trial might, for example, examine the effect of two different ways of conveying health promotion messages about smoking cessation to teenagers. Figure 3.3 shows a schematic diagram of a typical **randomized controlled trial** (RCT) considering the impact of an intervention on infection rates of patients coming for an operation.

RCTs are known as the 'gold standard' for a clinical trial and are considered by many to produce very 'strong', that is, valid and reliable, evidence about cause-and-effect relationships. This is because the investigator retains control over who does and does not receive the intervention – sometimes called the 'independent variable'. Table 3.2 provides a checklist of some features you should look out for when assessing the validity of RCTs. For a more detailed list, consider the Consolidated Standards of Reporting Trials (CONSORT)

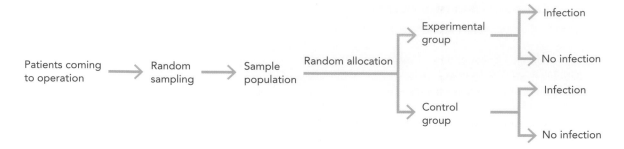

Figure 3.3 **Outline of a randomized controlled trial**
Source: Mulhall, 1996

statement developed in 1996 to improve the reporting of RCTs and most recently updated in 2010 (Campbell et al., 2010; Moher et al., 2010).

> **?** Consider a study to investigate whether patients washing with an antibacterial soap before an operation suffer fewer postoperative wound infections:
> - Why is it important to have two groups of participants?
> - Why is it important that the two groups are similar in characteristics, such as age, sex and disease severity?
> - What factors could influence the outcome of this study and make it hard to tell whether washing does reduce the incidence of postoperative infections?

Since in trials we are interested in trying to pinpoint the relationship between just two variables – the intervention and the outcome – it is important to try to minimize the effect of any other factors. For example, if the patients in the control group in Figure 3.3 were younger than those in the experimental group, they might naturally suffer fewer postoperative wound infections. This would then interfere with the design of the trial and bias its results. To prevent this happening, trialists attempt to assemble two groups of participants whose characteristics, such as age, sex and disease severity, closely resemble each other. This is achieved by randomly allocating people into either the experimental or the control group, hence the name randomized controlled trial (RCT).

One of the most contentious issues surrounding the use of experiments is informed consent – in other words, do people know what they are letting themselves in for when they agree to enter a trial? Although all good trials pay particular attention to this, the gap between the knowledge and language of healthcare professionals and laypeople often militates against the latter really gaining a good understanding. This is well illustrated in a study by Snowdon et al. (1997) that examined informed consent by exploring the parental reaction to a random allocation of their sick babies to treatment or control groups in the 'UK collaborative randomised trial of extracorporeal membrane oxygena-

Table 3.2 **Checklist for assessing the validity of RCTs**

- Is the randomization of the participants into each group blinded? If clinicians have a choice of which subjects enter which group in the trial, it is highly likely that the two groups that emerge will not be comparable

- Is the assignment of participants to the treatment groups random? Checking whether the two groups are roughly comparable in terms of various characteristics such as age, sex and so on helps to determine whether the two groups are similar

- Are those assessing outcomes blind to the treatment allocation? If clinicians and/or subjects are aware of which group they are in, this may bias the outcome results

- Are the groups treated identically other than for the named intervention? In all trials, it is important to try to prevent other factors interfering with the outcome of the trial

tion'. The researchers illustrated how the nature of the trial or the trial treatment, particularly the concept of randomization, was poorly understood by parents. In only 12 out of 21 interviews were they sure that at least one parent was aware of the random nature of the allocation of their baby to standard or trial treatment.

Observational studies

Observational studies involve studying population groups and events as they occur naturally. Thus, epidemiologists might take a group of people who have been exposed through the course of life events to a risk factor, say an occupational exposure to carcinogens, and compare them with another group who have not suffered such exposure to determine whether the exposed group have a higher incidence of cancer.

Epidemiologists undertake three main types of observational research: cohort studies, case control studies and prevalence studies. In each of these designs, attempts must be made to recognize, and deal with, the potential differences that might arise between comparison groups.

Cohort studies

Cohort studies are sometimes called 'longitudinal' or 'prospective' studies, indicating that they continue over a period of time and the participants are usually followed into the future. A **cohort** is a defined group of people who have a characteristic in common, for example the same disease, live in the same town or work for the same organization, who are then followed over time to find out what happens to them. Examples might be the survival rate for Hodgkin's disease, or the development of cardiovascular disease among Whitehall civil servants: the cohort study would be used to study prognosis in the case of Hodgkin's disease and risk factors for the development of cardiovascular disease in the study of civil servants. Cohort studies are often used to study the risk to our health from the way we live our lives, that is, the longer term risk of the things we do or expose ourselves to through the things we eat or the places we go. Predicting risk of adverse health outcomes may be one product of such studies. For example, the Framingham 'risk score' is a widely used cardiovascular risk assessment tool developed from the Framingham cohort study (Wilson et al., 1998; cvdrisk.nhlbi.nih.gov/calculator.asp).

Cohort studies provide the next best available evidence when it is not possible to undertake experiments. This is because the design of such studies aims to minimize the effect of the three types of bias (selection, measurement and confounding; see above). There are, however, disadvantages to cohort studies:

- the length of time that may be necessary to conduct the study

- the subsequent costs that will accrue

- the necessity for large-scale studies when the outcome of interest occurs infrequently; the Framingham Heart Study (Dawber, 1980), for example, followed 5,000 adults over many years.

As a result of these disadvantages, another type of research design for assessing risk – the case control study – has been developed.

Case control studies

In case control studies, a group of people with the particular condition of interest, for example brain tumours, are assembled (the cases) and compared with an otherwise similar group without the condition (the controls). Thus, in contrast to a cohort study, the cases already have the outcome of interest – a search being made for factors in the past that may explain the outcome. Case control studies are therefore always retrospective. Figure 3.4 outlines a typical case control study.

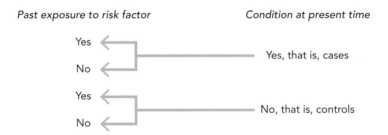

Figure 3.4 **Outline of the design of a case control study**
Source: Mulhall, 1996

The advantages of such a design are that the investigator identifies cases at the current time. This is simpler and economically cheaper than the situation in the cohort design where one has to observe a large group of unaffected individuals and wait for cases to occur. In other words, the natural frequency of the disease (which may be very low) does not constrain the identification of cases. A case control study is often the most practical study design for investigating potential causative agents in rare conditions. For example, case control studies have been used to investigate the risk of brain tumours in relation to mobile phone use (Interphone Study Group, 2010).

Case control studies are more prone to bias than cohort studies. Since the 'case' and 'control' groups are chosen by the investigator, selection bias may occur. It is important that cases and controls have had an equal chance of being exposed to the factor of interest. Furthermore, there is a strong chance of measurement bias, which may occur when cases recall exposure differently from non-cases. Unsurprisingly, sick people have generally reflected more than healthy controls on past events (either medical, for example drug history, or non-medical, for example working conditions) that may have affected their condition.

Table 3.3 lists some of the terms most commonly used in descriptive epidemiology.

Table 3.3 **Common rates used in epidemiology**

Crude rates	These refer to the entire population, for example the **mortality rate** for Greater Manchester, but tell us nothing of the characteristics of the underlying population
Specific rates	These measure the number of events occurring in a subgroup of the population, for example the mortality rate of female children in social class I in two different districts of Manchester
Standardized rates	These take account of the structure of a population. This is important when comparing rates because we know that certain characteristics of a population will affect the disease incidence; for example a population with a high proportion of elderly people will have a correspondingly high mortality rate. By determining how many deaths might be expected in a population and then comparing this with how many deaths actually occur, we can gain an idea of whether the experience of the population has been the same as the standard experience. The standardized mortality ratio is the ratio of: $$\frac{\text{number of observed deaths}}{\text{number of expected deaths}} \times 100\%$$ This figure is easy to understand since ratios over 100% indicate an unfavourable 'mortality experience', whereas those below 100% indicate a favourable experience. Coggan et al. (2003) provide a worked example of standardization

Prevalence studies

The final observational design is the cross-sectional or **prevalence** study. In a prevalence study, a defined population is surveyed and its disease status determined at one point in time. This gives us a 'snapshot' at a certain moment of who has and who has not got the condition of interest within a particular population (the point prevalence). This is different from incidence. Prevalence studies are particularly useful in planning healthcare services and informing policy issues.

Incidence is the proportion of a group free of a condition who develop it over a given period of time, for example a day, a year or a decade. It measures the rate at which new cases arise in a population, as opposed to prevalence, which measures the proportion of a population that have the condition at any one point in time.

case study trends in obesity

This case study illustrates how trends in obesity can be identified from routine data sources; how we can strengthen our argument about increasing trends in obesity by looking for replication of national patterns at local and international levels. From a health perspective, rising trends in obesity only become an important issue if they are accompanied by increases in ill health, so the case study will show how this can be investigated. Finally, to illustrate how some of the study designs discussed earlier can be put into action to tackle health problems, the case study will consider possible intervention studies and how they might change the trend.

How do we measure obesity?

If we are to examine trends in obesity over time, we need to consider how obesity is defined and measured and to be sure that measure is used in the same way over time and in different countries. The WHO (2000, p. 6) defines obesity as 'a condition of abnormal or excessive fat accumulation in adipose tissue, to the extent that health is impaired'. However, as discussed in Chapter 1, there is little consensus on how to measure fatness. Obesity is most commonly measured by body mass index (BMI), which is defined as weight (kg) divided by height squared (m^2). People with a BMI above 25 kg/m^2 are classified as overweight, while those people whose BMI exceeds 30 kg/m^2 are classified as obese. These categorizations are universally agreed and accord with WHO recommendations. BMI is a measure that has been consistently applied over time, so is useful for examining trends over time as we know we are looking at the same measure at each time point.

As BMI relies only on accurate measurement of height and weight, it is relatively simple to use and has been reliably collected for many years and in many countries. However, a difficulty with using BMI to measure fatness is that those people who exercise build up muscle mass and because muscle weighs more than fat, a super fit athlete may have a high BMI. In children, there are additional difficulties with interpreting BMI as a measure of fatness as it is complicated by growth. There is no universally accepted BMI-based categorization of obesity. In the UK, BMI measurement in children aged 2–20 years is related to the UK-WHO BMI growth charts (published by the Royal College of Paediatrics and Child Health in 2013 and adapted from 1990 growth charts) to give age and gender-specific information; a child above the 91st centile is classified as overweight and a child over the 98th centile as obese (www.rcpch.ac.uk/growthcharts). Thus, although BMI is the most widely used measure of obesity, it can be a misleading measure of fatness, particularly in children, so there may be a bias. Other measures of fatness can be used, such as skin fold thickness or waist-to-hip ratio, but these are more difficult to measure reliably and are less routinely measured than weight and height, so are usually only available in research studies.

Is obesity increasing?

To answer this question, we need to consider how we can access information about BMI for the population over several years. In the UK, height and weight are measures that general practice make for each patient usually when they register at the practice and then weight will be periodically measured. In theory, if all practices did this and we could gather the information from all GP practices, we could calculate BMI for a large proportion of the population. In reality, the data are not collected at a regular time and there is currently no way of pooling the data across practices, so this routine source will not be helpful for answering our question.

Fortunately, in the UK, a number of large national surveys are conducted each year, many of which gather some health measures and although this information is only on a sample of the population, we will be able to use this to examine national trends. The Health Survey for England (HSE) is an annual survey that began in 1991, and information about it is available from www.ucl.ac.uk/ hssrg/studies/hse and reports and data from the survey can be accessed through the Health and Social Care Information Centre (www. hscic.gov.uk/results). The HSE is conducted with a large stratified random sample of the population of England and BMI is part of the information collected. From the HSE, we know that in 1993, 13.2% of adult males and 16.4% of adult females in the England were obese (BMI > 30) and 44.4% of adult males and 32.2% of adult females were overweight (BMI 25–30). In the 2012 HSE, 24.4% of adult males and 25.1% of adult females in the England were obese and 42.2% of adult males and 32.1% of adult females were overweight. The trend in obesity for adult males and females is shown in Figure 3.5.

To consider the prevalence of obesity in local areas and compare this to the national picture, information is available through the local community health profile (www. apho.org.uk/default.aspx?QN=P_HEALTH_ PROFILES). Information in the community health profiles for 2013 is based on the HSE for the period 2006–08. The England average proportion of obese adults is 24.2% and the range for local authorities in England is 13.9– 30.7%, so there is evidence of significant local variation, even within a region. For example, the health profile for Lambeth in London for 2013 shows the proportion of obese adults is 20.5%. In neighbouring Southwark, the prevalence of adult obesity is 22.5%, both

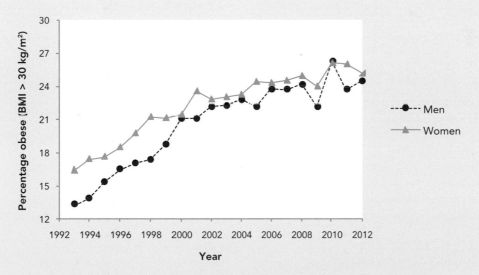

Figure 3.5 **Prevalence of obesity (BMI > 30 kg/m²) among adults in England by gender, 1993–2012**

Source: HSE, 2012

significantly below the average for England. However, in the London borough of Barking and Dagenham, the prevalence of adult obesity is 28.7%, significantly above the average for England. Local community health profiles first became available in 2006 and as this series has become established, it is becoming easier to monitor local trends over time.

Is there evidence of increasing trends in obesity in other countries?

National and state-based obesity prevalence data for America is available at www.cdc.gov, the website of the Centers for Disease Control and Prevention, based on data from the US National Health and Nutrition Examination Survey. In 1999–2000, the prevalence of obesity (BMI > 30) in adult men in the US was 27.5% and this had risen to 35.5% by 2010–11. In adult women in the US, the prevalence of obesity in 1999–2000 was 33.4%, and this had risen to 35.8% in 2010–11 (Flegal et al., 2012; Ogden et al., 2012). Finucane et al. (2011) provide an analysis of national, regional and global trends in BMI since 1980 for 199 countries, showing that the rate of increase varied substantially between nations. Many studies of individual countries have noted increases in childhood obesity in recent years. There are also reports of increasing obesity trends in older people; for example, Bulletin 12 from the Australian Institute of Health and Welfare (2004) showed that the rate of obesity among older Australians has trebled over the past 20 years. Even in low-income countries, malnutrition and obesity can coexist in the same communities due in part to high-fat and carbohydrate diets but also to the ways in which fatness is viewed favourably as a sign of socioeconomic status (Kruger et al., 2005; Ziraba et al., 2009).

The WHO Global Infobase (apps.who.int/infobase) allows comparison of obesity rates between different countries. While obesity rates are high in the UK compared to France, they are significantly lower than many other parts of the world. In 2010, the highest prevalence rates for obesity were in Nauru in the South Pacific, where 80.5% of women and 84.6% of men are obese (BMI > 30).

What has caused the increase in obesity?

While we cannot answer this sort of question definitively from cross-sectional survey data, if we examine information from surveys such as the HSE, we can look for trends over time in levels of physical activity and changing diet. This clearly indicates a pattern of decreasing levels of physical activity over the same period that Figure 3.5 indicates increasing levels of obesity. It is tempting to conclude that decreasing levels of physical activity cause the increase in obesity, but all that it is strictly possible to say from this cross-sectional data is that there is an association. To be able to say decreasing physical activity causes the rise in obesity, we would need to follow people through time and first see a decrease in their physical activity and then observe that this is followed by an increase in obesity in a cohort study. In addition, to be sure a drop in physical activity was the cause, we would need to carefully monitor their diet. If diet also changed, we will potentially have confounding variables and it will be difficult to identify whether the main cause is changing diet or changing physical activity unless we conduct an experiment.

What are the health effects of increasing obesity?

There is now considerable evidence that obesity is associated with a range of health problems (NAO, 2001). Table 3.4 shows the extent to which obesity increases the risk of developing a number of diseases relative to the non-obese population.

More recent evidence suggests the lifetime risk of developing diabetes substantially increased for those who are obese, particularly those who are obese at a young age. The lifetime diabetes risk at 18 years of

Table 3.4 Estimating increased risk for the obese of developing associated diseases, taken from international studies

Disease	Relative risk: women	Relative risk: men
Type 2 diabetes	12.7	5.2
Hypertension	4.2	2.6
Myocardial infarction	3.2	1.5
Cancer of the colon	2.7	3.0
Angina	1.8	1.8
Gall bladder diseases	1.8	1.8
Ovarian cancer	1.7	–
Osteoarthritis	1.4	1.9
Stroke	1.3	1.3

Source: National Audit Office, 2001

age increases from 17.1% in a female with BMI in the range of 18.5–25 to 74.4% for an 18-year-old female with BMI > 35 (Narayan et al., 2007).

If we examine diabetes and cardiovascular disease rates over time, we find that the increasing rates of diabetes and cardiovascular disease mirror the rises over time in the prevalence of obesity. If we look at the international pattern for rates of diabetes, we find that the countries with the highest rates of obesity also have the highest rates of diabetes. Nauru has the highest prevalence of obesity in the world and it also has the highest prevalence of diabetes in the world – almost a quarter of the adult population live with diabetes (Khambalia et al., 2011). This cross-sectional information can only indicate association and we require more complex studies to confirm that obesity is a major cause of diabetes.

Who is at risk?

The HSE 2004 found that those considered to be particularly at risk of obesity in the UK include black African, black Caribbean and Pakistani women and black Caribbean men (HSE, 2006). Also, children from families where one or both parents are overweight

or obese (Parsons et al., 1999) and those giving up smoking are at increased risk. High birth weight may also be associated with an increased risk of obesity later in life (Parsons et al., 1999). The risk of obesity is associated with social class and household income. The HSE 2012 estimated that 19% of women in the highest quintile of household income were obese compared with 33% in the 4th quintile and 31% in the lowest quintile of household income. Among men, 21% were obese in the highest quintile of household income and 24% were obese in the lowest quintile. In terms of household income, in 2012 the prevalence of obesity in women decreases as income increases, but the pattern is less clear for men (HSE, 2013).

What evidence is there of successful interventions?

Having established that there is a real increase in obesity and a related health problem, the next step is what to do about it. Interventions may focus on preventing obesity such as nutrition education with children, or focus on reducing the problem in those who are already obese in order to decrease their health risk. Evidence is needed to decide which interventions are most effective. RCTs are the best method for demonstrating effect. For example, Sahota et al. (2001) carried out an RCT of a primary school-based intervention to reduce risk factors for obesity and Moore et al. (2003) carried out a cluster randomized trial of an intervention to improve the management of obesity in **primary care**. NICE has published national guidance on the prevention, identification, assessment and management of overweight and obesity in adults and children in England and Wales (www.nice.org. uk/guidance/cg 43). In common with many systematic reviews of the evidence relating to effective interventions, it concludes that many studies of interventions to prevent and manage obesity were of short duration, with little or no follow-up, were conducted outside the UK and were poorly reported.

Summary

- Epidemiology has traditionally relied on a medical model as its basis for theory and practice

- Its key questions are who becomes sick and why particular people become sick. From this, it is possible to identify the risk factors for diseases and the healthcare needs of the population

- It also questions how effective curative and preventive healthcare services are. From this, more effective strategies for health may be identified

- Epidemiology employs the scientific method of enquiry to answer these questions and uses a variety of large data sets

- Epidemiology is increasingly embracing different perspectives from the social sciences to arrive at a more complete picture of health needs

Questions for further discussion

1. How and should epidemiological data be used as the basis for government policy? Are epidemiological data objective?

2. How would you describe the impact of a disease or health problem on health and health services, either in the UK or internationally? How and by whom should healthcare priorities be determined?

Further reading and resources

Coggan, D., Barker, D.J. and Rose, G. (2003) *Epidemiology for the Uninitiated* (5th edn). London: BMJ Publishing.
Provides succinct explanations for the novice of the major concepts and research designs used in epidemiology. A quick reference guide.

Moon, G., Gould, M., Brown, T. et al. (2000) *Epidemiology: An Introduction*. Buckingham: Open University Press.
Clear and readable introduction to the principles and methods of epidemiology.

Somerville, M., Kumaran, K. and Anderson, R. (2012) *Public Health and Epidemiology at a Glance*. Chichester: John Wiley & Sons.
Accessible introduction to the key concepts of population-level disease prevention, helping you appreciate the determinants of health that impact on healthcare services and their effectiveness.

Webb, P.M. and Bain, C.J. (2010) *Essential Epidemiology. An Introduction for Students and Health Professionals* (2nd edn). Cambridge: Cambridge University Press.
Clear, practical introduction to all areas of epidemiology.

www.statistics.gov.uk and www.apho.org.uk
GOV.UK and Association of Public Health Observatories (now part of Public Health England) provide summaries and analyses of health trends

www.hscic.nhs.uk
The Health and Social Care Information Centre provides access to information from the Health Surveys for England and statistics relating to health and lifestyle from a variety of other sources

www.nice.org.uk and www.york.ac.uk/inst/crd
NICE and the Centre for Reviews and Dissemination, a part of National Institute for Health Research and a department at the University of York, provide current evidence on effective interventions and guidelines for management of health condition

References

Allmark, P. and Tod, A. (2006) 'How should public health professionals engage with lay epidemiology?' *Journal of Medical Ethics* 32(8): 460–3.

Australian Institute of Health and Welfare (2004) *Obesity Trends in Older Australians*, Bulletin 12. Canberra: Australian Institute of Health and Welfare.

Berkman, L.F. and Kawachi, I. (2000) A historical framework for social epidemiology, in L.F. Berkman and I. Kawachi (eds) *Social Epidemiology*. New York: Oxford University Press, pp. 3–12.

Birmingham City Council (2004) *Children's Nutrition: Obesity*. Report to the City Council, 4 May. Birmingham: Scrutiny Committee, Birmingham City Council.

Bowling, A. (2004) *Measuring Health: A Review of Quality of Life Measurement Scales* (3rd edn). Buckingham: Open University Press.

Bradford Hill, A. and Hill, I.D. (1991) *Bradford Hill's Principles of Medical Statistics* (12th edn). London: Edward Arnold.

Campbell, M.K., Piaggio, G., Elbourne, D.R., Altman, D.G. for the CONSORT Group (2010) 'Consort 2010 statement: extension to cluster randomised trials'. *British Medical Journal* 345(7881): 19–22.

Coggan, D., Barker, D.J.P. and Rose, G. (2003) *Epidemiology for the Uninitiated* (5th edn). London: BMJ Publishing.

Crow, R.A., Chapman, R.G., Roe, B. and Wilson, J. (1986) *A Study of Patients with an Indwelling Urethral Catheter and Related Nursing Practice*. Report to the Department of Health. London: DH.

Dawber, D.R. (1980) *The Framingham Study: The Epidemiology of Atherosclerotic Disease*. Cambridge, MA: Harvard University Press.

Dingwall, R. (1992) 'Don't mind him, he's from Barcelona': qualitative methods in health studies, in Daly, J., MacDonald, I. and Willis, E. (eds) *Researching in Health Care: Designs, Dilemmas and Disciplines*. London: Routledge, pp. 161–75.

Finkel, M.L. and Law, A. (2011) 'The rush to drill for natural gas: a public health cautionary tale'. *American Journal of Public Health* 101(5): 784–5.

Finucane, M.M., Stevens, G.A., Cowan, M.J. et al. (2011) 'National, regional, and global trends in body-mass index since 1980: systematic analysis of health examination surveys and epidemiological studies with 960 country-years and 9.1 million participants'. *Lancet* 377: 557–67.

Flegal, K.M., Carroll, M.D., Kit, B.K. and Ogden, C.L. (2012) 'Prevalence of obesity and trends in the distribution of body mass index among US adults, 1999–2010'. *Journal of American Medical Association* 307(5): 491–7.

Fletcher, R.H. and Fletcher, S.W. (2013) *Clinical Epidemiology: The Essentials* (5th edn). Philadelphia: Lippincott Williams & Wilkins.

Frankenberg, R. (1980) 'Medical anthropology and development: a theoretical perspective'. *Social Science and Medicine* 14B(4): 197–207.

HSE (2006) *Health Survey for England 2004, Health of Ethnic Minorities: Main Report*. Available at www.hscic.gov.uk/catalogue/PUB01170 (accessed 20/3/2014).

HSE (2012) Trend tables. Health and Social Care Information Centre. Available at www.hscic.gov.uk/catalogue/PUB13219 (accessed 20/3/2014).

HSE (2013) *Health Survey for England 2012*. Chapter 10, Adult anthropometric measures, overweight and obesity. Available at www.hscic.gov.uk/catalogue/PUB13218/HSE2012-Ch10-Adult-BMI.pdf (accessed 20/3/2014).

Hunt, K. and Emslie, C. (2001) 'Commentary: the prevention paradox in lay epidemiology – Rose revisited'. *International Journal of Epidemiology* 30(3): 442–6.

Hunt, K., Emslie, C. and Watt, G. (2001) 'Lay constructions of a family history of heart disease: Potential for misunderstandings in the clinical encounter?' *Lancet* 357: 1168–71.

Interphone Study Group (2010) 'Brain tumour risk in relation to mobile telephone use: results of the INTERPHONE international case-control study'. *International Journal of Epidemiology* 39: 675–94.

Keogh, B. (2011) *Poly Implant Prostheses (PIP) Breast Implants: Interim Report of the Expert Group*. Available at www.gov.uk/government/publications/pip-breast-implants-interim-report-of-the-expert-group (accessed 20/3/2014).

Keogh, B. (2012) *Poly Implant Prostheses (PIP) Breast Implants: Final Report of the Expert Group*. Available at www.gov.uk/government/publications/poly-implant-prothese-pip-breast-implants-final-report-of-the-expert-group (accessed 20/3/2014).

Khambalia, A., Phongsavan, P., Smith, B.J. et al. (2011) 'Prevalence and risk factors of diabetes and impaired fasting glucose in Nauru'. *BMC Public Health* 11: 719.

Krieger, N. (2001) 'A glossary for social epidemiology'. *Journal of Epidemiology and Community Health* 55: 693–700.

Kruger, H.S., Puoane, T., Senekal, M. and van der Merwe, M. (2005) 'Obesity in South Africa: challenges for government and health professionals'. *Public Health Nutrition* 8(5): 491–500.

Lawlor, D.A., Frankel, S., Shaw, M. et al. (2003) 'Smoking and ill health: Does lay epidemiology explain the failure of smoking cessation programs among deprived populations?' *American Journal of Public Health* 93(2): 266–70.

Lewis, G. (1993) Some studies of social causes of and cultural response to disease, in C.G. Mascie-Taylor (ed.) *The Anthropology of Disease*. Oxford: Oxford University Press, pp. 73–124.

Lilienfeld, D.E. and Stolley, P.D. (1994) *Foundations of Epidemiology* (3rd edn). New York: Oxford University Press.

McKeown, T. (1976) *The Role of Medicine: Dream, Mirage or Nemesis*. London: Nuffield Provincial Hospitals Trust.

Marmot, M., Allen, J., Goldblatt, P. et al. (2010) *Fair Society, Healthy Lives: Strategic Review of Health Inequalities in England Post-2010*. London: The Marmot Review.

Mettlin, C., Lee, F., Drago, J. and Murphy, G. (1991) 'Findings on the detection of early prostate cancer in 2425 men'. *Cancer* 67(12): 2949–58.

Moher, D., Hopewell, S., Schulz, K.F. et al. (2010) 'CONSORT 2010 explanation and elaboration: updated guidelines for reporting parallel group randomised trials'. *Journal of Clinical Epidemiology* 63(8): 1–37.

Moore, H., Summerbell, C., Greenwood, D. et al. (2003) 'Improving management of obesity in primary care: cluster randomised trial'. *British Medical Journal* 327(7423): 1085–8.

NAO (National Audit Office) (2001) *Tackling Obesity in England*. London: TSO.

Narayan, K.M.V., Boyle, J.P., Thompson, T.J. et al. (2007) 'Effect of BMI on lifetime risk for diabetes in the U.S'. *Diabetes Care* 30(6): 1562–6.

Ogden, C.L., Carroll, M.D., Kit, B.K. and Flegal, K.M. (2012) Prevalence of obesity in the United States, 2009–2010, NCHS Data Brief No. 82, January. Available from www.cdc.gov/nchs/data/databriefs/db82.htm (accessed 20/3/2014).

Parsons, T. (1951) *The Social System*. London: Routledge & Kegan Paul.

Parsons, T., Power, C., Logan, S. and Summerbell, C. (1999) 'Childhood predictors of adult obesity: a systematic review'. *International Journal of Obesity* 23: S1–107.

Percy, A.K., Norbrega, F.T., Okazaki, H. et al. (1971) 'Multiple sclerosis in Rochester, Minn: a 60 year appraisal'. *Archives of Neurology* 25(2): 105–11.

Sackett, D.L., Haynes, R.B., Guyatt, G. and Tugwell, P. (2004) *Clinical Epidemiology: A Basic Science for Clinical Medicine* (3rd edn). Philadelphia, PA: Lippincott Williams & Wilkins.

Sahota, P., Rudolf, M., Dixey, R. et al. (2001) 'Randomised controlled trial of primary school based intervention to reduce risk factors for obesity'. *British Medical Journal* 323(7320): 1027–9.

Scheper-Hughes, N. (1978) 'Saints, scholars and schizophrenics: madness and badness in rural Ireland'. *Medical Anthropology* 2(3): 59–93.

Seedhouse, D. (2002) *Health: The Foundations of Achievement* (2nd edn). Chichester: John Wiley & Sons.

Snowdon, C., Garcia, J. and Elbourne, D. (1997) 'Making sense of randomisation: responses of parents of critically ill babies to random allocation of treatment in a clinical trial'. *Social Science and Medicine* 45(9): 1337–55.

Spiegelhalter, D., Knight, S. and Sant, T. (2012) 'Breast implants: the scandal, the outcry, and assessing the risks'. *Significance* 9(6): 17–21.

Valanis, B. (1999) *Epidemiology and Health Care* (3rd edn). Stamford: Appleton Lange.

WHO (World Health Organization) (1946) *Preamble of the Constitution of the World Health Organization*. Geneva: WHO.

WHO (2000) *Obesity: Preventing and Managing the Global Epidemic*. Report of WHO consultation. WHO Technical Report Series 894(3), i-253, Geneva: WHO.

WHO (2002) *Reducing Risks, Promoting Healthy Life*. Geneva: WHO. Available at www.who.int/whr/2002/en/whr02_en.pdf?ua=1 (accessed 20/3/2014).

WHO (2007) *World Health Report 2007: A Safer Future: Global Public Health Security in the 21st Century*. Geneva: WHO. Available at www.who.int/whr/2007/whr07_en.pdf?ua=1 (accessed 20/3/2014).

Wilson, P.W., d'Agostino, R.B., Levy, D. et al. (1998) 'Prediction of coronary heart disease using risk factor categories'. *Circulation* 97(18): 1837–47.

Ziraba, A.K., Fotso, J.C. and Ochako, R. (2009) 'Overweight and obesity in urban Africa: A problem of the rich or the poor?' *BMC Public Health* 9: 465–74.

chapter

Health psychology

4

Overview   114

Introduction   114

Part 1 The contribution of psychology to health studies   115
Health beliefs and behaviours   117
Communication in health settings   124
The experience of being ill and the example of pain   127

Part 2 Theoretical and research approaches   134
The health belief model   135
The protection motivation theory   136
The theory of planned behaviour   138
The stages of change model   140
The self-regulatory model   141
Developing interventions to change health-related behaviour 144

Case study The impact of beliefs on behaviour: the example
of obesity and diet   147
Summary   149
Questions for further discussion   149
Further reading   150
References   150

Learning outcomes

This chapter will enable readers to:

- Understand and describe the basic principles of health psychology and how it differs from biomedicine
- Understand why the study of health behaviours is important
- Show an understanding of the role of health beliefs in predicting and potentially changing health behaviours, and how they relate to people's coping mechanisms when ill
- Illustrate the ways in which health professionals' beliefs may influence their interactions with patients
- Illustrate the role of psychology in the experience of illness, drawing on theories of pain and pain management

Overview

Psychology focuses on what people believe and how they behave; health psychology explores how these beliefs and behaviours relate to health and illness. This chapter focuses on the beliefs that individuals have relating to health and illness and how these beliefs relate to their health behaviours and subsequently their health status. Part 1 explores the contribution of psychology to studying health and illness, describing the background to psychology and highlighting the importance of beliefs concerning health and illness on the part of laypeople and health professionals. Pain is used as an example of the role of psychology in the experience of illness. Part 2 describes the models that have been developed within health psychology, in particular focusing on the structured models of health beliefs and the self-regulatory model of illness behaviour. Finally, the case study on diet, eating habits and obesity explores in depth how psychological theories can be applied to a topical health issue.

Introduction

The roots of psychology date from the beginning of the twentieth century and the work of psychoanalysts such as Freud and Jung, as well as behaviourists such as Pavlov and Skinner. The psychoanalysts worked as therapists and developed theories based on the patients they saw. In contrast, the behaviourists used strict experimental approaches and carried out laboratory studies, mostly on animals such as rats and pigeons. The two perspectives appear to be quite different, but they were based on the same fundamental questions that remain at the centre of modern-day psychology. Psychologists then and now ask:

- How do people think?

- What causes how people think?

- What changes how people think?

- How do people behave?

- What causes people's behaviour?

- What changes people's behaviour?

These questions form the basis of all the different branches of psychology from biological psychology, with its emphasis on brain chemicals and neurons, to social psychology and its emphasis on individuals and their social world, to cognitive psychology, with its focus on information-processing, problem-solving and language. Health psychology is a relatively new branch of psychology and draws on the theories and research of its predecessors. Furthermore, although it asks similar questions, it applies these to the study of health and illness. In particular, health psychology asks:

- How do people think about their health and illness?

- How do people behave with regard to their health and illness?

- What impact do such beliefs and behaviours have on their health and illness?

- What impact do health and illness have on their beliefs and behaviours?

Health psychology places itself alongside other branches of psychology. However, as it is concerned with health and illness, it is also important to understand its relationship to biomedicine. The biomedical model of medicine was developed in the nineteenth century and emphasized that man was a part of nature and could therefore be studied in the same way that nature was studied. Health psychology has developed out of the biomedical model but differs in terms of the questions it asks and the answers it gives.

According to the biomedical model of medicine, disease either came from outside the body, or invaded the body and caused physical changes within the body, or originated as internal involuntary physical changes. Such diseases may be caused by several factors, such as chemical imbalances, bacteria, viruses and genetic predisposition. Within the biomedical model, health and illness are seen as qualitatively different – you are either healthy or ill, there is no continuum between the two. Because illness is seen as arising from biological changes beyond their control, individuals are not seen as being responsible for their illness. The biomedical model seeks to address the manifestations of illness through surgery or drug treatments that aim to change the physical state of the body. According to the biomedical model of medicine, the mind and body function independently of each other, this perspective being comparable to a traditional dualistic model of the mind/body split.

| Chapter 1 discusses the biomedical model of health and illness in greater detail. | **connections** |

Part 1 The contribution of psychology to health studies

example 4.1

The application of health psychology to contemporary health issues

- When AIDS was first identified in 1986, it was an acute terminal illness in the West and thousands of people died within a short space of time. Now, it is a chronic illness and people with AIDS have an almost normal life expectancy. This is mostly due to the development of medication. But many people in the West do not take their medication as advised even though it can prolong their life. Health psychology explores ways to understand and improve medication compliance or adherence.

- An obesity epidemic has spread across much of the world over the past 20 years. In the main, this is because of overeating and a sedentary lifestyle due to changes in our environment and the ways in which food is manufactured and consumed. Health psychology provides an understanding of why people eat what and how much they eat and can help develop interventions to promote healthy eating and weight loss. It also provides a framework for encouraging people to be more active.

- Medical research constantly creates new medications, new screening tools and new ways to investigate illness. These are designed to detect illness at an earlier stage and improve prognosis. But they cannot work if people do not take their medicine or turn up for their investigations. Health psychology helps us understand why people do or do not seek help or take the advice of health professionals. It can then develop interventions to improve patient self-care.

- Medical interventions can help prolong life through treatments such as surgery, radiotherapy or chemotherapy. But a longer life is not always a better one. Health psychology can help explain why quality rather than quantity of life is important and develop ways to measure and promote a broader set of health outcomes rather than just years survived.

- In 1952, research suggested that smoking was bad for health, yet more than 60 years later, people still smoke even though they know it is bad for them. Health psychology provides a framework for understanding why people behave in unhealthy ways and sets the scene for encouraging healthier lifestyles.

- Some people just get colds while others take to their beds. Some get back pain, which means they need bed rest, while others stay mobile and their pain gets better. Symptoms used to be seen as sensations and reactions to damage but nowadays they are seen as perceptions that are influenced by psychological factors. Health psychology explores how people make sense of their symptoms and how this influences how they manage their health.

During the twentieth century, the emergence of psychosomatic medicine, behavioural health, behavioural medicine and, most recently, health psychology has posed challenges for the biomedical model. Health psychology suggests that human beings should be seen as complex systems and that illness is caused by a multitude of interacting factors rather than a single causative factor. Health psychology claims that illness can result from a combination of factors – biological, for example a virus, psychological, for example behaviours and beliefs, and social, for example employment. This approach reflects the biopsychosocial model of health and illness (Engel, 1977, 1980; see Figure 4.1).

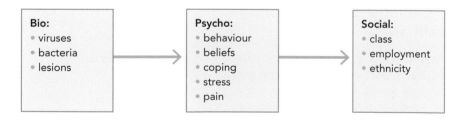

Figure 4.1 **The biopsychosocial model of health and illness**

Health psychology therefore differs from the biomedical model in several important respects:

- Individuals may be held more responsible, through their behaviours and beliefs, for the onset of illness and its management and cure

- Psychological factors are not solely a consequence of illness but may also contribute to its onset

- Treatment must be directed to the whole person rather than just their physical symptoms.

Health psychology emphasizes the role of psychological factors in the cause, progression and consequences of health and illness. Some of the key questions that health psychology tries to explore are:

- What is the role of psychology in the onset and development of illness?

- Should behaviour then be targeted for intervention?

- Can the study of beliefs predict unhealthy behaviour?

- Is it possible to change beliefs?

Health psychologists study the role of psychology in all areas of health and illness, including what people think about health and illness, the role of beliefs and behaviours in becoming ill, the experience of being ill in terms of adaptation to illness, contact with health professionals, coping with illness and compliance with a range of interventions, and the role of psychology in recovery from illness, quality of life and longevity. Health psychology therefore represents the study of the complex processes involved in the aetiology, impact and progression of illness.

Health beliefs and behaviours

It has been suggested that 50% of mortality from the 10 leading causes of death results from individual behaviour, indicating that behaviour and lifestyle have a potentially major effect on longevity. In particular, Doll and Peto (1981) estimated the contribution of different factors as a cause of all cancer deaths and concluded that tobacco consumption accounts for 30% of all cancer deaths, alcohol for 3%, diet for 35% and reproductive and sexual behaviour for 7%. From this estimate, approximately 75% of all deaths from cancer can be attributed to behaviour. More specifically, lung cancer, which is the most common form of cancer, accounts for 36% of all cancer deaths in men and 15% in women in the UK. It has been calculated that 90% of all lung cancer mortality is attributable to cigarette smoking, which is also linked to other illnesses such as cancer of the bladder, pancreas, mouth, larynx and oesophagus, and coronary heart disease. The relationship between mortality and behaviour is also illustrated by bowel cancer, which accounts for 11% of all cancer deaths in men and 14% in women. Research suggests that bowel cancer is linked to behaviours such as a diet high in total fat and meat and low in fibre.

Mokdad et al. (2004) explored the role of health behaviour in the deaths of 2.4 million people who had died in 2000 in the US. The results from this analysis showed the percentage of deaths caused by behaviours were as follows: tobacco: 18.1%, diet and inactivity: 16.6%, alcohol: 3.5%, motor vehicle: 1.8%, firearms: 1.2%, sexual behaviour: 0.8%, and illicit drug use: 0.7%. In 2008, data from a study in England also illustrated the impact of behaviour on mortality. Khaw et al. (2008) carried out a longitudinal study over 11 years in the UK of 20,244 men and women and concluded that death from all causes was related to four health behaviours: smoking, not being physically active, drinking more than moderate amounts of alcohol, and not eating five or more portions of fruit and vegetables per day. This study again supported the link between behaviour and mortality. In addition, it supports the role for a healthy lifestyle as mortality was predicted by the combined impact of these four behaviours, not just individual behaviours.

So, **health behaviours** in terms of smoking, drinking alcohol, diet and exercise seem to be important in predicting the mortality and longevity of individuals. Assuming that individuals behave in ways that are in line with their beliefs, health psychologists have therefore attempted to understand and predict health-related behaviours by studying **health beliefs**. For example, the belief that smoking is dangerous should be associated with non-smoking or smoking cessation; the belief that cervical cancer is preventable should be associated with attendance for cervical screening; and the belief that exercise is beneficial should be associated with increased physical activity. Health psychologists thus study what people believe and whether this relates to how they behave. In addition, they explore whether beliefs can be changed and whether any shifts in beliefs predict subsequent changes in behaviour. In particular, individuals have beliefs about:

- *causality and control:* what has contributed to their ill health and whether these factors are controllable

- *risk:* to what extent they feel susceptible to certain diseases or conditions

- *confidence:* whether they feel there are actions they can take that might affect the condition

- *beliefs about the illness:* what may have caused the illness, how long it might last and what they can do about it.

Beliefs about causality and control

Much work exploring people's beliefs relating to causality and control is based on Heider's **attribution theory** (Heider, 1958). Attribution theory states that people want to understand what causes events because this makes the world seem more predictable and controllable. Since its original formulation, attribution theory has been developed, differentiations having been made between self-attributions (attributions about one's own behaviour) and other attributions (those made about the behaviour of others). In addition, the dimensions of **attribution** have been defined as follows:

- *internal versus external:* 'My failure to give up smoking is due to my lack of willpower' versus 'Others persuade me to carry on smoking'

- *stable versus unstable:* 'The cause of my failure to give up smoking will always be around' versus 'Next time I might succeed in resisting or avoiding peer pressure'

- *global versus specific:* 'The cause of my failure to give up smoking reflects my lack of willpower generally' versus 'I lacked willpower at this specific time'

- *controllable versus uncontrollable:* 'The cause of my failure to stop smoking was controllable by me' versus 'It was uncontrollable by me'.

Attribution theory has been applied to the study of health and health-related behaviour. For example, Bradley et al. (1987) examined patients' attributions for responsibility for their diabetes and reported that perceived control over illness ('is the diabetes controllable by me or a powerful other?') influenced the choice of treatment by these patients. Patients could choose an insulin pump (a small mechanical device attached to the skin, which provides a continuous flow of insulin), intense conventional treatment, or a continuation of daily injections. The results indicated that the patients who chose an insulin pump showed decreased control over their diabetes and increased control attributed to powerful doctors. Therefore, if an individual attributed their illness externally and felt that they personally were not responsible for it, they were more likely to choose the insulin pump and were more likely to hand over responsibility to the doctors.

The internal versus external dimension of attribution theory has been specifically applied to health in terms of the concept of a health **locus of control**. People differ in terms of the extent to which they can make changes in their lives. Some people believe that what they do and what happens to them is up to them and regard events as personally controllable – an internal locus of control. Others, however, believe that events are largely not controlled by them – an external locus of control. Wallston and Wallston (1982) developed a measure of the health locus of control that evaluates whether individuals:

- regard their health as controllable by them, for example 'I am directly responsible for my health'

- believe that their health cannot be controlled by them but lies in the hands of fate, for example 'Whether or not I am well is a matter of luck'

- regard their health as under the control of powerful others, for example 'I can only do what my doctor tells me to do'.

In a study of young people with diabetes, Gillibrand and Stevenson (2006) reported that those with an internal locus of control rated the benefits of adhering to a self-care regimen as greater than the costs. Those with a stronger belief in powerful others, however, regarded their illness as less of a risk to their health.

> **?** How might locus of control be related to an individual's willingness to adopt a more healthy lifestyle?

People who generally have an external locus of control are less likely to take protective action regarding their health. Part of the work of health professionals may be to encourage them to take more control and set their own targets for change: merely expecting them to follow recommendations from a health professional is unlikely to be effective.

Beliefs about risk

People hold beliefs about their own susceptibility to a given problem and make judgements concerning the extent to which they are 'at risk'. Smokers, for example, may continue to smoke because although they understand that smoking is unhealthy, they do not consider themselves to be at risk of lung cancer. Likewise, a woman may not attend for a cervical smear because she believes that cervical cancer happens only to women who are not like her. People have ways of assessing their susceptibility to particular conditions, and this is not always a rational process. It has been suggested that individuals consistently estimate their risk of getting a health problem as less than that of others. Weinstein (1984) asked subjects to examine a list of health problems and to state 'compared to other people of your age and sex, are your chances of getting [the problem] greater than, about the same, or less than theirs?' The results of this study showed that most subjects believed that they were less likely than others to get the health problem. Weinstein called this phenomenon 'unrealistic optimism'; not everyone can be less likely to contract an illness. Weinstein (1987) suggested that people are likely to dismiss their risk and be unrealistically optimistic if:

- they have a lack of personal experience with the problem
- they believe that the problem is preventable by individual action
- they believe that if the problem has not yet appeared, it will not appear in the future
- the problem is infrequent.

Weinstein (1984) argued that individuals show selective focus by ignoring their own risk-increasing behaviour ('I may drink too much') and focusing primarily on their risk-reducing behaviour ('but at least I don't drink and drive'). He also argues that individuals tend to ignore others' risk-decreasing behaviour ('My friends all drink sensibly but that's irrelevant'). Individuals may therefore be unrealistically optimistic if they focus on the times when they drink in moderation when assessing their own risk and ignore the times when they do not, in addition focusing on the times when others around them drink to excess and ignoring the times when they are more sensible.

example 4.2

Impact of beliefs and behaviours on health: the example of stress

One of the reasons why stress has been studied so consistently is because of its potential effect on the health of the individual. Stress can affect health through either a behavioural or a physiological pathway. Most of the research into the stress–illness link has studied the physiological effects of stress. However, in support of the suggested behavioural pathway and in line with a psychological perspective, some recent research has examined the effect of stress on specific health-related behaviours and more general behavioural change (Krantz et al., 1981). Research, for example, suggests a link between stress and smoking behaviour in terms of smoking initiation, relapse and the amount smoked. Furthermore, not being able to smoke in a social situation can make the situation more stressful.

Contemporary definitions of stress regard external environmental stress, for example problems at work, as a *stressor*, the response to the stressor, for example the feeling of tension, as *stress* or *distress*, and the concept of stress as something that involves biochemical, physiological, behavioural and psychological changes. Researchers have also differentiated between stress that is harmful and damaging (distress) and stress that is positive and beneficial (*eustress*). The most commonly used definition of stress is that of a transactional model, stating that stress involves an interaction between the stressor and distress and therefore between people and their environment (Lazarus and Launier, 1978). This approach to stress provides a role for an individual's psychological state and is a departure from more medical perspectives, with their focus on physiology.

Over recent years, theories of stress have emphasized forms of self-control as important in understanding stress. This is illustrated in theories of self-efficacy, hardiness and feelings of mastery. In 1987, Lazarus and Folkman suggested that self-efficacy was a powerful factor for mediating the stress response. Self-efficacy refers to individuals' feelings of confidence that they can perform a desired action. Research indicates that self-efficacy may have a role in mediating stress-induced immunosuppression and physiological changes, such as those of blood pressure, heart rate and stress hormone levels. For example, the belief that 'I am confident I can succeed in this exam' may result in physiological changes that reduce the stress response. A belief in the ability to control one's behaviour may therefore relate to whether or not a potentially stressful event results in a stress response.

This shift towards emphasizing self-control is also illustrated by the concept of 'hardiness' (Maddi and Kobasa, 1984). Hardiness has been described as reflecting personal feelings of control, a desire to accept challenges, and commitment. It has been argued that the degree of hardiness influences an individual's appraisal of potential stressors and the resulting stress response. The term 'feelings of mastery' (Karasek and Theorell, 1990) reflects individuals' control over their stress response.

It has been argued that the degree of mastery may be related to the stress response. According to these recent developments, stress is conceptualized as a product of an individual's capacity for self-control. Successful coping and self-management eradicate stress, failed self-regulation results in a stress response, and stress-related illness is considered to be a consequence of prolonged failed self-management.

The relationship between stress and illness is not straightforward, and there is much evidence to suggest that several factors may mediate the stress–illness link. For example, how an individual copes with stress may reduce stress and subsequently decrease the chance of illness. In addition, increased social support has been related to a decreased stress response and a subsequent reduction in illness. Finally, the degree to which an individual feels in control of the stressor can influence the degree of stress experienced.

So, from a psychological perspective, an individual's state of mind relates to stress and the stress response in terms of:

- their appraisal of the external stressor – 'Is it stressful?'
- the degree of the stress response to this stressor – 'Do I feel stressed?'
- their ability to cope with and reduce this response – 'It's OK, I can talk this over with my friends'
- the degree of any subsequent changes in behaviour – 'I think I'll have a cigarette'.

Accordingly, each of these factors will in turn determine the extent of any resulting ill health.

Beliefs about confidence

Individuals also hold beliefs about their ability to carry out certain behaviours. Bandura (1977) has termed this **self-efficacy** to reflect the extent to which people feel confident that they can do whatever it is they wish to do. A smoker, for example, may feel they should stop smoking but have very little confidence they will be able to do so. Likewise, an overweight person may be convinced they should do more exercise but think this goal is unlikely to be achievable. These two examples would be said to have low self-efficacy. In contrast, a person who was motivated to attend for a health check, and felt confident they could, would be said to have high self-efficacy. Self-efficacy is defined not to reflect a personality trait, that is, this person always has high self-efficacy, but to describe a belief about a particular behaviour at a particular time, that is, this person shows high self-efficacy now in terms of changing this behaviour.

Beliefs about illness

Illness beliefs have been defined as 'a patient's own implicit common-sense beliefs about their illness' (Leventhal et al., 1980, 1997). Such beliefs provide individuals with a framework for coping with and understanding their illness, and for telling them what to look out for if they are becoming ill. There are five cognitive dimensions to these beliefs:

1. *Identity:* what label is given to the illness (the medical diagnosis) and the symptoms experienced, for example 'I have a chest infection (diagnosis) with a cough (symptoms)'

2. *The perceived cause of the illness:* causes may be biological or psychosocial. People may explain their illness as reflecting different causal models. One person may believe that 'My chest infection was caused by a virus', whereas another may believe that 'My chest infection was caused by stress and being run down'

3. *Timeline:* beliefs about how long the illness will last, that is, whether it is acute (short term) or chronic (long term), for example 'My chest infection will be over in a few days'

4. *Consequences:* perceptions of the possible effects of the illness on an individual's life. The consequences may be physical, for example pain and a lack of mobility, emotional, for example a loss of social contact or loneliness, or a combination of the two, for example 'My chest infection will prevent me going to college, which will prevent me seeing my friends'

5. *Curability and controllability:* individuals also represent illnesses in terms of whether they believe that the illness can be treated and cured, and the extent to which the outcome of their illness is controllable either by themselves or powerful others, for example 'If I rest, my chest infection will go away' or 'If I take my medication, my chest infection will go away'.

There is some evidence for a similar structure of illness representation in other cultures. Weller (1984) examined models of illness in English-speaking Americans and Spanish-speaking Guatemalans. The results indicated that illness was predominantly conceptualized in terms of contagion and severity. Lau (1995) argued that contagion is a version of the cause dimension, that is, the illness is caused by a virus, and severity is a combination of the magnitude of the perceived consequences and beliefs about the timeline, that is, how will the illness affect my life and how long will it last, dimensions that support those described by Leventhal et al.

Researchers in New Zealand and the UK have developed the illness perception questionnaire (Weinman et al., 1996). This asks subjects to rate a series of statements about their illness that reflect the dimensions identified by Leventhal et al. (1997). The questionnaire has been used to examine beliefs about illnesses such as chronic fatigue syndrome, diabetes and arthritis, and provides further support for the dimensions of illness beliefs.

Individuals have beliefs related to their health and illness. These beliefs influence their behaviours, which may in turn impact on how healthy they are. The decisions people make are not, however, wholly a product of their beliefs. It is not only laypeople who have such beliefs. Being healthy or ill can bring individuals into contact with a range of health professionals, including GPs, nurses, midwives, hospital doctors and alternative practitioners. These health professionals also have their own beliefs and behaviours.

Communication in health settings

The study of health professionals' beliefs developed from the examination of doctor–patient communication and the original focus on compliance. Haynes et al. (1979) defined **compliance** as 'the extent to which the patient's behaviour (in terms of taking medications, following diets or other lifestyle changes) coincides with medical or health advice'. Compliance has excited an enormous amount of clinical and academic interest over the past few decades, and it has been calculated that 3,200 English articles on compliance have been listed between 1979 and 1985 (Trostle, 1988). Nowadays, people tend to prefer the term 'adherence' to compliance as compliance is considered to describe the patient in a passive role. This chapter will, however, use the term 'compliance' as this is what is still often used in the literature.

Compliance is regarded as important primarily because following the recommendations of health professionals is considered to be essential to patient recovery. Studies estimate, however, that about half the patients with a chronic illness such as diabetes or hypertension are noncompliant with their medication regimens and that even compliance for a behaviour as apparently simple as using an inhaler for asthma is poor. Compliance also has financial implications: figures obtained from a patient compliance survey conducted in 2004 estimated the annual cost of noncompliance to be £60 billion (www.datamonitor.com).

?   What factors might contribute to a patient's compliance with a medical regimen?

Ley (1988) developed the cognitive hypothesis model of compliance. This claims that compliance can be predicted by a combination of:

- patient satisfaction with the process of the consultation
- understanding the information given
- recall of this information.

Several studies have been carried out to examine each element of the cognitive hypothesis model, illustrated in Figure 4.2.

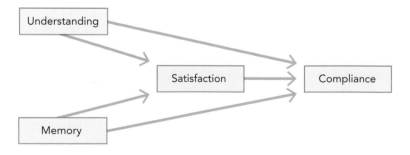

Figure 4.2 **Ley's model of compliance**

example 4.3

Health consultations

Numerous studies have looked at patients' understanding of what they have been told in a consultation, the extent to which they remember it and whether they feel satisfied with the consultation. Ley (1988) examined the extent of patient satisfaction with the consultation. He reviewed 21 studies of hospital patients and found that 41% of patients were dissatisfied with their treatment and 28% of general practice patients were similarly dissatisfied. Studies show that the level of patient satisfaction stems from various components of the consultation, in particular the affective aspects, for example emotional support and understanding, the behavioural aspects, for example adequate explanation and prescribing, and the competence, for example diagnosis and appropriateness of referral, of the health professional. Ley (1988) also reported that satisfaction is determined by the content of the consultation and that patients want to know as much information as possible, even if it is bad news. In studies looking at cancer diagnosis, for example, patients showed improved satisfaction if they were given a diagnosis of cancer rather than being protected from this information.

Several studies have also examined the extent to which patients understand the content of the consultation. One study by Boyle (1970) examined patients' definitions of different illnesses and reported that, when given a checklist, only 85% correctly defined arthritis, 77% jaundice, 52% palpitations and 80% bronchitis. Boyle further examined patients' perceptions of the location of organs and found that only 42% correctly located the heart, 20% the stomach and 49% the liver. This suggests that the understanding of the content of the consultation may well be low.

Further studies have examined the understanding of illness in terms of causality and seriousness. Roth (1979) asked what patients thought caused peptic ulcers and found a variety of responses, such as problems with the teeth and gums, food, digestive problems or excessive stomach acid. He also examined what individuals thought caused lung cancer and found that although the understanding of the causality of lung cancer was high in terms of smoking behaviour, 50% of individuals thought that lung cancer caused by smoking had a good prognosis.

Researchers have also examined the process of recall of the information given during the consultation. A study by Bain (1977) examined the recall from a sample of patients who had attended a GP consultation and found that 37% could not recall the name of the drug, 23% could not recall the frequency of the dose and 25% could not recall the duration of the treatment. A further study by Crichton et al. (1978) found that 22% of patients had forgotten the treatment regimen recommended by their doctors.

In a meta-analysis of research into the recall of consultation information, Ley (1988) found that recall is influenced by a multitude of factors, such as anxiety, medical knowledge, intellectual level, the importance of the statement, the primacy effect and the number of statements. He concluded, however, that recall is not influenced by the patient's age, contrary to some predictions of the effect of ageing on memory and some of the myths and counter-myths of the ageing process.

? What do these studies suggest about how patient compliance might be improved?

Traditional models of the communication between health professionals and patients have emphasized the transfer of knowledge from expert to layperson.

There are, however, several problems with this educational approach, which can be summarized as follows:

- It assumes that the communication from the health professional is from an expert whose knowledge base is one of objective knowledge and does not involve the health beliefs of that individual health professional

- Patient compliance is seen as positive and unproblematic

- Improved knowledge is predicted to improve the communication process

- The approach does not include a role for patient health beliefs.

Doctors are traditionally regarded as having an objective knowledge set that comes from their extensive medical education. If this were the case, it could be predicted that doctors with a similar level of knowledge and training would behave in a similar way. In addition, if doctors' behaviour were objective, it would also be consistent. Considerable variability has, however, been found among doctors in terms of different aspects of their practice. In particular, health professionals have been shown to vary in terms of their diagnosis of asthma, their prescribing behaviour, which ranged between 15% and 90% of patients being prescribed drugs, the methods used by doctors to measure blood pressure, and their treatment of diabetes (see Marteau and Johnston, 1990).

According to a traditional educational model of doctor–patient communication, this variability could be understood in terms of a differing level of knowledge and expertise: some individuals know more or less than others, and there is a correct way of behaving and a correct diagnosis that experts make successfully, whereas novices make errors. This variability can, however, also be understood by examining the health professionals' own health beliefs.

Patients are described as having **lay health beliefs** that are individual and variable, whereas health professionals are usually described as having professional beliefs that are often assumed to be consistent and predictable. If, however, health professionals vary in the diagnoses they make, the conclusions they reach and the treatments they prescribe, this suggests a role for the health professional's own health beliefs, which may vary as much as the patient's. In particular, these beliefs appear to play a central role in the development of a health professional's original hypothesis, for example 'This patient looks as if she has a chest infection', 'This patient is anxious but not physically ill', 'This patient wants to tell me something but is embarrassed' or 'This patient could have cancer'.

Health professionals have their own beliefs concerning health and illness, which influence their choice of hypothesis. Some may believe that health and illness are determined by biomedical factors, whereas others may view health and illness as relating to psychosocial factors. A patient suffering from tiredness may be seen by the former as anaemic and by the latter as suffering from stress. Health professionals will also hold beliefs about the prevalence and incidence of any given health problem. For example, whereas one doctor may regard appendicitis as a common childhood complaint and hypothesize that a child presenting with acute abdominal pain has appendicitis, another may consider appendicitis to be rare and not consider this hypothesis.

Health professionals also have beliefs about the seriousness and treatability of a disease and are particularly motivated to reach a correct diagnosis for serious but treatable conditions. A health professional may, for example, diagnose appendicitis in a child presenting with abdominal pain because appendicitis is both a serious and a treatable condition. There is a high 'pay-off' for a correct diagnosis of such conditions. A health professional's existing knowledge of the patient will also influence their original hypothesis. Such knowledge may include the patient's medical history, their psychological state, an understanding of their psychosocial environment, and a belief about why the patient uses the medical services. In addition, the development of the original hypothesis may be influenced by the health professional's stereotyped views concerning the class, ethnicity or physical appearance of a patient. Furthermore, health professionals' mood, their profile characteristics (such as age and sex), their geographical location and their previous experience may all affect the decision-making process. Therefore, the variability in health professionals' behaviour can be understood in terms of the many pre-existing factors involved in the decision-making process.

In summary, laypeople have beliefs about their health and illness. These can take the form of beliefs about cause and control, risk, confidence and the illness in question. However, it is not only laypeople who hold such beliefs. Research exploring health professionals' behaviour indicates that their beliefs are just as complex, particularly in areas related to decision-making and diagnosis. Beliefs are therefore central to the experience of being ill in terms of health-related behaviours, beliefs about illness and the beliefs of health professionals. The role of such psychological factors in the experience of illness is illustrated in the research on pain and the role of beliefs and behaviours in its increase and decrease.

The experience of being ill and the example of pain

Early models of pain described pain within a biomedical framework as an automatic response to an external factor. From this perspective, pain was seen as a response to a painful stimulus involving a direct pathway connecting the source of pain, for example a burnt finger, to the area of the brain that detected the painful sensation. Although psychological changes ('I feel anxious') were described as resulting from the pain, there was no room in these models for psychology in either the cause or the moderation of pain ('My pain feels better when I think about something else'). Psychology began to play an important part in understanding pain throughout the twentieth century. This was based on several observations:

1. Medical treatments for pain, for example drugs and surgery, were, in the main, useful only for treating acute pain, that is, pain of short duration. Such treatments were fairly ineffective for treating chronic pain, that is, pain that lasts for a long time. This suggested that there must be something else involved in the pain sensation that was not included in the simple stimulus–response models.

2. Individuals with the same degree of tissue damage differed in their reporting of the painful sensation and/or the pain response. Beecher (1956) observed soldiers' and civilians' requests for pain relief in a hospital during the Second World War. He reported that, although soldiers and civilians often showed the same degree of injury, soldiers requested less medication than civilians. He found that whereas 80% of the civilians requested medication, only 25% of the soldiers did. Beecher suggested that this reflected a role for the meaning of the injury in the experience of pain: for soldiers, the injury had a positive meaning as it indicated that their time at war was over. This meaning mediated the pain experience.

3. Between 5% and 10% of amputees tend to feel pain in an absent limb, known as 'phantom limb pain'. Their pain can get worse after the amputation and continue even after complete healing. Sometimes the pain can feel as if it is spreading at the site, often being described as that of a hand being clenched with the nails digging into the palm. Phantom limb pain has no physical basis because the limb is obviously missing. In addition, not everybody feels phantom limb pain, and those who do, do not experience it to the same extent.

---

example 4.4

The gate control theory of pain

Melzack and Wall (1965) developed the gate control theory of pain, which represented an attempt to introduce psychology into the understanding of pain. This model is illustrated in Figure 4.3. It suggested that although pain still could be understood in terms of a stimulus–response pathway, this pathway was complex and mediated by a network of interacting processes. The gate control theory thus integrated psychology into the traditional biomedical model of pain, not only describing a role for physiological causes and interventions, but also allowing for psychological causes and interventions.

Melzack and Wall (1965) suggested that there was a gate existing at spinal cord level, which received input from the peripheral nerve fibre, that is, the site of injury, descending central influences from the brain relating to the psychological state of the individual, in terms of, for example, attention, mood and previous experiences, and the large and small fibres that constitute part of the physiological input to pain perception. They argued that the gate integrates all the information from these different sources and produces an output. This output then sends information to an action system, which results in the perception of pain, the degree of pain relating to how open or closed the gate is.

Melzack and Wall suggested that several factors open the gate:

- physical factors, such as injury or activation of the large fibres
- emotional factors, such as anxiety, worry, tension and depression
- behavioural factors, such as focusing on the pain or boredom.

The gate control theory also suggests that certain factors close the gate:

- physical factors, such as medication or stimulation of the small fibres
- emotional factors, such as happiness, optimism or relaxation
- behavioural factors, such as concentration, distraction or an involvement in other activities.

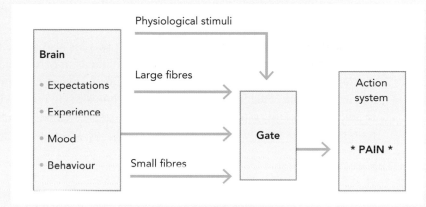

Figure 4.3 **The gate control theory of pain**

The gate control theory of pain was a development from previous theories, in that it allowed for the existence of mediating variables and emphasized active perception rather than passive sensation (Melzack and Wall, 1965). The gate control theory and subsequent attempts at evaluating the different components of pain perception reflect a three-process model of pain. The components of this model are:

1. physiological processes such as tissue damage

2. the release of endorphins and changes in heart rate

3. subjective-affective, cognitive and behavioural processes.

The latter sets of processes indicate a central role for psychological factors in pain perception and have been studied as follows.

Subjective-affective processes

Learning processes

- *Classical conditioning:* Research suggests that classical conditioning may have an effect on the perception of pain. As described by theories of associative learning, an individual may associate a particular environment with the experience of pain. For example, if an individual, because of past experience, associates the dentist with pain, pain perception may be enhanced when attending the dentist as a result of this expectation. In addition, because of the association between these two factors, the individual may experience increased anxiety when attending the dentist, which may also increase pain.

- *Operant conditioning:* Research suggests that there is also a role for operant conditioning in pain perception. Individuals may respond to pain by showing pain behaviour, for example resting, grimacing, limping or staying off work. Such pain behaviour may be positively reinforced by, for example, sympathy, attention and time off work, which may itself increase pain perception (see the section on Behavioural processes below).

The role of emotion

- *Anxiety:* Some research has explored how patients worry about their pain. For example, Eccleston et al. (2001) asked 34 male and female chronic pain patients to describe their experience of pain over a seven-day period. The results showed that the patients reported pain-related and non-pain-related worry and that these two forms of worry were qualitatively different. In particular, worry about chronic pain was seen as more difficult to dismiss, more distracting, more attention-grabbing, more intrusive, more distressing and less pleasant than non-pain-related worry.

    Other research has explored how anxiety relates to pain perception. Fordyce and Steger (1979) examined the relationship between anxiety and acute and chronic pain, reporting that anxiety has a different relationship to these two types of pain. In terms of acute pain, pain increases anxiety, the successful treatment of the pain then decreases the pain, which subsequently decreases the anxiety. This can then cause a further decrease in the pain level. Thus, with acute pain, because of the relative ease with which it can be treated, anxiety relates to this pain perception in terms of a cycle of pain reduction. The pattern is different for chronic pain. With chronic pain, pain increases anxiety, but the treatment of chronic pain is often not very effective, the pain then further increases anxiety, which further increases the pain. In terms of the relationship between anxiety and chronic pain, there is a cycle of pain increase.

- *Fear:* Many patients with an experience of pain can have extensive fear of increased pain or of the pain reoccurring, which can result in them avoiding a whole range of activities they perceive to be high risk. For example, patients can avoid moving in particular ways and exerting themselves to any extent. However, these patients often do not describe their experiences in terms of fear but in terms of what they can and cannot do. So, they do not report being frightened of making the pain worse by lifting a heavy object, but state that they can no longer lift heavy objects. Fear of pain and fear avoidance beliefs have been shown to be linked with the pain experience in terms of triggering pain in the first place. Vlaeyen and Linton (2000) measured fear avoidance beliefs in a large community sample of people who reported no spinal pain in the preceding year. The participants were then followed up after one year and the occurrence of a pain episode and their physical functioning was assessed. The results showed that 19% of the sample reported an episode of back pain at follow-up and that those with higher baseline scores of fear avoidance were twice as likely to report back pain and had a 1.7 times higher risk of lowered physical functioning. The authors argue that fear avoidance may relate to the early onset of pain.

  Some research also suggests that fear may be involved in exacerbating existing pain and turning acute pain into chronic pain. Crombez et al. (1999) explored the interrelationship between attention to pain and fear. They argued that pain functions by demanding attention, which results in a lowered ability to focus on other activities. Their results indicated that pain-related fear increased this attentional interference, suggesting that fear about pain increased the amount of attention demanded by the pain. They concluded that pain-related fear can create a hypervigilance towards pain, which could contribute to the progression from acute to chronic pain.

Cognitive processes

One of the most important factors that influences pain is the cognitive state of the individual. Beecher (1956), in his study of soldiers' and civilians' requests for medication, was one of the first people to examine this and ask the question: 'What does pain mean to the individual?' Beecher argued that differences in pain perception were related to the *meaning* of pain for the individual. In Beecher's study, the soldiers benefited from their pain. This has been described in terms of 'secondary gain', whereby the pain may have a positive reward for the individual. Pain research has identified a number of specific cognitive states that influence the pain experience.

Catastrophizing

Patients with pain, particularly chronic pain, often show 'catastrophizing'. Keefe et al. (2000) described catastrophizing as involving three components:

1. *Rumination:* a focus on threatening information, internal and external, for example 'I can feel my neck click whenever I move'

2. *Magnification:* overestimating the extent of the threat, for example 'The bones are crumbling and I will become paralysed'

3. *Helplessness:* underestimating personal and broader resources that might mitigate the danger and disastrous consequences, for example 'Nobody understands how to fix the problem and I just can't bear any more pain'.

Catastrophizing has been linked to the onset of pain and the development of longer term pain problems (Sullivan et al., 2001).

Attention

There has also been research exploring the impact of attention on pain, showing that attention to the pain can exacerbate pain, whereas distraction can reduce the pain experience. Eccleston and Crombez (1999) have carried out much work in this area. They illustrated how patients who attend to their pain experience more pain than those who are distracted. This association explains why patients suffering from back pain who take to their beds, and therefore focus on their pain, take longer to recover than those who carry on working and engaging with their lives. This association is also reflected in relatively recent changes in the general management approach to back pain problems – bed rest is no longer the main treatment option. In addition, Eccleston and Crombez (1999) provide a model of how pain and attention are related. They argue that pain interrupts and demands attention and that this interruption depends on pain-related characteristics, such as the threat value of the pain, and environmental demands such as emotional arousal. They argue that pain causes a shift in attention towards the pain as a way to encourage escape and action. The result of this shift in attention towards the pain is a reduced ability to focus on other tasks, resulting in attentional interference and disruption. This disruption has been shown in a series of experimental studies indicating that patients with high pain perform less well on difficult tasks that involve the greatest demand of their limited resources (Eccleston, 1994; Crombez et al., 1999).

Behavioural processes

The way in which an individual responds to the pain can itself increase or decrease the perception of the pain. In particular, research has looked at pain behaviours, which have been defined by Turk and colleagues (Turk and Rennert, 1981; Turk et al. 1985) as:

- facial or audible expressions, for example clenched teeth and moaning

- distorted posture or movement, for example limping or protecting the painful area

- negative affect, for example irritability and depression

- the avoidance of activity, for example not going to work or lying down.

It has been suggested that pain behaviours are reinforced by attention, the acknowledgement they receive, and secondary gains, such as not having to go to work. Positively reinforcing pain behaviour may increase pain perception. Pain behaviour can also cause a lack of activity, muscle wastage, a lack of social contact and a dearth of distraction, leading to the adoption of a sick role, which can also increase pain perception.

Pain treatment: a role for psychology?

If psychology is involved in the perception of pain, recent research has suggested that psychology can also be involved in the treatment of pain. There are several methods of pain treatment that reflect an interaction between psychology and physiological factors:

- *Biofeedback* has been used to enable individuals to exert voluntary control over their bodily functions. The technique aims to decrease anxiety and tension and so decrease pain.

- *Relaxation* methods are also used. These aim to decrease anxiety and stress, and thus decrease pain.

- *Operant conditioning* is related to an increased pain perception, thus it can also be used in pain treatment to reduce pain. Some aspects of pain treatment aim positively to reinforce compliance as a means to reduce pain and discourage pain behaviour, such as not walking or standing in ways that avoid pain. By doing so, it is hoped that people will avoid the secondary gains of pain, such as being let off normal duties or staying in bed, which could in turn make the pain worse.

- A *cognitive approach* to pain treatment involves factors such as attention diversion, encouraging the individual not to focus on the pain, and imagery, encouraging the individual to have positive, pleasant thoughts. Both factors appear to decrease pain.

- *Hypnosis* has also been shown to reduce pain. However, whether or not this is simply an effect of attention diversion is unclear.

Multidisciplinary pain clinics

Over recent years, multidisciplinary pain clinics have been set up to treat pain and attempt to challenge the factors that cause or exacerbate pain. The goals of these clinics include:

- improving physical and lifestyle functioning: this involves improving muscle tone, self-esteem, self-efficacy and distraction, and decreasing boredom, pain behaviour and secondary gains

- a decreasing reliance on drugs and medical services: this involves improving personal control, increasing self-efficacy, and decreasing the sick role

- increasing social support and family life: this aims to increase optimism and distraction, and decrease boredom, anxiety, sick role behaviour and secondary gains.

Part 2 Theoretical and research approaches

example 4.5

Examples of research in health psychology

- Quality of life: Much research within health psychology explores quality of life in terms of how it can be understood, the best ways to measure it and how it can be improved by health-related interventions. A focus on quality of life recognizes that quality rather than quantity of life is important
- Behaviour change: Nowadays, most people die from chronic rather than acute illnesses, such as cancer, coronary heart disease, diabetes, obesity or AIDS. These illnesses all show a strong link with health behaviours, including smoking, diet, exercise, sex, and medication compliance. Many health psychology researchers are involved in evaluating the mechanisms of behaviour change and developing effective interventions to encourage healthier lifestyles
- Compliance: Dieticians may develop the perfect diet for weight loss or the management of diabetes, drug companies may develop a new wonder drug to manage illness, and scientists may have discovered that smoking causes lung cancer. But none of these breakthrough discoveries are of any use unless people can be encouraged to behave in the way health professionals want them to. Health psychology researchers focus on the causes of noncompliance to advice and the ways in which people can be encouraged to become more compliant

- Pain management: Acute pain can be managed with painkillers and mostly disappears over time. Chronic pain is, however, much more difficult to treat and is exacerbated by a number of psychological factors, such as pain behaviour, focusing on the pain, faulty cognitions and fear. Research within health psychology addresses the factors that trigger and exacerbate pain and has developed pain management approaches to reduce the pain experience
- Stress and illness: Stress can cause illnesses either directly through changes in physiology or by promoting unhealthy behaviours such as smoking, excessive alcohol consumption, lack of sleep or poor diet. Research in health psychology uses laboratory methods to assess the impact of stress and develop stress management techniques to prevent stress responses to potential stressors

Health psychology draws on a range of **models** in its approach. These models help us to understand:

- people's views about the causes of ill health

- the extent to which people feel they can control their life and make changes

- how people explain their health and ill health, which is crucial to making sense of the strategies they adopt to promote health, prevent ill health and manage illness.

The health belief model

The health belief model (Figure 4.4) was initially formulated by Rosenstock in 1966. It is used to predict people's adoption of preventive health behaviours and in the behavioural response to medical treatment for illness.

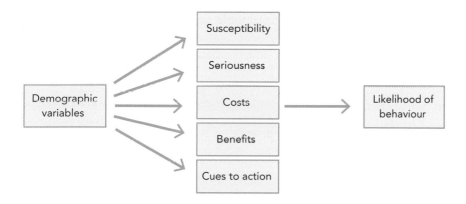

Figure 4.4 **The health belief model**

The health belief model predicts that behaviour is a result of a set of stable, core beliefs concerning:

- susceptibility to illness, for example 'My chances of having a heart attack are low'

- the seriousness of the illness, for example 'Heart disease is a serious illness'

- the costs involved in carrying out the behaviour, for example 'Eating less will be stressful and boring'

- the benefits involved in carrying out the behaviour, for example 'Eating more healthily will make me feel better'

- cues to action, which may be internal, such as the symptom of breathlessness, or external, such as information in the form of health education leaflets.

Becker and Rosenstock's (1987) revised health belief model includes:

- an assessment of sufficient motivation to make health issues salient or relevant

- the belief that change following a health recommendation will be beneficial to the individual at a level of acceptable cost.

> **?** How might the health belief model be used to predict the likelihood of a smoker giving up? What are the strengths and weaknesses of this model of behaviour change?

The health belief model would predict smoking cessation if an individual perceived that they were highly susceptible to lung cancer, lung cancer was a serious health threat, the benefits of stopping smoking, for example more money and less odour, were high and the costs of such action, for example potential weight gain or isolation in the peer group, were comparatively low. Furthermore, individuals are more likely to give up if subjected to cues to action that are external, such as a leaflet in the doctor's waiting room, or internal, such as the symptom of breathlessness perceived (correctly or otherwise) to be related to lung cancer.

The health belief model has been used in a wide range of studies to explain and predict behaviours such as screening uptake, smoking, dental health and dietary change (see Abraham and Sheeran, 2005, for a comprehensive review). In general, research shows that the different components of this model can predict different behaviours but that the links between beliefs and actual behaviour are often quite small.

The protection motivation theory

As a result of some of the criticisms of the health belief model and the emerging focus on self-efficacy, Rogers (1983) developed the protection motivation theory (see Figure 4.5), which expanded the health belief model to include additional factors. The protection motivation theory claims that health-related behaviours are a product of five components:

1. *Self-efficacy:* for example 'I am confident that I can attend for a cervical smear'

2. *Response effectiveness:* for example 'Having a smear will enable abnormalities to be detected early'

3. *Severity:* for example 'Cervical cancer is a serious illness'

4. *Vulnerability:* for example 'My chances of getting cervical cancer are high'

5. *Fear:* for example an emotional response in response to education or information.

These components predict behavioural intentions, for example 'I intend to change my behaviour', which are related to behaviour. Response effectiveness and self-efficacy relate to coping appraisal, that is, individual self-appraisal, whereas severity, vulnerability and fear relate to threat appraisal, that is, assessing the outside threat. Information, which can be either environmental, such as verbal persuasion or observational learning, or intrapersonal, such as prior experience, influences the five components of the protection motivation theory, giving rise to either an adaptive coping response, that is, behavioural intention, or a maladaptive coping response, for example avoidance or denial.

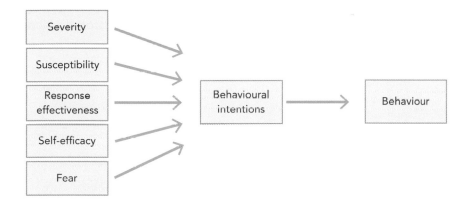

Figure 4.5 **The protection motivation theory**

? How might the protection motivation theory be applied to those thinking about taking up exercise?

Information on the contributory role of a poor fitness level to coronary heart disease would increase individuals' anxiety and their perception of how serious coronary heart disease was (perceived severity) and might also increase their belief that they were likely to have a heart attack (perceived vulnerability/susceptibility). If individuals also felt confident that they could change their level of physical activity (self-efficacy) and that this change would have a beneficial outcome (response effectiveness), such as weight loss, they would be more likely to change their behaviour (behavioural intentions). This would be seen as an adaptive coping response to the information. Alternatively, they might not perceive themselves to be unfit and might therefore deny that the information had any relevance to them. This would be seen as a maladaptive coping response.

The protection motivation theory has been used to predict a range of behaviours including exercise, binge drinking, breast self-examination and children's compliance to wearing an eye patch (e.g. Norman et al., 2003; Plotnikoff et al., 2010). The fear component has been useful for focusing on the role of emotions in behaviour, but similar to the health belief model, the links between beliefs and behaviour are often quite weak.

The theory of planned behaviour

The theory of reasoned action (Fishbein and Ajzen, 1975) suggests that people's beliefs relate to their social world, and that the expectations of others who are important to them will affect their behaviour. The theory of reasoned action therefore sees the individual within a social context and, in contrast to the traditional approach in which behaviour is seen as rational, includes a role for values. The theory of planned behaviour (see Figure 4.6) was developed by Ajzen (1988) and represented a progression from the theory of reasoned action.

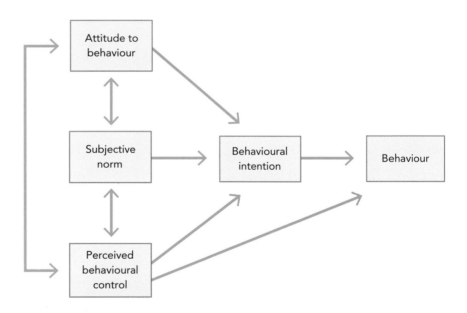

Figure 4.6 **The theory of planned behaviour**

This theory views intentions as 'plans of action in pursuit of behavioural goals'. These intentions are the result of the following beliefs:

- **Attitude** *towards a behaviour:* this is composed of a positive or a negative evaluation of a particular behaviour and the beliefs about the outcome of the behaviour, for example 'Dieting is boring but will improve my health'.

- *Subjective norm:* this includes the perception of social norms and pressures to perform a behaviour, and an evaluation of the individual's motivation to comply with this pressure, for example 'People who are important to me will approve if I stop smoking and I want their approval'.

- *Perceived behavioural control:* this reflects individuals' beliefs that they can carry out a particular behaviour. It is derived from internal control factors, for example skills, abilities and information, and external control factors, for example obstacles such as a lack of time, money or opportunity, both relating to past behaviour.

These three factors predict behavioural intentions, which are then linked to behaviour. The theory of planned behaviour also states that perceived behavioural control could have a direct effect on behaviour without the mediating effect of behavioural intentions.

> **?** How might the theory of planned behaviour be applied to someone who wanted to reduce their drinking?

The theory of planned behaviour would make the following predictions. If an individual believed that cutting down on drinking would make their life more productive and would be beneficial to their health (the attitude to the behaviour), and believed that the important people in their life wanted them to stop (subjective norm), as well as believing that they were capable of reducing or stopping drinking because of their past behaviour and an evaluation of internal and external control factors (high behavioural control), this would predict a high intention to stop drinking (behavioural intention). The model also predicts that perceived behavioural control could predict behaviour without the influence of intentions. For example, if someone believed that they could not stop drinking because they were dependent on alcohol, this would be a better predictor of their behaviour than would their intention to stop drinking.

The theory of planned behaviour has been used to predict behaviours such as condom use, blood donation, smoking, exercise during pregnancy, walking and suicidality (see Connor and Norman, 2005 for a review). Perceived behavioural control appears to be the most effective factor for predicting behaviour, although research consistently identifies the intention–behaviour gap, with many people's intentions to perform certain behaviours not actually turning into behaviour (Connor and Norman, 2005).

The stages of change model

The stages of change model (also known as the 'transtheoretical model of behaviour') was originally developed by Prochaska and DiClemente (1982). Unlike other models of beliefs and behaviours, this model does not try to explain what contributes to a decision to change but describes how the change might take place.

Prochaska and DiClemente's model of behaviour change is based on the following stages:

1. *Precontemplation:* not intending to make any changes

2. *Contemplation:* considering a change

3. *Preparation:* making small changes

4. *Action:* actively engaging in a new behaviour

5. *Maintenance:* sustaining the change over time.

The model is cyclic and bidirectional. In other words, an individual may move to the preparation stage and then back to the contemplation stage several times before progressing to the action stage. Furthermore, even when an individual has reached the maintenance stage, they may slip back to the contemplation stage over time. Many smokers, for example, contemplate stopping smoking, stop smoking for a while, start smoking again with no intention to stop and then start contemplating cessation again.

An individual may not have an awareness of contemplating, actioning and maintaining change but will at different stages focus on either the costs of a behaviour, for example 'Taking up exercise will mean that I have less time with my children', or the benefits of the behaviour, for example 'Exercise will make me feel fitter'.

The stages of change model has been applied to several health-related behaviours, such as smoking, alcohol use, exercise and screening behaviour (see Marshall and Biddle, 2001 for a comprehensive meta-analysis). In general, research indicates that the stages of change model has provided a useful framework for assessing patients for interventions and describing the process of change, but that it is less effective for predicting change and may not be any more useful than simply asking people: 'Do you want to stop smoking?'

> **thinking about** Imagine that you were trying to convince a friend to stop smoking. What beliefs do you think you would have to change in order to be successful? How would you go about doing this? Consider this, bearing in mind the models described above.

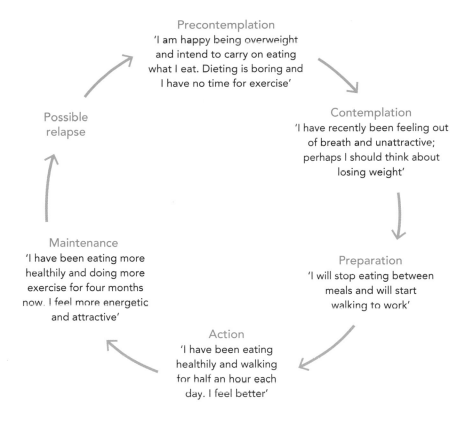

Figure 4.7 **Model of behaviour change**
Source: Prochaska and DiClemente, 1982

The self-regulatory model

The above models tend to be used to explore the predictors of health-related behaviours. In contrast, the self-regulatory model is commonly used to examine how individuals adjust to illness (Leventhal et al., 1985, 1997). In particular, the self-regulatory model suggests that illness and symptoms are dealt with by individuals in the same way as other problems (Figure 4.8). Thus, if an individual is usually healthy, any onset of illness will be interpreted as a problem, and the individual will be motivated to re-establish their state of health. To do this, an individual needs first to make sense of the problem and then to cope with it. The stages of the self-regulatory model are described below.

Stage 1: interpretation

An individual may be confronted with the problem of a potential illness through two channels: symptom perception and social messages.

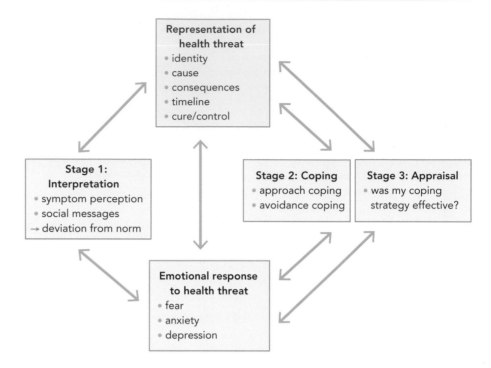

Figure 4.8 **Self-regulatory model of illness behaviour**

Symptom perception

Symptom perception ('I am feeling breathless') is not a straightforward process but is influenced by individual difference, mood and cognitions. Pennebaker (1982) argues that individuals vary in the amount of attention they pay to their internal state. In addition, being more internally focused does not necessarily mean being more accurate in terms of symptom perception. In a study evaluating the accuracy of detecting changes in heart rate, Pennebaker (1982) reported that individuals who were more focused on their internal state tended to overestimate any changes in their heart rate compared with subjects who were externally focused. Being internally focused has also been shown to relate to a perception of a slower recovery from illness. Being internally focused may result in an exaggerated perception of symptom change rather than a more accurate one.

Symptom perception is also influenced by mood. For example, studies show that higher stress levels are associated with a higher number of reported physical symptoms (Cropley and Steptoe, 2005), and that asthma patients with low mood report more symptoms and are more likely to attribute a wider range of symptoms to their asthma (Mora et al., 2007).

An individual's cognitive state may also influence their symptom perception. Ruble (1977) carried out a study in which she manipulated women's expectations of when they were due to start menstruating. She gave subjects an 'accurate physiological test' and told women either that their period was due shortly or that it was at least a week away. The women were then asked to report any premenstrual symptoms. The results showed that believing they were about to start menstruating (even though they were not) increased the number of reported premenstrual symptoms. This indicates an association between cognitive state and symptom perception.

The factors contributing to symptom perception can be illustrated by a condition known as 'medical students' disease', described by Mechanic (1962). A large component of the medical curriculum involves learning about the symptoms associated with a multitude of different illnesses. More than two-thirds of medical students incorrectly report that, at some time, they have had the symptoms they are being taught about. This phenomenon can perhaps be understood in terms of mood, cognition and social norms. Medical students, for example, become quite anxious as a result of their workload, which may heighten their awareness of any physiological changes, making them more internally focused. In addition, medical students are thinking about symptoms as part of their course, which may result in a focus on their own internal state. Furthermore, once one student starts to perceive symptoms, others may model themselves on this behaviour. Therefore, symptom perception influences how an individual interprets the problem of illness.

Social messages

Information about illness also comes from other people, in the form of a formal diagnosis from a health professional ('The doctor has diagnosed this breath-lessness as asthma'), or a positive test result from a routine health check. Such messages may or may not be a consequence of symptom perception. In addition, information about illness may come from individuals who are not health professionals. Before (and often after) consulting a health professional, people often access their social network – their 'lay referral system' (colleagues, friends and family) – and seek their information and advice. For example, someone with a sore throat may speak to another friend who had a similar condition or may take up a suggestion of a favoured home remedy. Such social messages will influence how the individual interprets the 'problem' of illness.

Individuals may receive information about the possibility of illness through either symptom perception or social messages. This information influences how an individual makes sense of the problem and the development of illness cognitions that will be constructed according to the dimensions of identity, cause, consequences, timeline and cure/control (see above). These cognitive representations of the 'problem' will give the problem meaning and enable the individual to develop and consider suitable coping strategies.

Stage 2: coping

People cope with illness in many different ways, but, broadly speaking, coping can be considered in terms of two main categories:

1. *Approach coping:* such as taking pills, going to the doctor, resting and talking to friends about emotions

2. *Avoidance coping:* which involves denial and wishful thinking.

Taylor (1983) examined how individuals adjust to threatening events including illness and rape. Taylor suggested that coping consists of:

- a search for meaning – 'Why did it happen to me?'

- a search for mastery – 'How can I prevent it happening again?'

- a process of self-enhancement – 'I am better off than a lot of people'.

Taylor argued that these three processes are central to developing and maintaining illusions that constitute a process of cognitive adaptation.

Stage 3: appraisal

Appraisal involves individuals evaluating the effectiveness of the coping strategy to determine whether to continue with this strategy or try an alternative one.

The model is self-regulatory because its three components (interpretation, coping and appraisal) interrelate in order to maintain the status quo, that is, they regulate the self. Thus, if the individual's normal state (health) is disrupted (by illness), the model proposes that the individual is motivated to return the balance to normality. This self-regulation involves the three processes interrelating in an ongoing and dynamic fashion.

> **thinking about** Some people are always seriously ill and frequently visit their GP – 'I have bronchitis', 'I have tonsillitis', 'I have a migraine'. Others have only mild complaints – 'I have a cough', 'I have a sore throat', 'I have a headache'. How might this relate to the way in which they make sense of their symptoms?

Developing interventions to change health-related behaviour

Health psychology theory provides a framework for understanding behaviour and beliefs and exploring how these factors may relate to illnesses. These theories draw on social cognition models, implementation intentions, and the self-regulatory model to inform interventions aiming to change behaviours and beliefs.

Using social cognition models

Social cognition models have been developed to describe and predict health behaviours such as smoking, screening, eating and exercise. In recent years, there has been a call towards using these models to inform and develop interventions to change behaviours. This has been based on two observations:

1. Many interventions designed to change behaviour were only minimally effective. For example, reviews of early interventions to change sexual behaviour concluded that these interventions had only small effects (Oakley et al., 1995) and dietary interventions for weight loss may result in weight loss in the short term but the majority show a return to baseline by follow-up (NHS Centre for Reviews and Dissemination, 1997).

2. Many interventions were not based on any theoretical framework nor were they drawing on research that had identified which factors were correlated with the particular behaviour.

Some researchers have therefore outlined how theory can be translated into interventions. In particular, Sutton (2002) describes a series of steps that can be followed to develop an intervention:

● identify target behaviour and target population

● identify the most salient beliefs about the target behaviour in the target population using open-ended questions

● conduct a study involving closed questions to determine which beliefs are the best predictors of behavioural intention. Choose the best predictor as the target belief

● analyse the data to determine the beliefs that best discriminate between intenders and non-intenders. These are further target beliefs

● develop an intervention to change these target beliefs.

Over recent years, an increasing number of behavioural interventions have drawn on a theory of behaviour change to change behaviours such as condom use, sun cream use and cervical cancer screening. For example, Quine et al. (2001) followed the steps outlined above to identify salient beliefs about safety helmet wearing for children. They then developed an intervention based on persuasion to change these salient beliefs. The results showed that after the intervention, the children showed more positive beliefs about safety helmet wearing than the control group and were more likely to wear a helmet at five months follow-up.

Using implementation intentions

Social cognition models emphasize the relationship between the intention to behave in a certain way and actual behaviour. Research indicates, however, that intentions do not always translate into behaviour. Gollwitzer's (1993)

notion of implementation intentions has been employed to strengthen this association. Gollwitzer regards carrying out an intention as involving the development of specific plans as to what an individual will do, given a specific set of environmental factors. Implementation intentions describe the 'what' and the 'when' of a particular behaviour. For example, the intention 'I intend to stop smoking' will be more likely to be translated into 'I have stopped smoking' if the individual makes the implementation intention 'I intend to stop smoking tomorrow at 12.00 when I have finished my last packet'. Some experimental research has shown that encouraging individuals to make implementation intentions can actually increase the correlation between intentions and behaviour for behaviours such as reducing dietary fat. Gollwitzer and Sheeran (2006) carried out a meta-analysis of 94 independent tests of the impact of implementation intentions on a range of behavioural goals, including eating a low-fat diet, using public transport, exercise and a range of personal goals. The results from this analysis indicated that implementation intentions had a medium to large effect on goal attainment. By tapping into variables such as implementation intentions, it is argued that the models may become better predictors of actual behaviour.

Using the self-regulatory model

Research indicates that patients' beliefs about their illness may relate to a range of health outcomes in terms of compliance or adherence to medication, attendance at rehabilitation, return to work and adjustment. Interventions have therefore been developed to change beliefs and promote more positive outcomes. For example, Petrie et al. (2002) aimed to change illness cognitions and examined the subsequent impact on a range of patient outcomes. The intervention consisted of three sessions of about 40 minutes with a psychologist and was designed to address and change patients' beliefs about their myocardial infarction (MI). Throughout the intervention, the information and discussion were targeted to the specific beliefs and concerns of the patient. The results showed that patients who had received the intervention reported more positive views about their MI at follow-up in terms of beliefs about consequences, timeline, control/cure and symptom distress. They were also better prepared to leave hospital, returned to work at a faster rate, and reported a lower rate of angina symptoms. Thus the intervention appeared to change cognitions and improve patients' functional outcome after MI. The study of beliefs and behaviour related to food and diet is illustrated in the following case study.

connections	Chapter 1 discusses the biological processes involved in weight gain.

case study the impact of beliefs on behaviour: the example of obesity and diet

The increase in adult and child obesity has been well documented. As a means to explain this increase, researchers have focused their attention on the role of the obesogenic environment and have highlighted the importance of factors such as the food industry, food advertising, food labelling, the availability of energy-dense foods, and an environment increasingly designed to encourage a sedentary lifestyle through the use of cars, computers and television. Central to this change is a shift in two key behaviours; eating behaviour and physical activity. We will focus on the links between obesity and diet and explore why people eat what they eat and how this relates to obesity onset and maintenance.

Research exploring how much and what obese people eat is problematic due to the difficulty in measuring diet without changing it. However, there is evidence that obese people eat relatively more fat than non-obese people, while the very process of weight gain indicates that they are eating more than their body requires (see Ogden, 2010).

Within psychological research, there are three main theories of eating behaviour that can help us understand why some people eat differently and more than others, and why some may become overweight and obese. These are the cognitive approach, the developmental model and the impact of dieting on eating behaviour.

A cognitive approach to diet

Most research using a cognitive approach has drawn on social cognition models to predict eating behaviour. For example, attitudes have been found to predict fat intake, table salt use, eating in fast-food restaurants, consuming low-fat milk and healthy eating, conceptualized as high levels of fibre, fruit and vegetables and low levels of fat (Povey et al., 2000). A cognitive approach to eating behaviour emphasizes the role of cognitions and explores how these cognitions predict what we eat. From this perspective, we eat food because we have positive thoughts about it. The obese may overeat because they have more positive thoughts about foods that are then translated into behaviour.

A developmental approach

In contrast, a developmental approach to eating behaviour emphasizes the importance of learning in terms of operant and classical conditioning and focuses on the development of food preferences in childhood. Social learning describes the impact of observing other people's behaviour on one's own behaviour and is sometimes referred to as 'modelling' or 'observational learning'. In one study, peer modelling was used to change children's preference for vegetables (Birch, 1980). For four consecutive days, the target children were placed at lunch next to other children who preferred a different vegetable to themselves (peas versus carrots). By the end of the study, the children showed a shift in their vegetable preference that persisted at a follow-up assessment several weeks later. The impact of social learning has also been shown in an intervention study designed to change children's eating behaviour using video-based peer modelling (Lowe et al., 1998). Food preferences therefore change through watching others eat. In terms of obesity, some people may overeat or eat more unhealthily because they have watched others close to them doing so.

Parental attitudes to food and eating behaviours are also central to the process of social learning. Olivera et al. (1992) reported a correlation between mother's and children's food intakes for most nutrients in preschool children. Contento et al. (1993) found a relationship between mothers' health motivations and the quality of children's diets, while Brown and Ogden (2004) reported consistent correlations between parents and their children in terms of reported snack food intake and eating motivations. Obesity clearly runs in families. This may reflect the transmission of eating-related attitudes and behaviours from parent to child.

Associative learning refers to the impact of contingent factors on behaviour. Some research has examined the effect of rewarding eating behaviour as in 'if you eat your vegetables, I will be pleased with you'. Birch et al. (1982) showed that if food was given to children in association with positive adult attention, the preference for the food increased. Rewarding eating behaviour seems to improve food preferences. Other research has explored the impact of using food as a reward. For these studies, gaining access to the food is contingent on another behaviour, as in 'if you are well behaved, you can have a biscuit'. Birch et al. (1982) presented children with foods either as a reward, as a snack or in a non-social situation (the control). The results showed that food acceptance increased if the foods were presented as a reward but that the more neutral conditions had no effect. This suggests that using food as a reward increases the preference for that food.

The relationship between food and rewards, however, appears to be more complicated than this. In an early study, Lepper et al. (1982) told children stories about children eating imaginary foods called 'hupe' and 'hule', in which the child in the story could only eat one if they had finished the other. This is analogous to saying 'if you eat your vegetables, you can eat your pudding'. Although parents use this approach to encourage their children to eat vegetables, the evidence indicates that this may be increasing their children's preference for pudding even further as pairing two foods results in the 'reward' food being seen as more positive than the 'access' food. In terms of obesity, people may overeat and become obese because they have learned that higher fat, unhealthier foods are more rewarding than others and/or because their parents used unhealthier foods as rewards for eating the healthier foods.

The role of dieting

The final theoretical perspective that may illuminate why some people become obese is the focus on dieting and restraint theory (see Ogden, 2010). Dieting is the conscious attempt to cognitively control food intake. Many people who are already obese diet as a means to lose weight. Dieting, however, may not only be a consequence of obesity but also a cause, as there is evidence that dieting is often characterized by periods of overeating, precipitated by factors such as lowered mood and eating a high-calorie food. From this perspective, it has been argued that attempting to eat less paradoxically causes overeating, as the process of denial and self-control makes food more attractive and creates a situation whereby the individual becomes increasingly preoccupied with eating. There is also some evidence that overeating is reflected in weight gain, particularly in women. For example, French et al. (1994) reported the results from a cross-sectional and longitudinal study of 1,639 men and 1,913 women who were involved in a worksite intervention study for smoking cessation and weight control. The cross-sectional analysis showed that a history of dieting, current dieting and previous involvement in a formal weight-loss programme were related to a higher body weight in men and women. Similarly, the prospective analysis showed that baseline measures of involvement in a formal weight-loss programme and dieting predicted increases in body weight at follow-up. However, this was for women only. In particular, women who were dieting or who had been involved in a formal weight-loss programme at baseline gained nearly 1 kg more than those who had not. Klesges et al. (1992) reported similar results in their study of 141 men and 146 women who were followed up after one year. This showed that the dieting men and women were heavier than their non-dieting counterparts at baseline. Higher baseline weight and higher restraint scores at baseline also predicted greater weight gain at follow-up in women. If dieters perceive themselves to be overweight, but are not necessarily obese, and if dieting causes overeating and subsequent weight gain, then dieting could predictably play a causal role in the development of obesity. It is possible that dieting also results in the relative overconsumption of high-fat foods as these are the foods that dieters try to avoid.

Obesity is on the increase in adults and children and research suggests a clear role for changes in behaviour, particularly diet. Psychological theories focusing on cognitions, learning and the role of dieting suggest that overeating may be a result of their beliefs about food, how and what they have seen others eat, how food was presented to them in their childhood, and their subsequent attempts to diet and reduce their food intake.

Summary

- Health psychologists are interested in how people think about their health and their health-related attitudes and beliefs
- Health psychologists have developed various models to explain the relationship between attitudes, beliefs and behaviours, as well as to predict the decisions people make
- The study of individual beliefs provides an insight into people's health-related behaviour and how unhealthy behaviours can be changed
- Health psychologists study how people make sense of illness and how these beliefs may contribute to the onset, progression and possible treatment of illness
- Understanding the role of psychological factors may help people to adopt preventive health beliefs and behaviours and reduce the impact of being ill

Questions for further discussion

1. Why do people continue to behave in unhealthy ways? Discuss with reference to smoking, diet, exercise or alcohol.
2. There is no such thing as a physical illness: all illnesses have a psychological component. Discuss.
3. Why is patient compliance or adherence to medical treatment regimes so low? How might it be increased?

Further reading

Connor, M. and Norman, P. (eds) (2005) *Predicting Health Behaviours* (2nd edn). Buckingham: Open University Press.
Thorough description of social cognition models and the extent to which they predict health-related behaviour.

Ogden, J (2010) *The Psychology of Eating: From Healthy to Disordered Behaviour* (2nd edn). Oxford: Wiley-Blackwell.
Detailed account of the relevant literature, if you are particularly interested in eating behaviour, eating disorders or obesity.

Ogden, J. (2012) *Health Psychology: A Textbook* (5th edn). Buckingham: Open University Press.
Comprehensive overview of health psychology covering a range of health psychology areas of research and theory. The current chapter was based on this book.

References

Abraham, C. and Sheeran, P. (2005) The health belief model, in M. Conner and P. Norman (eds) *Predicting Health Behaviour: Research and Practice with Social Cognition Models* (2nd edn). Buckingham: Open University Press, pp. 28–81.

Ajzen, I. (1988) *Attitudes, Personality and Behaviour*. Chicago: Dorsey Press.

Bain, D.J. (1977) 'Patient knowledge and the content of the consultation in general practice'. *Medical Education* 11: 347–50.

Bandura, A. (1977) 'Self efficacy: toward a unifying theory of behavior change'. *Psychological Review* 84: 191–215.

Becker, M.H. and Rosenstock, I.M. (1987) Comparing social learning theory and the health belief model, in W.B. Ward (ed.) *Advances in Health Education and Promotion*. Greenwich, CT: JAI Press, pp. 245–9.

Beecher, H.K. (1956) 'Relationship of significance of wound to the pain experienced'. *Journal of the American Medical Association* 161: 1609–13.

Birch, L.L. (1980) 'Effects of peer models' food choices and eating behaviors on preschoolers' food preferences'. *Child Development* 51: 489–96.

Birch, L.L., Birch, D., Marlin, D. and Kramer, L. (1982) 'Effects of instrumental eating on children's food preferences'. *Appetite*, 3: 125–34.

Boyle, C.M. (1970) 'Differences between patients' and doctors' interpretations of common medical terms'. *British Medical Journal* 2: 286–9.

Bradley, C., Gamsu, D.S., Moses, J.L. et al. (1987) 'The use of diabetes-specific perceived control and health belief measures to predict treatment choice and efficacy in a feasibility study of continuous subcutaneous insulin infusion pumps'. *Psychology and Health* 1: 133–46.

Brown, R. and Ogden, J. (2004) 'Children's eating attitudes and behaviour: a study of the modelling and control theories of parental influence'. *Health Education and Research* 19(3): 261–71.

Connor, M. and Norman, P. (eds) (2005) *Predicting Health Behaviours* (2nd edn). Buckingham: Open University Press.

Contento, I.R., Basch, C., Shea, S. et al. (1993) 'Relationship of mothers' food choice criteria to food intake of pre-school children: identification of family subgroups'. *Health Education Quarterly* 20: 243–59.

Crichton, E.F., Smith, D.L. and Demanuele, F. (1978) 'Patients' recall of medication information'. *Drug Intelligence and Clinical Pharmacy* 12: 591–9.

Crombez, G., Eccleston, C., Baeyens, F. et al. (1999) 'Attention to chronic pain is dependent upon pain-related fear'. *Journal of Psychosomatic Research* 47(5): 403–10.

Cropley, M. and Steptoe, A. (2005) 'Social support, life events and physical symptoms: A prospective study of chronic and recent life stress in men and women'. *Psychology, Health & Medicine* 10(4): 317–25.

Doll, R. and Peto, R. (1981) *The Causes of Cancer*. New York: Oxford University Press.

Eccleston, C. (1994) 'Chronic pain and attention: a cognitive approach'. *British Journal of Clinical Psychology* 33(4): 535–47.

Eccleston, C. and Crombez, G. (1999) 'Pain demands attention: a cognitive-affective model of the interruptive function of pain'. *Psychological Bulletin* 125(3): 356–66.

Eccleston, C., Crombez, G., Aldrich, A. and Stannard, C. (2001) 'Worry and chronic pain patients: a description and analysis of individual differences'. *European Journal of Pain* 5: 309–18.

Engel, G.I. (1977) 'The need for a new medical model: a challenge for biomedicine'. *Science* 196: 129–35.

Engel, G.L. (1980) 'The clinical application of the biopsychosocial model'. *American Journal of Psychiatry* 137: 535–44.

Fishbein, M. and Ajzen, I. (1975) *Belief, Attitude, Intentional Behaviour: An Introduction to Theory and Research*. Reading, MA: Addison-Wesley.

Fordyce, W.E. and Steger, J.C. (1979) Chronic pain, in O.F. Pomerleau and J.P. Brady (eds) *Behavioural Medicine: Theory and Practice*. Baltimore: Williams & Wilkins, pp. 125–53.

French, S.A., Jeffery, R.W., Forster, J.L. et al. (1994) 'Predictors of weight change over two years among a population of working adults: the healthy worker project'. *International Journal of Obesity* 18: 145–54.

Gillibrand, R. and Stevenson, J. (2006) 'The extended health belief model applied to the experience of diabetes in young people'. *British Journal of Health Psychology* 11: 155–69.

Gollwitzer, P.M. (1993) Goal achievement: the role of intentions, in W. Stroebe and M. Hewstone (eds) *European Review of Social Psychology* 4: 141–85.

Gollwitzer, P.M. and Sheeran, P. (2006) 'Implementation intentions and goal achievement: A meta-analysis of effects and processes'. *Advances in Experimental Social Psychology* 38: 69–119.

Haynes, R.B., Sackett, D.L. and Taylor, D.W. (eds) (1979) *Compliance in Health Care*. Baltimore: Johns Hopkins University Press.

Heider, F. (1958) *The Psychology of Interpersonal Relations*. New York: John Wiley & Sons.

Karasek, R. and Theorell, T. (1990) *Healthy Work. Stress, Productivity and the Reconstruction of Working Life*. New York: Basic Books.

Keefe, F.J., Lefebvre, J.C., Egert, J.R. et al. (2000) 'The relationship of gender to pain, pain behaviour and disability in osteoarthritis patients: the role of catastrophizing'. *Pain* 87: 325–34.

Khaw, K.T., Wareham, N., Bingham, S. et al. (2008) Combined impact of health behaviours and mortality in men and women: the EPIC-Norfolk prospective population study'. *PLoS Medicine* 5(1): e12.

Klesges, R.C., Isbell, T.R. and Klesges, L.M. (1992) 'Relationship between dietary restraint, energy intake, physical activity, and body weight: a prospective analysis'. *Journal of Abnormal Psychology* 101: 668–74.

Krantz, D.S., Glass, D.C., Contrada, R. and Miller, N.E. (1981) *Behavior and Health: National Science Foundations Second Five Year Outlook on Science and Technology*. Washington, DC: US Government Printing Office.

Lau, R.R. (1995) Cognitive representations of health and illness, in D. Gochman (ed.) *Handbook of Health Behaviour Research*, vol. I. New York: Plenum Press, pp. 51–71.

Lazarus, R.S. and Folkman, S. (1987) 'Transactional theory and research on emotions and coping'. *European Journal of Personality* 1: 141–70.

Lazarus, R.S. and Launier, R. (1978) Stress related transactions between person and environment, in L.A. Pervin and M. Lewis (eds) *Perspectives in International Psychology*. New York: Plenum Press, pp. 287–327.

Lepper, M., Sagotsky, G., Dafoe, J.L. and Greene, D. (1982) 'Consequences of superfluous social constraints: effects on young children's social inferences and subsequent intrinsic interest'. *Journal of Personality and Social Psychology* 42: 51–65.

Leventhal, H., Meyer, D. and Nerenz, D. (1980) 'The common sense representation of illness danger', in S. Rachman (ed.) *Contributions to Medical Psychology* 2. Oxford: Pergamon Press, pp. 7–30.

Leventhal, H., Prohaska, T.R. and Hirschman, R.S. (1985) Preventive health behaviour across the life span, in J.C. Rosen and L.J. Solomon (eds) *Prevention in Health Psychology*. Hanover, NH: University Press of New England, pp. 191–235.

Leventhal, H., Benyamini, Y., Brownlee, S. et al. (1997) Illness representations: theoretical foundations, in K.J. Petrie and J.A. Weinman (eds) *Perceptions of Health and Illness: Current Research and Applications*. Amsterdam: Harwood Academic, pp. 19–45.

Ley, P. (1988) *Communicating with Patients*. London: Croom Helm.

Lowe, C.F., Dowey, A. and Horne, P. (1998) Changing what children eat, in A. Murcott (ed.) *The Nation's Diet: The Social Science of Food Choice*. Harlow: Addison Wesley Longman, pp. 57–80.

Maddi, S. and Kobasa, S.G. (1984) *The Hardy Executive: Health Under Stress*. Homewood, IL: Dow Jones-Irwin.

Marteau, T.M. and Johnston, M. (1990) 'Health professionals: a source of variance in health outcomes'. *Psychology and Health* 5: 47–58.

Marshall, S.J. and Biddle, S.J.H. (2001) 'The transtheortical model of behaviour change: a meta analysis of applications to physical activity and exercise'. *Annals of Behavioural Medicine* 23: 229–46.

Mechanic, D. (1962) *Students under Stress: A Study in the Social Psychology of Adaptation*. Glencoe, IL: Free Press.

Melzack, R. and Wall, P.D. (1965) 'Pain mechanisms: a new theory'. *Science* 150: 971–9.

Mokdad, A.H., Marks, J.S., Stroup, D.F. and Gerberding, J.L. (2004) 'Actual causes of death in the United States, 200'. *Journal of the American Medical Association* 10(29): 1238–45.

Mora, P.A., Halm, E., Leventhal, H. and Ceric, F. (2007) 'Elucidating the relationship between negative affectivity and symptoms: the role of illness specific affective responses'. *Annals of Behavioural Medicine* 34: 77–86.

NHS Centre for Reviews and Dissemination (1997) *Systematic Review of Interventions in the Treatment and Prevention of Obesity*. York: University of York.

Norman, P., Searle, A., Harrad, R. and Vedhara, K. (2003) 'Predicting adherence to eye patching in children with amblyopia: an application of protection motivation theory'. *British Journal of Health Psychology* 8: 67–82.

Oakley, A., Fullerton, D., Holland, J. et al. (1995) 'Sexual health education interventions for young people: a methodological review'. *British Medical Journal* 310: 158–62.

Ogden, J. (2010) *The Psychology of Eating: From Healthy to Disordered Behaviour* (2nd edn). Oxford: Blackwell.

Olivera, S.A., Ellison, R.C., Moore, L.L. et al. (1992) 'Parent-child relationships in nutrient intake: the Framingham Children's Study'. *American Journal of Clinical Nutrition* 56: 593–8.

Pennebaker, J. (1982) *The Psychology of Physical Symptoms*. New York: Springer Verlag.

Petrie, K.J.,Cameron, L.D., Ellis, C.J. et al. (2002) 'Changing illness perceptions after myocardial infraction: an early intervention randomized controlled trial'. *Psychosomatic Medicine* 64: 580–6.

Plotnikoff, R.C., Lippke, S., Trinh, L. et al. (2010) 'Protection motivation theory and the prediction of physical activity among adults with type 1 or type 2 diabetes in a large population sample'. *British Journal of Health Psychology* 15(3): 643–61.

Povey, R., Conner, M., Sparks, P. et al. (2000) 'The theory of planned behaviour and healthy eating: examining additive and moderating effects of social influence variables'. *Psychology and Health* 14: 991–1006.

Prochaska, J.O. and DiClemente, C.C.D. (1982) 'Transtheorctical therapy: toward a more integrative model of change'. *Psychotherapy: Theory Research and Practice* 19: 276–88.

Quine, L., Rutter, D.R. and Arnold, L. (2001) 'Persuading school-age cyclist to use safety helmets: effectiveness of an intervention based on the theory of planned behaviour'. *British Journal of Health Psychology* 6: 327–45.

Rogers, R.W. (1983) Cognitive and physiological processes in fear appeals and attitude change: a revised theory of protection motivation, in J. Cacioppo and R. Petty (eds) *Social Psychophysiology*. New York: Guilford Press, pp. 153–77.

Roth, H.P. (1979) Problems in conducting a study of the effects of patient compliance of teaching the rationale for antacid therapy, in S.J. Cohen (ed.) *New Directions in Patient Compliance*. Lexington, MA: Lexington Books, pp. 111–26.

Ruble, D.N. (1977) 'Premenstrual symptoms: a reinterpretation'. *Science* 197: 291–2.

Sullivan, M.J., Thorn, B., Haythornthwaite, J.A. et al. (2001) 'Theoretical perspectives on the relation between catastrophizing and pain'. *Clinical Journal of Pain* 17(1): 52–64.

Sutton, S. (2002) Using social cognition models to develop health behaviour interventions: problems and assumptions, in D. Rutter and L. Quine (eds) *Changing Health Behaviour: Intervention and Research with Social Cognition Models*. Buckingham: Open University Press, pp. 193–208.

Taylor, S.E. (1983) 'Adjustment to threatening events: a theory of cognitive adaptation'. *American Psychologist* 38: 1161–73.

Trostle, J.A. (1988) 'Medical compliance as an ideology'. *Social Science and Medicine* 27: 1299–308.

Turk, D.C. and Rennert, K. (1981) Pain and the terminally ill cancer patient: a cognitive social learning perspective, in H. Sobel (ed.) *Behaviour Therapy in Terminal Care*. Cambridge, MA: Ballinger, pp. 95–124.

Turk, D.C., Wack, J.T. and Kerns, R.D. (1985) 'An empirical examination of the 'pain-behaviour' construct'. *Journal of Behavioral Medicine* 8: 119–30.

Vlaeyen, J.W. and Linton, S.J. (2000) Fear-avoidance and its consequences in chronic musculoskeletal pain: a state of the art. *Pain* 85(3): 317–32.

Wallston, K.A. and Wallston, B.S. (1982) Who is responsible for your health? The construct of health locus of control, in G.S. Sanders and J. Suls (eds) *Social Psychology of Health and Illness*. Hillsdale, NJ: Laurence Erlbaum, pp. 65–95.

Weinman, J., Petrie, K.J., Moss-Morris, R. and Horne, R. (1996) 'The illness perception questionnaire: a new method for assessing the cognitive representation of illness'. *Psychology and Health* 11: 431–46.

Weinstein, N. (1984) 'Why it won't happen to me: perceptions of risk factors and susceptibility'. *Health Psychology* 3: 431–57.

Weinstein, N. (1987) 'Unrealistic optimism about illness susceptibility: conclusions from a community-wide sample'. *Journal of Behavioural Medicine* 10: 481–500.

Weller, S.S. (1984) 'Cross cultural concepts of illness: variables and validation'. *American Anthropologist* 86: 341–51.

MAT JONES and NORMA DAYKIN

Sociology and health

chapter

5

Overview 156

Introduction 156

Part 1 The contribution of sociology to health studies 157
Socioeconomic inequalities in health 159
Explaining health inequalities 161
Gender and health 165
Explaining gender inequalities in health 167
'Race', ethnicity and health 169

Part 2 Theoretical and research approaches 172
The sociology of lay–professional relationships: functionalist approaches 173
Medicalization and social control 175
Marxist and political economy perspectives 176
Health professions and interprofessional relationships 178
Interactionist perspectives and the experience of illness 179
Sociology of the body 180
Social constructionist perspectives and beyond 181

Case study The social determinants and social construction
of diet 183
Summary 187
Questions for further discussion 187
Further reading 187
References 188

Learning outcomes

This chapter will enable readers to:

- Identify the key characteristics of sociology as a discipline
- Understand key sociological concepts and debate their relevance to health and healthcare
- Understand research evidence exploring the social patterning of health and disease
- Debate various theoretical explanations for the social patterning of health and disease
- Understand theories and concepts relating to the social impact of healthcare and the social roles of the healthcare professions

Overview

When we become ill, it sometimes seems that bad luck has singled us out for special attention, yet an extensive body of evidence suggests that health and disease are patterned in complex ways that defy notions of luck or chance, indicating a more systematic process of disease causation. In Part 1, the social patterning of health and illness is explored. Evidence linking social divisions, such as class, gender and ethnicity, with experiences of health and healthcare is examined. Finding adequate explanations for the persistence of social inequalities, as well as strategies to eliminate or reduce them, is an important goal of health policy, and one to which sociology can make a distinctive contribution. Part 2 explores the methodological approaches of sociology to understanding the ways in which people interpret and manage ill health in their lives. The attempts of health professionals to manage and cure ill health have come under sociological scrutiny. In particular, sociologists have looked beyond the altruism often assumed of health professionals to examine the individual, group and social impact of professional practice. Sociology relies on evidence and theory. In addition to a critical examination of the available sources of evidence, such as mortality rates, sociology involves the development and testing of theoretical frameworks and perspectives that seek to explain broad patterns of health and illness.

Introduction

In contrast to disciplines such as biology and psychology, which focus on health at the individual level, sociology examines the social dimensions of health, illness and healthcare. Sociology is a broad discipline including diverse approaches and perspectives. Some of the key questions addressed by sociologists researching health and illness include:

- What accounts for socioeconomic inequalities in health and illness?

- How do social structures, institutions and processes affect the health of individuals?

- What are the characteristics of healthcare work?

- What is the nature of professional–client relationships?

- How do ordinary people make sense of health and illness?

- What impact do healthcare services have on individuals and society?

The ideas and practices surrounding Western scientific medicine have been a central concern within sociology. These ideas are often taken for granted as the basis on which much healthcare provision is organized. However, they only emerged alongside the economic and cultural changes brought about by the spread of industrial capitalism during the eighteenth and nineteenth centuries (Stacey, 1988). This period was characterized by urbanization and a changing class structure. The growth of the middle classes provided new markets for healthcare, which supported the newly established profession of medicine.

These events were underlined by a widespread support for the ideas as well as the practices of medicine. However, support for scientific medicine reached a peak in the postwar period and medicine's dominance in healthcare has since been challenged. Scientific medicine is seen as limited, in that it draws on the belief that mind and body are separate entities. This notion of 'Cartesian dualism', named after the philosopher Descartes, is seen as problematic for at least two reasons:

1. It leads to a rather mechanistic approach in which illness and disease are treated as mechanical malfunctions

2. It leads to a reductionist approach, that is, it reduces diseases to a single, usually physical, cause.

This form of scientific medicine is challenged by complex, chronic conditions that affect an increasing number of people. For example, there is no real agreement on the existence of physical causes for conditions such as repetitive strain injury and myalgic encephalomyelitis (ME). Scientific medicine has, however, always coexisted with a number of rival or alternative approaches. In recent years, the support for such alternatives seems to have grown, with an increasing number of people seeking help from complementary therapists as well as, or instead of, medical professionals.

Part 1 The contribution of sociology to health studies

example 5.1

Application of sociology to contemporary health issues

- Large-scale social upheavals often follow sudden changes in the global economy. For example, the 2008 collapse of international financial markets led to a rapid increase in rates of unemployment and poverty. Drawing on theories such as political economy, social capital and social solidarity, sociologists seek to explain how such changes impact on patterns of mental and physical health
- The care provided by healthcare professionals, for example nurses in hospital settings, is often under the public and political spotlight following reports of negligence or malpractice. In this context, a sociological approach might seek to explore how professionals manage their own everyday routines and behaviours. 'Self-surveillance' may have a greater bearing on practice than overt forms of control or sanction, and have implications for everyday interactions with patients
- Recent evidence in many Western countries suggests that rates of illegal drug use are falling among younger age groups.

This appears to be a reversal of a general upward trend since the 1970s. Sociologists are interested to explain the social processes at work that might account for this phenomenon. An intriguing parallel to this decline has been the rise of the internet and, in particular, social media. We might speculate that the use of social media is leading to changes in young people's health-related behaviour

- Rates of tuberculosis (TB) are increasing in high-income countries, having declined steadily throughout the twentieth century. Some commentators have suggested that this rise is partly due to migrants from low-income countries – particularly sub-Saharan Africa and the Indian subcontinent – who are more likely to carry the TB infection. Sociologists are interested not only in investigating the claims for this

link, but also in examining the implications for defining migrants as a 'risk group', including the potential for fuelling racial discrimination in healthcare

- Post-traumatic stress disorder (PTSD) has been used as a diagnostic category for people who are severely affected by major life events such as threat of injury, sexual assault or threat of death. Symptoms include chronic anxiety, distressing flashbacks and blocked memories. PTSD is increasingly applied to victims of recent military conflicts and natural disasters. Sociologists are interested in evidence of the societal risks that might lead to PTSD, but also examine how ideas of PTSD have become commonplace and the wider implications of this label for how we perceive and respond to risk more generally

Sociologists have sought to understand these diverse perspectives on health. They have examined the conditions of healthcare provision and the social relationships between healthcare providers and recipients. Healthcare institutions and their social context have been an important focus of study for sociologists. Social factors such as **gender**, for example, seem to exert a powerful influence on the makeup of the various health professions, particularly nursing and medicine.

Sociology provides a number of well-established approaches to questions such as those about the social patterning of health and disease and the social impact of healthcare interventions. While sociology overlaps with other disciplines such as epidemiology, psychology and social policy, sociology is also a distinct discipline with its own theoretical and methodological frameworks. For example, while sociologists draw on epidemiological data to analyse patterns of health and illness, they are concerned to understand the social processes affecting illness and healthcare rather than mapping the aggregate population risk. Similarly, while sociologists increasingly share with psychologists a concern with subjective experiences of ill health, they emphasize social and cultural rather than individual aspects of these.

Sociological writings are infused with key concepts such as social class, social context, social structure and social process. There is no single shared understanding among sociologists about the definitions of these concepts, although notions of power are central to many sociological accounts of health and illness. Recently, in response to wider socioeconomic and cultural changes, new debates and perspectives have emerged. Changing experiences of work, the impact of globalization on economic and cultural life, and changing ideas about gender roles and emerging patterns of family life have all influenced sociological writings. The debate is reflected in increasing concerns with, for example, identity, consumption, the body and the emotions. Sociologists have also debated whether these changes reflect an intensified late modern society or herald a new postmodern condition. At the same time, central themes such as social divisions of **class**, gender and **ethnicity** remain central to the sociology of health and illness.

Socioeconomic inequalities in health

A key area that sociology has investigated in relation to health is that of **social inequalities** and their impact on health. During the last century, life expectancy in relatively affluent countries such as the UK, the US and Europe has risen steadily, yet there remains a strong inverse relationship between mortality and morbidity rates and socioeconomic status (Townsend and Davidson, 1982; Adler et al., 1994; Roberts and Power, 1996; Drever and Bunting, 1997; Acheson, 1998; Kunst et al., 1998; van Rossum et al. 2000; Lantz et al., 2001; Marmot et al., 2010; Mackenbach, 2012). Such inequalities in health exist not only within high-income countries but are a recurrent feature between social groups in all national settings (WHO, 2008).

See Chapter 3 for more details about data collection and the interpretation of epidemiological data.   **connections**

In the UK, the Report of the Working Group on Inequalities in Health, known as the Black Report (Townsend and Davidson, 1982), examined standardized mortality ratios for different social classes in order to assess the scale of inequality and monitor changes over time. The working group used occupational class as a measure of inequality, adopting the Registrar General's classification of social class 1 (professional occupations) to social class V (unskilled manual occupations). The well-known findings of the Black Report include a marked and persistent difference in mortality rates between the occupational classes, for both sexes and at all ages. A steep class gradient, showing that the risk of death increases with lower social class, was observed for most causes of death. The pattern for respiratory diseases was particularly strong. Babies born to parents in social class V were found to be at double the risk of death in the first month of life compared with the babies of professional class parents.

The authors concluded that the introduction of the NHS, which aimed to provide free healthcare to all regardless of income or social status, had not eliminated health inequalities. Furthermore, patterns of relative inequality seemed to have changed little over time despite an overall improvement in life expectancy. In relation to infant mortality, social class differences had actually increased during key periods. Mortality alone was acknowledged as a crude indicator of population health. Evidence from sources such as the General

Household Survey was presented to show that patterns of morbidity followed a similar class gradient to that of mortality, with people in lower socioeconomic groups reporting higher levels of ill health than those in higher socioeconomic groups. Finally, inequalities were also found to exist in the utilization of health services, with working-class people making less use of services and receiving less good care than their middle-class counterparts.

The original report (1980) received a rather frosty reception by the then Conservative government, which seemed reluctant to embrace the notion of health inequality. More recently, the changing public health agenda has encouraged a renewed focus on socioeconomic influences on health. This has been underlined by a concern with widening income inequalities and the growing problems of poverty and homelessness. Subsequent independent inquiries, notably the Acheson Report (1998) and the Marmot Review (Marmot et al., 2010), found that inequalities in health have not only persisted but have, in some cases, become greater. Other factors, such as ethnicity and housing status, were also found to be associated with increased risk of mortality and morbidity. Socioeconomic status is also linked to health-related behaviours such as cigarette smoking and dietary habits. For example, the Acheson Report found that the percentage of smokers among men in the unskilled manual classes was more than two and a half times that seen in the professional classes.

Table 5.1 shows trends in life expectancy at birth in England and Wales for the years 1982–86, 1992–96 and 2002–06 from the Office of National Statistics' Longitudinal Survey. During the period 1982–2006, socioeconomic inequalities in male and female life expectancy increased despite improvements over time

Table 5.1 **Life expectancy at birth by gender and NS-SEC class, 1982–86, 1992–96 and 2002–06**

Analytic classes	1982–86		1992–96		2002–06	
	Males	Females	Males	Females	Males	Females
1. Higher managerial and professional	75.6	80.9	77.5	82.3	80.4	83.9
2. Lower managerial and professional	74.3	79.7	76.5	81.2	79.6	83.4
3. Intermediate	73.3	79.6	75.3	81.4	78.5	82.7
4. Small employers and own a/c workers	73.6	79.1	75.6	80.7	77.8	82.6
5. Lower supervisory and technical	72.3	78.5	73.8	79.4	76.8	80.4
6. Semi-routine	71.3	78.1	72.4	79.2	75.1	80.6
7. Routine	70.7	77.1	71.6	78.3	74.6	79.7
All	71.7	77.4	73.8	79.2	77.0	81.1
Range highest-lowest	4.9	3.8	5.9	4.0	5.8	4.2

Source: ONS, 2011a

for all classes. Put another way, the greatest growth in life expectancy was experienced by those classified in the highest two classes, and the least growth in life expectancy was experienced by those in the two least advantaged classes. In 2000, the system of classification changed from the previous Registrar General's classification based on occupation to the National Statistics Socio-economic Classification (NS-SEC). NS-SEC has been constructed to measure the employment relations and conditions of occupations in modern societies. In the period 2002–06, a boy born into the 'higher managerial and professional' class, such as directors of major organizations, doctors and lawyers, could expect to live almost six years longer than a boy born to parents classified as having 'routine' occupations such as labourers and cleaners.

The additional years gained from increased life expectancy are not always lived in good health. Data from the 2011 General Lifestyle Survey (ONS, 2013a) included the following:

- 32% of adults aged 16 and over in private households in Great Britain reported having a limiting long-standing illness (LLSI) or disability

- The proportions reporting an LLSI increased with age: 12% (aged 16–44), 25% (aged 45–64), 36% (aged 65–74) and 47% (aged 75 and over)

- The lowest rate of LLSI is found among those working in managerial and professional occupations (13% of males and 15% of females), compared with 23% of males and 26% of females for those working in routine and manual occupations

- People who had never worked or were long-term unemployed had the highest rate of LLSI (38%) of any socioeconomic group.

Explaining health inequalities

Sociologists are not interested simply in mapping patterns of health inequality: they also seek to provide explanations for these patterns. These explanations have important implications for the planning and delivery of health and social services.

> **?** What accounts for the socioeconomic patterns of health and disease?

A range of different explanations was debated in the Black Report and subsequent publications. The debate centred on four types of explanation for inequalities in health: artefact, social selection, cultural, and material/structural.

The artefact explanation

Following the publication of the Black Report (Townsend and Davidson, 1982), there was a debate on the nature, definition and measurement of social class. For some, the apparent widening of health inequalities was a product of the methods of measurement used (Illsley, 1986). This approach questions the validity of comparing death rates between social class groupings whose size and composition are changing over time. Economic developments and changes in employment have led to the diminishing size of social class V, which contains traditional unskilled groups such as manual workers.

In order to overcome the difficulties suggested by the artefact explanation, several studies have adopted alternative methodologies and drawn on different data sets to examine the evidence (Bartley et al., 1998; Shaw et al., 2000). Researchers have increasingly made use of longitudinal data to explore the relationships between deprivation and health over the life course (Bartley, 2004). The evidence suggests that there is a persistent inverse relationship between health and socioeconomic status regardless of how socioeconomic status is measured.

> **thinking about** Do you think people's health affects their employment? If so, in what ways?

The social selection explanation

The social selection explanation suggests that the poorer health status of those in the lower social classes reflects a tendency towards downward mobility of people with ill health rather than an outcome of class inequality The healthiest members of each socioeconomic group may be absorbed into higher groups, leaving those with the greatest number of health problems behind.

Longitudinal research, which follows people over a long period in order to identify which emerges first, ill health or downward social mobility, is needed to test this theory. Such research suggests a complex relationship between health and social mobility (Bartley et al., 1998; Bartley, 2004). Poor health can often serve to disadvantage people in employment and other areas. However, the selection explanation cannot account for the whole pattern of health inequality, and selection processes themselves may apply differently to different groups. People in more advantageous social positions, with more resources and support, seem to be better able to overcome the effects of early health problems than those in disadvantaged circumstances.

Cultural explanations

Cultural explanations suggest that the social distribution of ill health is linked to differences in health behaviours, such as smoking and alcohol consumption, and different groups' attitudes to their health. These behaviours are complex and situated in particular circumstances. For example, cigarette smoking may be a response to specific needs arising from poverty and deprivation, as Hilary Graham's (1987, 1988) work with mothers caring for young children has shown. The authors of the Black Report did not accept cultural factors as an adequate explanation for health inequalities.

Materialist/structural explanations

The authors of the Black Report favoured explanations of health inequalities that focused on the **material** causes of ill health, such as living and working conditions. This generated research on the impact of factors such as nutrition, housing, transport, environmental and occupational hazards on health. This research took as its starting point that these impacts are a product of the way society is organized, the result of material deprivation and structural inequality. Deprivation is absolute (the inability to obtain a defined level of resources necessary to sustain health) and relative (the inability to obtain socially valued resources and to participate in society), and both are important influences on health.

The debate since the 1990s

Are there social inequalities in health?

The debate about the relative merits of these explanations, particularly between cultural and materialist explanations, became somewhat polarized during the 1990s. For many, the lifestyle explanations favoured by some politicians were seen as overemphasizing personal responsibility for health. This polarization was in part a response to the entrenched nature of politics in the years (1979–90) of the Thatcher government (Williams, 2003). By the late 1990s, a shift in public policy under the New Labour government of the time (1997–2010) heralded a greater willingness to recognize the impact of poverty and deprivation as well as lifestyle choices on health inequalities (DH, 1999). While the post-2010 Conservative/Liberal Democrat coalition government introduced health spending restrictions, there was broad acceptance of the findings of the independent Marmot Review (Marmot et al., 2010) on the case for tackling inequalities in health.

How important is social class in explaining differences in modern society?

Although there is now little doubt about the evidence of inequalities in health in all national contexts where data are available, there remains an ongoing debate about how to theorize health inequalities and address these in practice (WHO, 2010). This stems in part from different understandings of social inequality. While the notion of social class is central to the study of socioeconomic inequalities in health, there are diverse perspectives among sociologists about what class is and how it can be measured (Drever and Whitehead, 1997; Williams, 2003).

Marxist sociologists such as Navarro (2004) view class as a relational concept based on exploitation. However, in many empirical studies that shape policy, social class is loosely defined and is used as a summary indicator of a range of dimensions of inequality such as income, housing status and educational level.

How do inequalities impact on health?

The years after 1990 and Thatcher's retirement also saw a greater willingness among researchers to recognize the complex relationships between material and cultural factors affecting health. For example, Wilkinson (1996) has offered a psychosocial explanation of health inequalities that identifies connections between stress, health and relative inequality. The data presented by Wilkinson mapped levels of life expectancy against the gross national product (GNP) of advanced capitalist societies, indicating that the rate of health improvement attained by a particular country is not determined simply by its level of development. Rather, health outcomes are influenced by the extent of income and status differentials in a particular country. More egalitarian societies characterized by a narrow income differential enjoy a greater improvement in overall life expectancy than more unequal societies at a comparable stage of economic development. This may be because unequal societies are characterized by chronic social stress, while societies with a narrow income differential are characterized by greater levels of social cohesion and community support. Subsequently, Wilson and Pickett (2009) extended the scope of this analysis to argue that per capita income can reach a threshold after which increased income does not lead to longer life or contribute to societal wellbeing.

What is the impact of social structures on health?

Other authors have also explored the influence of status, social cohesion and self-esteem on health outcomes (Marmot, 2004). These studies have opened the way for a neo-Durkheimian exploration of the role of social cohesion and the impact of social structures on patterns of health (Williams, 2003). One example of this is the increasing use of the concept of **social capital** in relation to health.

> **thinking about** What do you understand by social capital and how important do you think this is in explaining differences in modern society?

The notion of social capital has its origins in Durkheim's (1952) findings that a lack of social integration was associated with an increased risk of suicide. Recent proponents of social capital include Coleman, Bourdieu and Putnam. Bourdieu defines social capital in terms of the actual or potential resources that are linked to membership of a group (Everingham, 2001). Putnam (1995, p. 66) defines social capital positively as 'features of social organization such as networks, norms and trust, that facilitate coordination and cooperation for mutual benefit'. Coleman's definition of social capital is anything that facilitates individual or collective action (in Portes, 1998). Authors therefore use different definitions, ranging from subjective perceptions of engagement to tangible economic resources. While most authors see social capital as a positive force, it is not inevitably so, and several authors call for caution in addressing the issue (Baum, 1999; Lynch et al., 2000). The Mafia and the 'old boys' network' are two examples of strongly cohesive groups with high social capital that are not necessarily beneficial for health and may actively operate to reduce the health status of others outside the network.

Kawachi et al. (1997) contend that it is social capital (in this case defined as levels of trust and networking) rather than income that is responsible for improved health status, or vice versa. Any positive effects of social capital on health are hard to demonstrate, given the dominance of the individual and the randomized controlled trial in medical trials and evidence bases. However, a growing body of research and evidence strongly indicates that social capital is linked to improved health, and that strategies to support social capital may be more cost-effective than the traditional manipulation of individual **lifestyles** and behaviours.

Do life events and social determinants have a longer term influence on health?

A further perspective has emphasized the importance of time and timing to understand the causal links between events and the individual life course. This life course explanation focuses on how the social determinants of health operate at every level of development – from infancy, childhood, adolescence, young adulthood and into older age (Ben-Shlomo and Kuh, 2002). These determinants have an immediate influence and longer term influences on health and provide the basis for illness – or wellness – later in life. Within this approach, the critical periods model has examined how a harmful exposure, such as poor nutrition, acts at a specific point in time, for example in infancy, to have lasting or lifelong effects. Meanwhile, the accumulation of risk model suggests that factors that raise disease risk or promote good health may accumulate gradually over the life course. These explanations have been underpinned by the availability of longitudinal and comprehensive data on birth cohorts from the 1930s in the UK (Davey Smith, 2003).

Gender and health

thinking about How do you explain the apparent paradox that although women tend to live longer than men, they seem to experience higher levels of ill health?

Recent trends suggest that these patterns are not fixed and that the relationships between sex, gender and health are increasingly complex. Early research on gender and health also focused on women's health. The debate in the 1970s and 80s was largely driven by activism by women to improve their health and healthcare (Doyal, 2001). This approach was a response to long-standing imbalances that had led to male health concerns dominating research and policy interventions. There is evidence that gender bias continues to affect contemporary research and health policy. For example, conditions such as coronary heart disease and stroke are often assumed to be 'male' diseases, despite their significance for women in industrialized and developing countries (Doyal, 1995). More recently, men have begun to focus on the implications of masculinity and gender for their health.

Life expectancy

In most countries, women's life expectancy exceeds that of men, although levels of socioeconomic development and the degree of discrimination against women also impact on this finding (Arber and Thomas, 2001). Statistics for 2011 show that in some countries, for example Sierra Leone, where life expectancy at birth is 47.5 years, there is very little difference in life expectancy at birth between males (46) and females (47); whereas in the Russian Federation, female life expectancy exceeds that of males by 12 years (WHO, 2014). In developed countries such as the UK, women's life expectancy exceeds that of men by about 3 years (WHO, 2014), and this pattern is now apparent in some developing countries.

> **?** What might account for the narrowing of the gap in life expectancy of men and women in developed societies?

This may be as a consequence of changing patterns of employment as well as the increasing adoption by women of 'risk' behaviours such as smoking and alcohol consumption. In industrial countries like the UK, male deaths from circulatory diseases (including heart disease and stroke) have tended to exceed those of women, particularly between the 1950s and 1980s (Lawlor et al., 2001). However, circulatory diseases along with cancer are the commonest cause of death for both sexes (ONS, 2014a). Cancer death rates among females rose to a peak in the late 1980s, declining during the 1990s, while among males rates increased substantially to the late 1970s and then declined more rapidly from the 1990s (ONS, 2014a).

Differences in ill health

The differences in ill health between men and women show complex interactions between sex, age and socioeconomic status (Bartley et al., 2004). In the 2011 census, males were somewhat more likely than females to report good health; however, self-reported rates of good health decrease steadily with age, with 40% of those identifying themselves as not in good health being aged 65 and over. The overall difference between the sexes was small once the age distribution of the population was taken into account. Similarly, up to age 59, there were few differences in the rates of LLSI between males and females. However, in the 60–74 age group, males had a higher prevalence of LLSI than females; while the situation was reversed for those aged 75 and over, with more females than males reporting an LLSI (ONS, 2013b). These data suggest that as a consequence of their greater life expectancy, women in developed countries are more likely than men to experience a range of conditions that lead to chronic impairment and disability. While ageing does not inevitably lead to ill health and a loss of independence, older women are more likely than older men to suffer from disabling conditions and need help in performing basic activities such as bathing and shopping (Arber, 1998).

Mental health

Other areas where gender differences have been examined are mental health (Payne, 1998), the use of health services (Doyal, 1998) and patterns of health-related behaviour. In relation to mental health, the prevalence of the most common mental health conditions, neurotic disorders, are higher among women than men. On the other hand, suicide rates are higher among men (ONS, 2014b). In relation to use of health services, data from the 2009 General Lifestyle Survey on GP consultation rates show that consultations tend to be higher among women; around 1 in 16 females attended a GP consultation compared with 1 in 25 males in the 14 days prior to interview (ONS, 2011b). However, these differences disappear in the oldest age groups.

Health-related behaviour

Data from the General Lifestyle Survey 2011 (ONS, 2013a) show that there is a convergence in some male and female health behaviour patterns. In 1974, there was a 10% difference between men and women – 51% of men smoked cigarettes compared with 41% of women – whereas in 2011, there was only a 2% difference between them – 21% of men compared with 19% of women.

> **?** What do you think accounts for gender differences in health status and reported ill health?

Explaining gender inequalities in health

As in the case of socioeconomic inequalities in health, a number of explanations for gender differences in health have been put forward. These include biological, materialist and structural, and cultural and social constructionist accounts.

Biological explanations

Biological explanations focus on the different reproductive roles of men and women, which impact on health. Sociologists traditionally tended to reject biologically based notions of gender identity. More recently, however, they have begun to engage more critically with notions of the body, which has led to a more inclusive focus and an engagement with biological discourse. This shift is also reflected in feminist research, which has explored the interaction between biology and society and the influence of biological factors on male and female health (Doyal, 1995, 2001).

Materialist/structural explanations

Materialist and structural explanations look at health outcomes for men and women, and how these may be determined by social factors. Researchers have drawn attention to differences in the social roles of men and women as well as differences in their access to resources such as income, employment, housing and leisure. Such research has uncovered persistent inequalities that can influence health. For example, segregation in the labour market means that women continue to be concentrated in low-paid employment and roles such as caring and service work (Doyal, 1995; Arber and Khlat, 2002). They also continue to bear the bulk of responsibility for unpaid caring and domestic work (Lloyd, 1999; Moss, 2002). This means not only that women have less access than men to health-promoting resources, but that women and men may face different hazards and risks in paid and unpaid work settings.

Cultural explanations and social constructionist accounts

Cultural explanations focus on the way in which health outcomes are influenced by roles, relationships, norms and expectations at macro- and micro-levels (Moss, 2002). Social constructionist accounts of gender go further than this, implying that gender is not a fixed category and questioning the notion that traits associated with masculinity and femininity are *essential* characteristics inherited at birth. Instead, gender roles are seen as being continuously negotiated (Cameron and Bernades, 1998). Thus, creating and performing an appropriate gender identity is a continuous task, and masculinity and femininity may both be associated to a varying degree with individual men and women (Annandale and Hunt, 1990).

> **thinking about** Can you think of an example where how you feel about your gender has impacted on your health or health-related behaviour?

Research has explored the impact on health of expectations, attitudes and behaviours concerning approved forms of gender identity. A key area is that of sexual health: expectations about gender clearly help shape interactions and the negotiation of sexual activity. The social construction of gender therefore provides the context for, and sometimes constrains, strategies to reduce a number of risks, for example unwanted pregnancy and sexually transmitted disease. For example, one study found that young men's conversations about sexual health focused primarily around their sexual encounters ('guy talk') or expressions of hypermasculine power ('manning up'), with the effect of shutting down communication about wider sexual health issues with peers and sex partners (Knight et al., 2012).

Earlier research explored the effects of stereotyping of female patients in healthcare services (Doyal, 1998; Payne, 1998). More recently, it is suggested that certain notions of masculinity may have a negative effect on men's health. This research distinguishes between different forms of masculinity. Traditional or hegemonic masculinity, with its emphasis on risk-taking, self-reliance and dominance, is viewed as potentially dangerous, for example it can discourage men from seeking help for health problems (Cameron and Bernades,

1998). These issues have been explored in studies of the relationship between masculine identities, risk-taking and health promotion (Courtenay, 2000; de Visser and Smith, 2006; Gough and Conner, 2006; Robertson, 2006). Finally, research has identified emerging trends in women's health that have arisen as a consequence of the adoption by women of traditional 'masculine' practices such as cigarette smoking (Graham, 1998) and alcohol consumption (Bloomfield et al., 2006; Wilsnack et al., 2006).

The different explanations of gender inequalities in health are not necessarily mutually exclusive, rather they focus on different aspects of gender, such as the impact of reproductive roles, psychosocial factors, occupational factors, cultural trends and social structuring (Arber and Thomas, 2001). Health outcomes are increasingly recognized as part of a complex relationship between macro- and micro-level social factors spanning the geopolitical environment and cultural norms that shape the distribution of risks and resources within households (Moss, 2002).

example 5.2

Changing patterns of risk in HIV/AIDS

The impact of gender on HIV/AIDS risk is discussed by Türmen (2003). In the early stages of the pandemic, infection was predominantly among men but by the early years of the twenty-first century, women represented 48% of new infections and, in developing countries, 67% of newly infected individuals aged 15–24. This shift is attributed to a number of factors, including women's greater biological susceptibility to infection than that of men, as well as social and cultural factors that increase the risk of HIV infection among women. These include high levels of sexual violence against women, a lack of education and knowledge about risks, poverty and dependence on male partners, and a lack of negotiating power in relation to safe sexual behaviour.

'Race', ethnicity and health

thinking about What do you understand as the difference between the concepts of 'race' and 'ethnicity'?

Since the 1970s, a growing body of research has examined the patterning of health by 'race' and ethnicity. This debate is complicated by problems of terminology and measurement. Like the notion of gender, 'race' is often taken to stand for biological differences between people rather than being understood as a socially constructed notion. Medicine has played a key role in the establishment of 'racial' differences. Alongside its treatment and curative role, medicine contributes to processes of labelling, racialization and social exclusion. This can be clearly illustrated by examining the debate on ethnicity, racism and health. During the nineteenth century, 'scientific' support was provided for the belief that human beings could be categorized according to skin colour and other physical characteristics. During slavery, medicine even provided labels such as 'drapetomania', the supposedly pathological desire of slaves to run away from their master (Ahmad, 1993).

While this notion of 'race' is now discredited in academic and scientific circles, the concept of race continues to influence the beliefs of ordinary people and has significant consequences, including social and economic discrimination and the stereotyping of black and minority ethnic patients by healthcare workers. Unsurprisingly, the quest to identify distinctive patterns of health and disease for different ethnic groups arouses scepticism among some critics.

In order to measure these effects without reinforcing racist discourse, some researchers adopt the notion of ethnicity. Ethnicity refers to shared experiences such as religion, language, history and culture. Ethnicity applies to white as well as black people, thereby avoiding the assumption that only the ethnicity of black people needs to be examined. In practice, however, the term 'ethnicity' is often used as a euphemism for 'race', and most studies of ethnicity and health focus only on ethnic minorities.

---

example 5.3

'Race', ethnicity and health

- The evidence linking ethnicity with health is complex and apparently contradictory, the picture being further limited by a number of methodological problems. UK studies have, however, shown excess mortality for men born in Bangladesh, Ireland, Scotland and West/South Africa (Davey Smith et al., 2002)
- An excess coronary heart disease mortality has been found in people born in the Indian subcontinent, and a relatively high mortality from stroke has been found among people of African-Caribbean origin. Research has examined ethnic differences in risk factors, especially in relation to alcohol use in the white population and weight in the black population (Dundas et al., 2001)

- The mortality rates of common types of cancer, such as breast and lung cancer, appear to be relatively low among people from the Caribbean and the Indian subcontinent (Harding and Rosato, 1999). A higher rate of infant mortality is found for most migrant groups, a particularly high level being seen among the babies of Pakistan-born mothers (Davey Smith et al., 2002)
- The members of most minority ethnic groups perceive their health in poorer terms than do the general population (ONS, 2013c). Middle-aged Irish and Pakistani men and older Indian and Pakistani women show significantly higher rates of common mental disorders than their white English counterparts (Weich et al., 2004)

A number of explanations for ethnic minority differences in health have been put forward. These include artefact, biological, and materialist and structural explanations.

Artefact explanations

The Black Report's framework, developed by Davey Smith et al. (2002), has been used as a starting point to explain these data. As with social class, artefact explanations focus on the problems caused by the use of particular measurement tools (Manly, 2006). Challenges in ethnicity and health research stem from the problematic use of country of birth as a measure of ethnicity, with half of the UK's ethnic minorities having been born in the UK. Other problems include treating ethnicity and class separately, and failing to recognize the heterogeneous nature of ethnic majority populations.

Biological explanations

Biological explanations focus on factors such as genetic variations and the role of inherited conditions such as blood disorders in relation to conditions like thalassaemia. These explanations have been criticized for overestimating the impact of genetic factors on the causation of disease and reinforcing biological conceptualizations of 'race' (Frank, 2001). Cultural explanations tend to focus on particular lifestyles, behaviours, religious practices and beliefs associated with different ethnic groups. On the one hand, the increasing diversity of societies like the UK and the US has stimulated demands for 'culturally and linguistically competent healthcare' (Shaw-Taylor, 2002). On the other hand, the focus on cultural differences as a cause of health outcomes has been challenged. The cultural characteristics of minority ethnic groups are often portrayed in negative terms, and the positive influences of culture on health are sometimes overlooked.

Material and structural explanations

Material and structural explanations emphasize the direct effects of socioeconomic factors, such as poor housing and unemployment, on members of minority ethnic groups (Nazroo, 1997). Members of minority ethnic groups are disproportionately represented in lower socioeconomic groups. While material disadvantage impacts negatively on the health of minority ethnic groups, it is unlikely that social class alone can explain the excess mortality observed in minority ethnic groups (Nazroo, 2001).

Racism has been used to explain patterns of ethnicity and health. Racism can affect the health of minority ethnic groups through several pathways, including:

- restricted access to social resources, such as employment, housing, healthcare and education

- increased exposure to risk factors, such as unnecessary contact with the criminal justice system

- reduced uptake of healthy behaviours (e.g. exercise)

- increased adoption of unhealthy behaviours (e.g. substance misuse) either directly as stress-coping or indirectly via reduced self-regulation

- direct physical injury caused by racist violence (Priest et al., 2013).

Such impacts often start early in life. Priest et al. (2013) found that there were significant associations between racial discrimination and children's mental health in three-quarters of the 121 research studies they identified in a global systematic review.

Part 2 Theoretical and research approaches

example 5.4

Examples of research in sociology and health

- Social structural research exploring issues such as poverty and its impact on health, the social patterning of health and illness, and access to health services
- Research exploring the subjective lived experience of people with a particular condition, such as AIDS or sickle cell disease

- Studies of the role of volunteers and laypeople in providing social support networks for people with chronic illnesses
- Investigation of the role and status of healthcare professionals in managing the disruptive effects of illness as well as its clinical manifestations
- Exploration of the body as a field of discourse

Sociology – the study of human social life – involves a conscious distancing of the sociologist from the object of study, whether that involves personal emotions (e.g. bereavement or ill health), social institutions (e.g. the family or healthcare services) or group life (e.g. health professionals peer group norms and pressures). Sociological study often involves investigating what appears at first sight to be natural, universal or common sense, only to discover that such behaviours or practices are fundamentally affected by specific social factors and influences. Sociology offers a wide range of theoretical and methodological approaches for the study of health. This brief introduction presents an overview of selected issues in the sociology of health that illustrate key theoretical and methodological approaches.

These approaches begin with different starting points when considering issues such as the impact of health services. While health services seem self-evidently beneficial, some have questioned this, even arguing that the harm done by modern medicine outweighs the benefits. We can explore this debate by distinguishing between consensus and conflict approaches. Both acknowledge that health professionals, particularly doctors, enjoy a significant amount of power. They can sanction a number of benefits such as employees' sick leave, claimants' eligibility for welfare payments, and patients' entitlement to services. They also endorse controlling and restraining actions such as the incarceration of individuals defined as mentally ill.

Consensus approaches accept the necessity of these functions for the smooth running of modern societies. Furthermore, they suggest that because of their extensive training and commitment to ethical conduct, members of regulated professions are well placed to carry them out. In contrast, conflict perspectives question professional power, highlighting issues of professional domination and social control, and the oppressive impact of some practices.

Recent developments, such as the advancement of nursing and other professions, increased managerialism in the NHS and the growth of complementary therapies, suggest that power, particularly medical power, is not exercised without challenge and resistance. Theorizing these trends, recent accounts suggest that traditional approaches may be limited by a rather narrow and mechanistic understanding of power. Rather than being delegated by society or imposed on individuals and groups, power is increasingly viewed as fluid and diffuse, capable of being mobilized in many ways and from a range of sources.

The sociology of lay–professional relationships: functionalist approaches

The **functionalist** sociology of Parsons (1951, 1975) provides a well-known and influential example of a consensus model. Parsons was concerned to demonstrate the ways in which practices such as medicine contribute to the maintenance of the social order. Illness not only disturbs individual functioning, but is also socially dysfunctional, undermining the values, activities and roles that support productivity and social stability. In order to prevent such a disruption, mechanisms are needed that render illness an undesirable and temporary social state. Parsons identified such a mechanism in the form of the **sick role**, into which people ideally enter when they become ill. The sick role confers both rights and obligations. The rights are:

- an exemption from responsibilities such as work and social obligations, which needs to be legitimized by a physician in order to be valid

- the sick individual avoids any blame or responsibility for their condition.

The two obligations are:

- the sick person must want to get better

- the sick person must seek competent help, usually from a trained physician.

> ? How adequate is the sick role in accounting for:
> - someone with food poisoning?
> - someone with depression?
> - someone with asthma?
> - someone who is HIV positive?

Sociologists have debated the relevance of the concept of the sick role in relation to contemporary patterns of health and illness. One of the issues that arises is that access to the sick role may not be enjoyed equally by all. The sick role concept may apply relatively closely to acute illnesses such as influenza, but even in these cases there are some social obligations (such as caring for others) from which exemption may be difficult to gain. In the case of chronic conditions, the rights associated with the sick role concept apply less clearly, and social obligations may be difficult to escape in the longer term. Furthermore, some conditions, for example HIV/AIDS, carry a stigma. This means that assumptions of responsibility and blame may influence how the person is seen and treated by others.

The obligations associated with the sick role concept are also more complex than at first appears. These obligations render the doctor much more powerful than the patient in professional–client interactions. Functionalists such as Parsons accept the asymmetrical nature of the doctor–patient relationship on the grounds that doctors, as modern professionals, are required to be altruistic and ethical practitioners as well as knowledgeable. These attributes are seen as ensuring that a doctor's personal feelings towards a patient do not influence the consultation or treatment offered. The physician is expected to put the welfare of the patient above any personal interest.

connections   Chapter 12 discusses the ethical principles underlying professional practice and the layperson's obligations.

The power imbalance between doctors and patients becomes more problematic if professionals are seen as a group seeking to influence the organization of services and rewards. Further, patients can often become experts in their condition and may feel frustrated if they are not listened to by doctors. A more critical perspective would suggest that professionals' interests may conflict with those of service users, and would question the degree of trust that society grants to doctors – evidenced by their high degree of autonomy and the lack of external surveillance of many procedures.

Hence, Parsons' concept of the sick role has been criticized as being naive in relation to issues of power, although the debate continues. The **empowerment** model (Crossley, 1998) has developed as an alternative way of conceptualizing professional–client relationships. This model suggests that doctors' technical competence may be more limited than traditional beliefs concerning the efficacy of scientific medicine suggest. This can be seen in relation to conditions such as repetitive strain injury or ME for which there appears to be little medical consensus on the cause of the problem or appropriate treatment, or HIV, in which there is little possibility of a cure. The obligation to seek technically competent help from a physician makes little sense if technical competence is beyond the physician's scope. Instead, the empowerment model seeks to enhance the status and authority of the experiential knowledge of the sufferer in the face of doctors' limited capacity to respond to complex chronic conditions.

Crossley (1998) warns, however, that the 'empowerment' perspective underestimates the benefits of medicine. Whereas scientific medicine has not been able to provide a cure for many conditions, the medical management of chronic illness is constantly developing. Furthermore, the empowerment model is seen as offering a weak basis for practice because it lacks any notion of duty or social obligation to accompany the 'rights' associated with chronic illness.

The sick role concept, although criticized, has provided useful insights into the experience of illness and the role of medicine, and has paved the way for a broader debate on the nature of medical authority and the relationship between medicine and social control.

Chapter 4 discusses individual adoption of the sick role in response to pain and health conditions.

connections

Medicalization and social control

During the 1960s and 70s, a number of critical perspectives on medical power emerged. These often drew on the **medicalization** thesis, in which medicine is seen as expanding its social jurisdiction and replacing earlier mechanisms of social control such as religion. While Parson's functionalist model emphasized the benign and productive aspects of medical power, critical perspectives have identified some undesirable social costs of medical expansion.

The medicalization of society has been seen as taking place at a number of levels (Zola, 1972):

- Medicine has expanded its concerns to encompass areas of life not previously regarded as illness

- Medicalization has resulted in the concentration of control over technical procedures among doctors

- Doctors' authority has expanded to encompass areas of moral decision-making.

Medicalization involves the pursuit of medical, individual and technical solutions to an expanding range of problems. Where these problems are social in origin, medicalization can be seen as obscuring their social causes, inhibiting the development of alternative solutions.

example 5.5

Medicine as a threat to health

In one well-known critique, Illich (1977) described medicalization as a major threat to health. Modern medicine was portrayed as generating iatrogenic disease, that is, illness that would not have come about without medical intervention. It was also suggested that society would be better off without professions such as medicine, which encourage dependency rather than self-reliance.

During the 1990s, feminist researchers highlighted the negative impact of conventional healthcare on women, suggesting that the benefits of modern medicine to women are oversold and its harmful effects understated (Foster, 1995). As patients, women are constrained in their ability to make rational choices, partly because doctors are themselves unaware of many of the risks attached to accepted forms of medical treatment. Furthermore, when doctors are aware of the risks, they may assume that female patients will not be able to cope with the information, and therefore keep their knowledge to themselves.

The notion of medicine as a threat to health remains influential. Contemporary journalism often seeks to expose the 'dangers of modern medicine', while the increasing popularity of complementary therapies and self-help sources such as the internet reveals apparent widespread disillusionment with conventional medical approaches (McTaggart, 1996).

While it is important not to overstate the benefits of medical practice, these theories may understate medicine's benefits; empirical evidence is needed in order to evaluate the impact of different health interventions. Without such evidence, these theories could potentially undermine efforts to improve health and reduce health inequalities. Given that, for many people in the world, access to basic healthcare remains limited, it seems important to emphasize the widening access to beneficial practices and resources as well as re-examine questionable aspects of medical practice.

These theories do, however, highlight the impact of medical decision-making and point towards the need for a greater involvement of patients and laypeople in such activity. In the face of such challenging claims about medicine, it seems that consumers need to make more and more complex and difficult choices concerning their healthcare. This theme is explored in the following sections, which examine a number of different approaches to understanding the relationships between medicine, the health professions and society.

connections   Chapter 8 reviews policies designed to increase service user involvement in health and social care provision.

Marxist and political economy perspectives

Marxist and political economy perspectives also highlight the negative impact of medical power. However, rather than seeing professionals as the main problem, Marxist theory suggests that professional power is a product of a deeper set of power relations. Political economy perspectives draw on Marxist theory to suggest that the structuring of society around the needs of capitalism as an economic system is the starting point of any analysis of health and healthcare. This theory suggests that capitalist societies are organized around the generation of profit, which is created by the exploitation of labour power.

Political economy writers such as Navarro (1979) drew broadly on this theory and applied it to health in a number of ways:

- The processes of industrial capitalism cause ill health directly, for example through occupational disease, industrial accidents and the manufacturing and marketing of harmful consumer products, such as tobacco

- This burden of disease is disproportionately felt by those in lower socioeconomic groups

- Society does not do enough to prevent these problems or promote health because society's resources are channelled towards the maintenance of production over and above the social goal of securing and improving public health.

> **?** Consider the political economy of tobacco. How do you account for its continued manufacture and advertising?

Governments' reluctance to ban the manufacture and advertising of this dangerous product could be explained in terms of the dominance of the interests of tobacco producers over those of other groups and the economic benefits derived by governments from tobacco tax.

The political economy perspective also offers a critique of the role of medical and health services. According to Navarro (1979), doctors are often seen as serving the interests of the dominant class, because of their own class position and social role. Hence, the role of medicine is seen as helping minimize disruption to the economic functioning of society, even if this means supporting exploitative and oppressive economic and social relationships.

> **?** How relevant is the view that capitalism is a major threat to population health?

The global nature of capitalism perhaps makes it impossible to identify examples of societies and cultures unaffected by it. However, critics have argued that other (non-economic) social processes are equally influential. These include the cultural discourse of ideas and concepts. Furthermore, critics have argued that Marxism places too much emphasis on class divisions as the driving force of social change, ignoring the independent impact of other social relations, including gender and ethnicity.

> Chapter 7 discusses the cultural construction of concepts of health and illness.   **connections**

In response to these criticisms, political economy perspectives have taken a broader view than those of traditional Marxism, widening their scope to examine other aspects of power relationships such as gender and ethnicity. Political economy perspectives have exercised a strong influence over the sociology of health and illness, although this influence declined during the 1980s and 90s as new economic and social trends, such as changes in employment, leisure and lifestyle, emerged to challenge core assumptions concerning identity and class. Political economy perspectives may still evolve to meet these challenges. In the meantime, however, their legacy can still be seen, for example in relation to the inequalities in health debate, where material and structural explanations continue to hold sway.

Health professions and interprofessional relationships

Since the 1970s, a great deal of attention has been given to the role of health professions, with early discussions focusing on whether it is possible to identify core traits, such as knowledge, training, practices of regulation and autonomy, that set a 'profession' apart from other occupational groups (Freidson, 1970). Much of this research focused on the profession of medicine. Subsequently, the scope of the discussion has widened to include the roles and relationships between other groups including nurses (Davies, 1995; Porter, 1999).

Some of this writing has been influenced by neo-Weberian approaches, which focus on the characteristics of different professional groups in relation to social class and other hierarchies, as well as examining the strategies adopted by occupational groups to gain influence and control (Johnson, 1993). These professionalization projects involve professional groups in negotiating their relationship with the state as well as with other professional groups in situations where healthcare resources are increasingly limited (Witz, 1992; Johnson, 1993, 1995). Professionalization strategies have been identified such as that of 'dual closure' (Witz, 1992). This has two elements: usurpation to renegotiate role boundaries with more powerful groups; and demarcation to organize their relationships with less powerful groups. Foucauldian perspectives have also been brought to bear on this debate, identifying ways in which the discourses of health, illness and care are used to shape professional roles and interprofessional relationships (Foucault, 1976; Armstrong 1995; Lupton 1995; Martin et al., 2013).

---

example 5.6

Professionalization in the NHS

These issues were explored in a study by Daykin and Clarke (2000) of interprofessional relationships between nurses and healthcare assistants in the NHS. A training programme sought to enhance the roles of healthcare assistants, providing them with the skills to undertake tasks previously undertaken by nurses such as bedside observations. At the same time, staffing ratios were to be changed to reduce the number of qualified nurses on the wards. The project was in part a response by managers to ongoing difficulties of recruitment and retention of qualified nursing staff and an attempt to reduce the rising costs of employing agency nurses to cover the work of this group.

The nursing and care staff had mixed views about the project, with some welcoming the changes and others seeing them as a dilution and fragmentation of care. For these nurses, the training of healthcare assistants was a 'task-oriented' approach that undermined the more holistic 'nursing process' discourse (Porter, 1992), which was key to their professional identity and job satisfaction. Others recognized the importance of the division of labour in healthcare and saw the changes as an opportunity for themselves and the healthcare assistants to enhance their roles (Witz, 1992). The research identified among nurses a dual closure strategy of usurption in relation to doctors and demarcation in relation to healthcare assistants. Some participants saw managers as being able to bridge these differences and divisions in order to overcome resistance to the changes in care they proposed and avoid the challenge of providing adequate resources to support alternative solutions to the problems of care delivery.

Interactionist perspectives and the experience of illness

The perspectives discussed so far concentrate on the impact of illness, health and healthcare on society as whole. Sociologists have also examined the nature and meanings of the illness experience at the individual level, analysing this experience in the context of the interaction between people and exploring its implication for notions of identity and self. This tradition draws on the work of Mead (1934), who saw human beings as distinctive, in that they are able to reflect on their own thoughts and actions. This approach, sometimes referred to as 'symbolic **interactionism**', emphasizes the ways in which people gain a shared understanding of the meanings attached to objects and phenomena. Meanings are not seen as pre-existing or intrinsic, but emerge from an inter- pretative process between people in which language is an important element. A nurse's uniform, for example, suggests femininity, caring, altruism and sacri- fice – meanings reaffirmed by countless media portrayals.

Sociologists have applied these insights to the study of changes in iden- tity, which occur when people become chronically ill or impaired. Goffman's work on stigma (1963) provides a well-known example of such an approach. According to Goffman, a person's sense of identity is formed in interaction with others and is reflected back to the individual through verbal and nonver- bal communication. When someone possesses a distinguishing attribute that is perceived negatively by others, their identity is to some extent 'spoiled' or stigmatized. People attribute a range of negative characteristics, unrelated to the original attribute, to the individual. Wheelchair users, for example, are often assumed to be physically and intellectually dependent. Stigma may be attributed to people on the basis of physical attributes or personal and social characteristics, such as being gay or lesbian.

Goffman suggested that stigmatized individuals may react in a number of ways. They may attempt to 'pass', maintaining a performance of self in which the stigmatized attribute is disguised or hidden. They may also respond in ways that seem to confirm society's stereotyped views. Alternatively, they may create meanings that turn their experience into a positive one, for example reflecting on the lessons that their experiences have taught them. They may feel that they have grown in wisdom or sensitivity or somehow become a 'better person' because of their circumstances.

Goffman's theory was developed during the early 1960s and reflects the social values and norms of that time. In contemporary society, it seems that a wider range of options is available to stigmatized groups. These include activism and campaigning to transform social attitudes and end discrimination. Examples of this can be seen in the disability rights movement and the responses of the gay community, which have challenged negative social attitudes and found collective sources of solidarity.

Interactionist perspectives may be limited, in that they focus attention on the victim rather than examining the reasons for discrimination against particular groups. Nevertheless, they do draw attention to the stress that can accompany stigmatizing experiences, including illness and disability. They also highlight the need for coping strategies in response to the challenges to identity that these experiences may represent. As a consequence, interactionist perspectives have had a strong influence on research in medical sociology, much of which is focused on interactions between professionals and patients, and the experiences of people with particular conditions.

Questions of identity and illness are increasingly important in sociological research. Increasing life expectancy and technological advances mean that an increasing number of people are surviving for a longer period, and are more likely to be living with a chronic condition. This in turn means that an increasing number of people may find that they cannot sustain the values of independence and achievement that they assumed would carry them through adult life. The onset of chronic illness may represent a profound threat to personal identity. Bury (1982, 2001) illustrates this through the notion of illness as a 'biographical disruption', disrupting the patterns of daily life and social relationships, and generating a range of tasks. These tasks may relate to practical needs such as symptom management, but also to maintaining a sense of identity and preserving one's cultural competence in the eyes of others. This rethinking of biography following the onset of chronic illness can often be understood as an interactive or co-created process between individuals. For example, Radcliffe et al. (2013) explore the shared creation of meanings among older stroke survivors and their spouses and the implications for individual and couple identity.

Sociology of the body

The intimate relationship between illness and identity has led to a rethink of the body from a sociological standpoint. Evidently, our bodies form the physical locus within which we experience and interpret health and illness. Sociology has traditionally been highly 'disembodied', seeing the body as a matter of intellectual concern for biology and biomedicine. At the same time, sociologists have also questioned whether there are any essential physical experiences that are not mediated by culture and social context. In this way, the body had almost become invisible within sociological discourse. Authors such as Frank (1991) have argued for a renewed focus on the body drawing on the concept of 'embodiment' – the lived experience of our bodies in the world. A concern with embodiment provides a bridge between structure and agency, between macro-social processes and micro-personal experience. For example, tiredness is clearly a physical sensation of the body. From an embodied perspective, tiredness can be seen to encompass a temporary exit from a productive, socially structured role and a loss of willpower. While an episode of tiredness will hold specific personal biographical meaning, it is also the bodily expression of patterned and value-laden ideas current in society.

Chapter 1 focuses on the physical concepts of health and disease.	connections

Recent interest in the body is unsurprising in the context of modern consumer society. What we eat, what we wear and whether we are fit are all cultural markers, locating our identities. Frost (2003) suggests that the emphasis on individualistic models of health, for example the focus on personal responsibility for a healthy diet and fitness, has made the body the object of self-discipline. While this disciplining of the body may seem to imply a continuous round of self-denial in order to restrain any appetite for excess, it also opens the way for more tangible forms of consumption. The plethora of health and fitness magazines, slimming aids, sportswear and membership of gym clubs are but a few of the goods and services available to assist the quest for a managed body. Giddens (1991) argues that the pace of social change is such that people lack traditional reference points for identity within a fragmented and shifting social order. Instead, the self, or body, becomes a project, the seat of identity and a source of stability, albeit in an ever-changing and unfinished form.

Social constructionist perspectives and beyond

So far, we have explored perspectives that examine the impact of social processes on the meanings of phenomena such as health and illness. These perspectives suggest that health and illness cannot be understood as fixed and unchanging entities. Instead, the meanings attributed to health and illness may differ at different historical periods and between different cultures. Within Western medicine, for example, homosexuality is no longer perceived as a disease. At the same time, new diseases and syndromes such as 'attention deficit disorder' and 'premenstrual syndrome' describe behaviour that would in previous decades have been understood in very different terms.

Sociologists have also explored the formation of ideas about health and illness, examining the role of different groups, such as professionals and scientists, in the production of discourses of health. These debates have implications for the study of lay perspectives, which may differ significantly from scientific and professional views. There has been a general shift away from approaches assuming that medical science is 'right' and other views 'wrong'.

Instead, there is a growing recognition that professional and lay views are both socially constructed, meaning that they cannot easily be categorized as 'right' or 'wrong' because they both arise from the experiences and circumstances of different groups within society.

The writings of Foucault (1976, 1979a) have been studied by sociologists seeking to explore further this process of the social construction of medical knowledge. The notion of the 'gaze' has been used to explain the processes that enabled a medical understanding of the body to emerge during the eighteenth century. This perspective draws attention to the surveillance and control that are exercised through medical practices. Today, the bodies of healthy as well as sick people are seen as being increasingly under surveillance. Medical practice is no longer concerned with just the treatment of disease but has been extended into new areas such as prevention and health promotion. These practices, while apparently beneficial, may have negative consequences. While apparently exercising care, health professionals may also be exercising power and control.

Sociologists of late modernity have focused on the ways in which social control and surveillance has spread throughout society. Beck (1992) first coined the term 'risk society' to describe the expansion of risk within modernized societies. Modernization is linked to particular risks as temporal and spatial limits no longer apply. Global climate change is a good example of the increased risks associated with modernization.

One response to the perception of increased risk is to try to control and avoid exposure to risk (Jones, 2004). The most effective strategy is to persuade people to practise risk avoidance voluntarily rather than try to enforce it. Foucault (1979b) used the notion of the gaze and surveillance to describe the modern trend for self-regulation and control. This has its origins in the panopticon, Bentham's late eighteenth-century prison design incorporating a central watchtower. The argument was that prisoners would not know if they were being watched, so would develop self-discipline. Today, modern society is increasingly under surveillance, with computerization opening up new avenues for monitoring and regulation. The increased use of CCTV is often cited as symptomatic of modern life. Increasingly, people have been persuaded that surveillance is a good thing, to the extent that they voluntarily take on the task, and self-surveillance and self-monitoring in all aspects of life is rapidly escalating. Examples of this include routine monitoring of blood pressure at home, self-monitoring regarding alcohol intake, and parental use of mobile phones to monitor the activities of children and young people. There is also general compliance with the increased levels of surveillance, evident in everything from the use of pin codes on bank cards to the routine recording and playing back of phone calls to businesses.

thinking about What examples of surveillance in professional life can you think of? Do you think this degree of surveillance is positive or negative? Why?

This degree of monitoring and self-regulation is often linked to the 'risk-averse' nature of society. It has been argued that this process is unhelpful and leads to negative outcomes. For example, risk aversion has been linked to professional defensiveness, as the fear of litigation in cases of negligence or unprofessional practice spurs greater professional closure. The result of this process is arguably greater social distance between practitioners and patients. It also leads to more resources being directed towards providing evidence of actions taken and consent procedures (the audit trail), at the expense of direct action undertaken to care for clients and patients.

case study the social determinants and social construction of diet

There seems little doubt that diets and eating practices in the West are undergoing major transformations. Caraher and Coveney (2004, p. 592) suggest that 'we in the developed world can expect to eat a different and better diet than did our predecessors 100 years ago'. Dietary improvements have meant that we live longer, are taller and rarely suffer diseases of deprivation.

Furthermore, consumers live in an environment that appears to offer unprecedented food security. The major retail stores offer thousands of food lines, reliably sourced on the global market and with little seasonal variation. For those lacking time or inclination, there is an expanding market for eating out and eating in with ready-prepared foods. Average households have greater disposable incomes, and food expenditure in real terms accounts for a smaller slice of personal spending than it did two decades ago (Hitcham et al., 2002). Given these conditions, we examine how two perplexing issues have attracted sociological enquiry: why diet-related health inequalities continue to exist in the West; and what accounts for the high level of social anxieties surrounding food and eating practices.

These two areas can be used to illustrate different traditions of sociological thought:

1. The *social causation* perspective is drawn on to understand food insecurity and social inequalities in diets. This approach is similar to the materialist/structural approach developed by the authors of the Black Report (Townsend and Davidson, 1982) and is adopted by researchers working within a Marxist or political economy perspective.

2. The *social constructionist* perspective is adopted to explore perceptions of risk, trust and anxiety in relation to food. This approach is concerned to explore the conditions under which ideas and meanings are generated. Social constructionism therefore builds on the interactionist tradition in sociology, and questions commonplace assumptions about the relationship between language and objective knowledge.

Social causation of food insecurity and dietary inequalities

Research from a variety of Western nations indicates that there are clear socioeconomic differences in diets and diet-related ill health. Lower income groups tend to eat less fruit, vegetables and food rich in dietary fibre, have a lower intake of foods containing antioxidants, some minerals and vitamins, and have higher salt intake. As part of a general social trend, lower income groups increasingly consume processed and energy-dense foods (high-sugar, high-fat foods). These dietary patterns are strongly linked to higher rates of obesity, increased risk of coronary heart disease and circulatory problems, some diet-related cancers and dental decay (Acheson, 1998; Shaw et al., 2000; Cummins and Macintyre, 2006; Kamphuis et al., 2006). Social causation perspectives have sought to explain these patterns with reference to a variety of societal processes. These draw together the changing character of global and local economic systems and the material conditions of people on low incomes in industrialized countries.

Lang and colleagues (Lang and Heasman, 2004; Lang, 2005) hold that global transformations of the food industry account, in part, for contemporary inequalities in diets. Lang (2005) argues that there has been a revolution within the food system in all aspects, from production, processing, distribution and retail through to consumption. Within this system, leading retailers assume a pivotal position. For example, in 15 EU states, 3.2 million farmers feed 250 million consumers, but this supply and demand is funnelled through only 600 supermarket chains with 110 key buying desks (Lang, 2005).

Retailers, along with a small number of leading brand processing corporations, now exercise unprecedented leverage over consumer tastes. Investment in marketing and promotion by these organizations considerably outstrips the health promotion budgets of national governments (Lang, 2005). The two leading commercial ad-spend budgets of the world each amount to $1.7 billion a year, which is vastly more than the entire health education budgets of governments (Lang, 2005).

According to Lang, weak government controls have allowed a largely unfettered promotion of highly processed and energy-dense foods. These changes have had greater impact on the diets of lower income groups. In part this is because high-fat, high-sugar and high-salt foods have been marketed at a lower cost than 'healthier alternatives'. But the effects are amplified for poorer groups because of links with other social processes. Since the 1970s, the retail geography

of industrialized countries has changed dramatically. The decline of high-street and neighbourhood food retailers has been mirrored by an expansion of large, often out-of-town supermarkets. These changes have left many low-income communities with a dearth of retail outlets (Caraher and Coveney, 2004). Given that low-income households are less likely to own a car, these groups may encounter additional difficulties accessing supermarkets with poor public transport links.

The decline of local retail outlets has given rise to the claim that many low-income neighbourhoods in industrialized countries have become 'food deserts'. Cummins and Macintyre's (2006) review of food availability and pricing studies found that American and Canadian 'healthier' foods were less available and more costly in low-income neighbourhoods. In the US, income inequalities also appear to coincide with racial divisions. One study found that supermarkets were on average 1.15 miles further away for residents in black compared to white neighbourhoods (Cummins and Macintyre, 2006). However, these associations are less clear in other industrialized countries such as the UK, Australia and the Netherlands. For example, a Glasgow study found that 57 foods representing 'a modest but adequate diet' were slightly more available in areas of deprivation and that prices varied little by area, but it was also notable that high-fat and high-sugar foods were cheaper in poorer areas of the city (Cummins and Macintyre, 2002).

While many low-income areas have seen a decline in retail grocery outlets, fast-food outlets appear to have become more prevalent and more accessible in comparison to affluent areas (Cummins and Macintyre, 2006). Fast food is becoming an increasingly important part of people's diets in industrialized countries (Millstone and Lang, 2003). This has dietary implications because these foods tend to be high in animal fats and are up to 65% more energy dense than the average diet. In England and Scotland, MacDonald's restaurants are more likely to be located in areas of social deprivation (Cummins et al., 2005). There is some evidence to suggest that these associations may explain higher rates of obesity in these neighbourhoods.

Other studies emphasize how food accessibility is more than just a question of proximity to shops. Hitcham et al.'s (2002) London-based study found that people on low incomes in the same streets had very different levels of access and patterns of shopping. Older people's diets were particularly sensitive to local shop closures. Given the personal nature of local shops, their closure also represented the loss of a social resource, which in turn reduced their everyday support networks. Street crime, vandalism and personal threats deterred older people from using public transport and shopping further afield. Dietary inequalities therefore connect to wider social issues. Hitcham et al. (2002, p. 9) argue that 'the geography of food poverty cannot simply be drawn on a map'.

Poor diets and food insecurity also have a relationship to gender dynamics within low-income households. While women have increasingly become active in the labour market, gender roles around domestic work have been slower to change. British Social Attitudes surveys show that in 70% of households, women make the evening meal and continue to do the majority of routine shopping (Lupton, 2000).

The interviewees who took part in Hitcham et al.'s study (2002) often suggested that men were unskilled at shopping efficiently within a budget. Regular and often unsociable working hours for many working women on low incomes meant it was difficult to prepare and coordinate regular family meals. Participants also reported how these pressures combined with the demands of family members to meet individual taste preferences. Hitcham et al. (2002, p. 9) found that cooks (usually women) did not lack awareness of 'healthy diets', nor did they lack skills in food preparation, but that 'achieving a nutritious diet on a low income requires

extraordinary levels of persistence, flexibility and awareness'. The social causation perspective has therefore sought to identify the sum of social influences that determine poor diets in industrialized countries.

Social constructionist perspectives on food, risk and insecurity

The second group of theoretical approaches has been concerned with the social meaning of diets and eating practices. Here, we consider how this approach has been used to explore perceptions of diet-related choice and food anxieties.

Giddens (1991) has noted how, for many people in the West, diets involve a bewildering array of choices of what and where to buy, how to cook and how to consume. Increasingly, these choices are not informed by tradition but are perceived to be 'expressions of identity': eating has become one very visible aspect of personal decision-making. While these choices appear to present unparalleled possibilities for self-expression, Giddens and, in a similar vein, Beck (1992) argue that they also entail new forms of insecurity. For example, eating disorders among young people could be seen to have their origins in the profound opportunities *and* strains of contemporary life. According to Frost (2003), eating practices, especially for young women, have become intimately associated with creating an ideal body image and moral strength of character. Yet, the very freedom to self-create the body – and by inference one's identity – carries a burden that propels some young people into dietary disorders and self-starvation.

Where established beliefs and practices are less salient, it also becomes less clear where we invest trust. For Beck and Giddens, individuals under conditions of late modernity have become increasingly conscious of food hazards produced by the technologies of the era. Food scares associated with, for example, BSE, genetically modified foods and salmonella mean that everyday foods are associated with health threats. Given that many of these risks are not readily perceptible, our food decisions are reliant on expert – and often medical – advice. Lupton (2005, p. 449) suggests that food advice has become 'deeply medicalized in its association with health, illness and disease'. However, this advice is often difficult to interpret or inconsistent in nature. For example, it may be difficult to make dietary choices based on complex information about 'good' and 'bad' fats, or the glycaemic index of carbohydrates.

Thus, our management of food hazards involves the individual in complex assessments and the balancing of diverse sets of 'risks' and benefits. We have to eat, but it can feel like a risky business. Clear decisions cannot readily be reached simply through the application of more knowledge or greater scientific awareness. Under these circumstances, social constructionists have sought to explore how people interpret food risks as part of everyday experience. Green et al. (2003) found that overt expressions of insecurity were exceptions rather than the norm. Everyday decision-making around food safety was presented as a routine endeavour, aided by a number of 'short cuts' or 'rules of thumb'. Similarly, Shaw's study (2004) of microbiological safety and BSE found that participants were able to locate their decisions in different contexts and, in so doing, brought competing logic to bear on risk decisions.

Discourse that surrounds food uncertainties can also be seen to serve ideological functions. Green et al. (2003) suggests that the language of safety was recurrently used by white study participants to explain reasons for avoiding 'ethnic (that is, Indian and Chinese) restaurants'. The researchers suggest that this 'risk speak' provided an apparently neutral framework for expressing disparaging and often racialized judgements of other social groups.

Food risk discourses are therefore often based in what Bourdieu (1984) described as 'processes of distinction', that is, they act as vehicles for marking out and making judgements of group identity. Thus Green et

al. (2003, p. 50) found that older age groups expressed active unconcern about risks:

> For older consumers, demonstrating their resistance to risk ... contributed to their rhetorical construction of 'modernity' as overly concerned and anxious about risk, and themselves as 'survivors' who were to some extent invulnerable to risk.

Although a lot of social constructionist work has concentrated on individual perceptions of food risks, more recent studies have explored interpersonal negotiations and, notably, family dynamics of dietary behaviours. Drawing on parental perceptions and understandings of 'normal weight' and 'overweight' young teenagers living in poorer socioeconomic circumstances, Backett-Milburn et al. (2006) explored the negotiations between parents and their children, arguing that parents lacked a discourse to talk about weight and overweight among their teenage children. Dietary issues were 'a fairly low priority in the hierarchy of health-relevant and other risks facing their teenagers' (Backett-Milburn et al., 2006, p. 624). Their study illustrates how social constructionist approaches can complement social causation theory. For many people on low incomes, weight-related issues have to be understood in the context of other risks that are perceived to be of greater importance.

Conclusion

This case study has provided a discussion of the ways in which sociological perspectives might apply to the study of food and diets. Although there are considerable differences, social causation and social constructionist approaches share some concerns common to most sociological enquiry. Both have an interest in the socially patterned nature of food consumption and the socially embedded character of individual choice. While it is commonplace to believe that dietary beliefs and practices are essentially personal matters, sociological accounts have sought to locate them in a wider social context.

Summary

- Sociology – the study of human social life – has addressed many issues concerning people's experiences of health and illness, and the organization of healthcare services

- A key theme in this area is the social patterning of health, ill health and premature death. Groups with less access to money and other material resources experience poorer health and a higher premature death rate. Societies with more egalitarian structures enjoy better health than more unequal societies

- There are several different sociological perspectives, ranging from those such as functionalism, which emphasizes the value of social consensus and continuity, to those such as Marxism and political economy, which emphasize the sources of social conflict and change

- Sociologists have explored the links between medical power and other social stratification variables such as gender and ethnicity

- Sociology involves the critical examination of data, such as mortality rates, and the testing of theoretical frameworks and propositions

Questions for further discussion

1. Analyse the emergence of HIV/AIDS as a health issue using social causation and social constructionist approaches.

2. Think back to recent encounters with the medical establishment. Critically analyse these encounters using sociological concepts.

3. To what extent are health-related behaviours socially determined? Illustrate your answer with reference to a specific behaviour, for example alcohol consumption or exercise patterns.

Further reading

The sociology of health and illness is an extensive subject and this brief introduction can only indicate some of the central concerns, trends and debates in sociological research. The following list includes general texts on the sociology of health and illness as well as writings on specific topics that are well worth the effort of reading.

Annandale, E. (2014) *The Sociology of Health and Medicine* (2nd edn). Oxford: Polity. Excellent account of the relationship between critical social theory and medical sociology. Quite wide ranging, with particularly useful sections on health status, social stratification and health inequalities.

Bartley, M. (2004) *Health Inequality: An Introduction to Theories, Concepts and Methods*. Cambridge: Polity.
Useful resource for understanding key theories of health inequality and the methods employed by researchers in this field. Seeks to bridge some of the disciplinary divides between sociology, psychology and biology and show how all can contribute to the study of health inequalities.

Blaxter, M. (2004) *Health*. Cambridge: Polity.
Discusses how health is defined, constructed, experienced and acted out, drawing on a range of empirical data and theoretical approaches for Western countries.

Cockerham, W.C. (2013) *Social Causes of Health and Disease* (2nd edn). Cambridge: Polity.
Stimulating argument that social factors such as stress, poverty, unhealthy lifestyles and unpleasant living and work conditions have direct causal effects on health and many diseases.

Daykin, N. and Doyal, L. (eds) (1999) *Work and Health: Critical Perspectives*. Basingstoke: Macmillan.
Edited collection of articles that set out to redefine the traditional boundaries of occupational health and work. Shows how a sociological approach can broaden commonsense understandings of what we mean by 'work' and 'health'.

Doyal, L. (1995) *What Makes Women Sick? Gender and the Political Economy of Women's Health*. Basingstoke: Macmillan.
Key text devoted to sociology and gender issues. Explores the structuralist and materialist perspectives on gender inequalities in society, with a particular focus on why women report more ill health than men, despite their greater longevity.

Frank, A. (1995) *The Wounded Storyteller: Body, Illness and Ethics*. Chicago: University of Chicago Press.
Suggests that ill people are more than victims of disease or patients of medicine; they are wounded storytellers. Uses a biographical approach to show how people tell stories to make sense of their suffering and argues that, when they turn their diseases into stories, they find healing.

Gabe, J., Kelleher, D. and Williams, G. (eds) (2006) *Challenging Medicine* (2nd edn). London: Routledge.
Appraisal of changes to the health service and their effects on the status and practice of health professionals. Draws on debates around the expertise of medical professionals in the context of a rapidly changing social environment.

Lupton, D. and Tulloch, J. (2003) *Risk and Everyday Life*. London: Sage.
The study of risk has become closely connected to health studies. This book explores how people respond to, experience and think about risk as part of their everyday lives. Shows how sociological theory can provide a bridge between private and wider public concerns.

Nettleton, S. (2013) *The Sociology of Health and Illness* (2nd edn). Cambridge: Polity.
Accessible text providing a wide-ranging overview of the field. Gives clear explanations of concepts, theories and debates. Good use is made of contemporary research evidence.

Finally, it is important to remember that sociological research often appears in journals before it is described in books. Relevant journals include the *Sociology of Health and Illness*, *Social Science and Medicine*, *Women's Studies International Forum*, *Health Promotion International* and the *International Journal of Health Services*.

References

Acheson, D. (1998) *Independent Inquiry into Inequalities in Health Report*. London: TSO.

Adler, N., Boyce, T., Chesney, M. et al. (1994) 'Socioeconomic status and health: the challenge of the gradient'. *American Psychologist* 49: 15–24.

Ahmad, W.I. (1993) Making black people sick: 'race', ideology and health research, in W.I. Ahmad (ed.) *'Race' and Health in Contemporary Britain*. Milton Keynes: Open University Press, pp. 11–13.

Annandale, E. and Hunt, K. (1990) 'Masculinity, femininity and sex: an exploration of their relative contribution to explaining gender differences in health'. *Sociology of Health and Illness* 12: 24–46.

Arber, S. (1998) Health, ageing and older women, in L. Doyal (ed.) *Women and Health Services: An Agenda for Change*. Buckingham: Open University Press, pp. 54–68.

Arber, S. and Khlat, M. (2002) 'Introduction to "social and economic patterning of women's health in a changing world"'. *Social Science and Medicine* 54(5): 643–7.

Arber, S. and Thomas, H. (2001) From women's health to gender analysis of health, in W.C. Cockerham (ed.) *The Blackwell Companion to Medical Sociology*. Oxford: Blackwell, pp. 94–113.

Armstrong, D. (1995) 'The rise of surveillance medicine'. *Sociology of Health and Illness* 17(3): 393–404.

Backett-Milburn, K., Wills, W., Gregory, S. and Lawton, J. (2006) 'Making sense of eating, weight and risk in the early teenage years: views and concerns of parents in poorer socio-economic circumstances'. *Social Science and Medicine* 63(3): 624–35.

Bartley, M. (2004) *Health Inequality: An Introduction to Theories, Concepts and Methods*. Cambridge: Polity.

Bartley, M., Blane, D. and Davey Smith, G. (1998) 'Introduction: beyond the Black Report'. *Sociology of Health and Illness* 20(5): 563–77.

Bartley, M., Sacker, A. and Clarke, P. (2004) 'Employment status, employment conditions, and limiting illness: prospective evidence from the British household panel survey 1991–2001'. *Journal of Epidemiology and Community Health* 58(6): 501–6.

Baum, F. (1999) 'Social capital: is it good for your health? Issues for a public health agenda'. *Journal of Epidemiology and Community Health* 53: 195–6.

Beck, U. (1992) *Risk Society: Towards a New Modernity*. London: Sage.

Ben-Shlomo, Y. and Kuh, D. (2002) 'A life course approach to chronic disease epidemiology: conceptual models, empirical challenges and interdisciplinary perspectives'. *International Journal of Epidemiology* 31(2): 285–93.

Bloomfield, K., Grittner, U., Kramer, S. and Gmel, G. (2006) 'Social inequalities in alcohol consumption and alcohol-related problems in the study countries of the EU concerted action Gender, Culture and Alcohol Problems: A Multi-National Study'. *Alcohol and Alcoholism* 41(suppl. 1): i26–36.

Bourdieu, P. (1984) *Distinction: A Social Critique of the Judgement of Taste*. London: Routledge.

Bury, M. (1982) 'Chronic illness as biographical disruption'. *Sociology of Health and Illness* 4(2): 167–82.

Bury, M. (2001) 'Illness narratives: fact or fiction?' *Sociology of Health and Illness* 23(3): 263–85.

Cameron, E. and Bernades, J. (1998) 'Gender and disadvantage in health: men's health for a change'. *Sociology of Health and Illness* 20(5): 673–93.

Caraher, M. and Coveney, J. (2004) 'Public health nutrition and food policy'. *Public Health Nutrition* 7(5): 591–8.

Courtenay, W.H. (2000) 'Constructions of masculinity and their influence on men's well-being: a theory of gender and health'. *Social Science and Medicine* 50(10): 1385–401.

Crossley, M. (1998) '"Sick role" or "empowerment": the ambiguities of life with an HIV positive diagnosis'. *Sociology of Health and Illness* 20(4): 507–31.

Cummins, S. and Macintyre, S. (2002) 'A systematic study of an urban landscape: the price and availability of food in Greater Glasgow'. *Urban Studies* 39(21): 195–7.

Cummins, S. and Macintyre, S. (2006) 'Food environments and obesity: Neighbourhood or nation?' *International Journal of Epidemiology* 35(1): 100–4.

Cummins, S., McKay, L. and Macintyre, S. (2005) 'McDonald's restaurants and neighborhood deprivation in Scotland and England'. *American Journal of Preventive Medicine* 29(4): 308–10.

Davey Smith, G. (ed.) (2003) *Health Inequalities: Lifecourse Approaches*. Cambridge: Polity.

Davey Smith, G., Dorling, D., Mitchell, R. and Shaw, M. (2002) 'Health inequalities in Britain: continuing increases up to the end of the 20th century'. *Journal of Epidemiology and Community Health* 56, 434–5.

Davies, C. (1995) *Gender and the Professional Predicament in Nursing*. Buckingham: Open University Press.

Daykin, N. and Clarke, B. (2000) '"They'll still get the bodily care". Discourses of care and relationships between nurses and health care assistants in the NHS'. *Sociology of Health and Illness* 22(3): 349–63.

De Visser, R. and Smith, J.A. (2006) 'Mister in-between: a case study of masculine identity and health-related behaviour'. *Journal of Health Psychology* 11(5): 685–95.

DH (Department of Health) (1999) *Saving Lives: Our Healthier Nation*. London: TSO.

Doyal, L. (1995) *What Makes Women Sick? Gender and the Political Economy of Health*. Basingstoke: Macmillan – now Palgrave Macmillan.

Doyal, L. (ed.) (1998) *Women and Health Services: An Agenda for Change*. Buckingham: Open University Press.

Doyal, L. (2001) 'Sex, gender and health: the need for a new approach'. *British Medical Journal* 323(7320): 1061–3.

Drever, F. and Bunting, J. (1997) Patterns and trends in male mortality, in F. Drever and M. Whitehead (eds) *Health Inequalities*. Decennial Supplement. ONS, Series DS No. 15. London: TSO, pp. 95–107.

Drever, F. and Whitehead, M. (eds) (1997) *Health Inequalities*. Decennial Supplement. ONS, Series DS No. 15. London: TSO.

Dundas, R., Morgan, M., Redfern, J. et al. (2001) 'Ethnic differences in behavioural risk factors for stroke: implications for health promotion'. *Ethnicity and Health* 6(2): 95–103.

Durkheim, E. (1952) *Suicide*. London: Routledge & Kegan Paul.

Everingham, C. (2001) 'Reconstituting community: social justice, social order and the politics of community'. *Australian Journal of Social Issues* 36(2): 105–22.

Foster, P. (1995) *Women and the Health Care Industry: An Unhealthy Relationship?* Buckingham: Open University Press.

Foucault, M. (1976) *The Birth of the Clinic: An Archaeology of Medical Perception*. London: Tavistock.

Foucault, M. (1979a) *The History of Sexuality*, vol. 1. London: Allen Lane.

Foucault, M. (1979b) *Discipline and Punish: The Birth of the Prison*. New York: Vintage.

Frank, A.W. (1991) For a sociology of the body: an analytical review, in M. Featherstone, M. Hepworth and B.S. Turner (eds) *The Body: Social Process, Cultural Theory*. London: Sage, pp. 36–103.

Frank, R. (2001) 'A reconceptualization of the role of biology in contributing to race/ethnic disparities in health outcomes'. *Population Research and Policy Review* 20(6): 441–55.

Freidson, E. (1970) *Professional Dominance*. New York: Atherton.

Frost, L. (2003) 'Doing bodies differently? Gender, youth, appearance and damage'. *Journal of Youth Studies* 6(1): 55–70.

Giddens, A. (1991) *Modernity and Self-identity: A Study of Comparative Sociology*. London: Polity.

Goffman, E. (1963) *Stigma*. London: Penguin.

Gough, B. and Conner, M.T. (2006) 'Barriers to healthy eating amongst men: a qualitative analysis'. *Social Science and Medicine* 62(2): 387–95.

Graham, H. (1987) 'Women's smoking and family health'. *Social Science and Medicine* 25(1): 47–56.

Graham, H. (1998) Health at risk: poverty and national health strategies, in L. Doyal (ed.) *Women and Health Services: An Agenda for Change*. Buckingham: Open University Press, pp. 22–38.

Green, J., Draper, A. and Dowler, E. (2003) 'Short cuts to safety: risk and "rules of thumb" in accounts of food choice'. *Health, Risk and Society* 5(1): 33–52.

Harding, S. and Rosato, M. (1999) 'Cancer incidence among first generation Scottish, Irish, West Indian and South Asian migrants living in England and Wales'. *Ethnicity and Health* 4(1/2): 83–92.

Hitcham, C., Christie, I., Harrison, M. and Lang, T. (2002) *Inconvenience Food: The Struggle to Eat Well on a Low Income*. London: Demos

Illich, I. (1977) *The Limits to Medicine*. Harmondsworth: Penguin.

Illsley, R. (1986) 'Occupational class, selection and the production of inequalities in health'. *Quarterly Journal of Social Affairs* 2(2): 151–65.

Johnson, T. (1993) Expertise and the state, in M. Gane and T. Johnson (eds) *Foucault's New Domains*. London: Routledge, pp. 139–53.

Johnson, T. (1995) Governmentality and the institutionalisation of expertise, in T. Johnson, G. Larkin and M. Saks (eds) *Professions and the State in Europe*. London: Routledge, pp. 7–24.

Jones, M. (2004) 'Anxiety and containment in the risk society: theorising young people's drugs policy'. *International Journal of Drug Policy* 15: 367–76.

Kamphuis, C., Giskes, K., de Bruijn, G. et al. (2006) 'Environmental determinants of fruit and vegetable consumption among adults: a systematic review'. *British Journal of Nutrition* 96(4): 620–35.

Kawachi, I., Kennedy, B.P. Lochner, K. et al. (1997) 'Social capital, income inequality, and mortality'. *American Journal of Public Health* 87(9): 1491–9.

Knight, R., Shoveller, J.A., Oliffe, J.L. et al. (2012) 'Masculinities, "guy talk" and "manning up": a discourse analysis of how young men talk about sexual health'. *Sociology of Health and Illness* 34(8): 1246–61.

Kunst, A.E., Feikje, G., Mackenbach, J.P. and the EU Working Group on Socioeconomic Inequalities in Health (1998) 'Mortality by occupational class among men 30–64 years in 11 European countries'. *Social Science and Medicine* 46(11): 1459–76.

Lang, T. (2005) 'Food control or food democracy? Re-engaging nutrition with society and the environment'. *Public Health Nutrition* 8(1): 730–7.

Lang, T. and Heasman, M. (2004) *Food Wars the Global Battle for Mouths, Minds and Markets*. London: Earthscan.

Lantz, P., Lynch, J., House, J. et al. (2001) 'Socio-economic disparities in health change in a longitudinal study of US adults: the role of health-risk behaviours'. *Social Science and Medicine* 53(1): 29–40.

Lawlor, D.A., Ebrahim, S. and Davey Smith, G. (2001) 'Sex matters: secular and geographical trends in sex differences in coronary heart disease mortality'. *British Medical Journal* 323(7312): 541–5.

Lloyd, L. (1999) The wellbeing of carers: an occupational health concern, in N. Daykin and L. Doyal (eds) *Health and Work: Critical Perspectives*. Basingstoke: Macmillan – now Palgrave Macmillan, pp. 54–70.

Lupton, D. (1995) *The Imperative of Health: Public Health and the Regulated Body*. London: Sage.

Lupton, D. (2000) Food, risk and subjectivity, in S. Williams, J. Gabe and M. Calnan (eds) *Health, Medicine and Society: Key Theories, Future Agendas*. London: Routledge, pp. 425–35.

Lupton, D. (2005) 'Lay discourses and beliefs related to food risks: an Australian perspective'. *Sociology of Health and Illness* 27(4): 448–67.

Lynch, J., Due, P., Muntaner, C. and Davey Smith, G. (2000) 'Social capital: Is it a good investment strategy for public health?' *Journal of Epidemiology and Community Health* 54(6): 404–8.

Mackenbach, J.P. (2012) 'The persistence of health inequalities in modern welfare states: the explanation of a paradox'. *Social Science and Medicine* 75(4): 761–9.

McTaggart, L. (1996) *What Doctors Don't Tell You: The Truth about the Dangers of Modern Medicine*. London: Thorsons.

Manly, J.J. (2006) 'Deconstructing race and ethnicity: implications for measurement of health outcomes'. *Medical Care* 44(11): S10–16.

Marmot, M. (2004) *Status Syndrome: How your Social Standing Directly Affects your Health and your Life Expectancy*. London: Bloomsbury.

Marmot, M., Allen, J., Goldblatt, P. et al. (2010) *Fair Society, Healthy Lives: A Strategic Review of Health Inequalities in England Post-2010*. London: The Marmot Review.

Martin, G.P., Myles, L., Minion, J. et al. (2013) 'Between surveillance and subjectification: professionals and the governance of quality and patient safety in English hospitals'. *Social Science and Medicine* 99: 80–8.

Mead, G.H. (1934) *Mind, Self and Society from the Standpoint of Social Behaviourism*. Chicago: Chicago University Press.

Millstone, E. and Lang, T. (2003) *The Atlas of Food: Who Eats What, Where and Why*. Brighton: Earthscan.

Moss, N.E. (2002) 'Gender equity and socioeconomic inequality: a framework for the patterning of women's health'. *Social Science and Medicine* 54: 649–61.

Navarro, V. (1979) *Medicine under Capitalism*. London: Croom Helm.

Navarro, V. (2004) 'The politics of health inequalities research in the United States'. *International Journal of Health Services* 34(1): 87–99.

Nazroo, J.Y. (1997) *The Health of Britain's Ethnic Minorities: Findings from a National Survey*. London: Policy Studies Institute.

Nazroo, J.Y. (2001) *Ethnicity, Class and Health*. London: Policy Studies Institute.

ONS (Office for National Statistics) (2011a) *Trends in Life Expectancy by National Statistics Socio-economic Classification 1982–2006*. London: ONS.

ONS (2011b) *General Lifestyle Survey Overview: A Report on the 2009 General Lifestyle Survey*. London: ONS.

ONS (2013a) *General Health: Report on the 2011 General Lifestyle Survey*. London: ONS.

ONS (2013b) *Self-assessed General Health for Males and Females, England & Wales 2011*. London: ONS.

ONS (2013c) *Ethnic Variations in General Health and Unpaid Care Provision 2011*. London: ONS.

ONS (2014a) *Mortality Rates*. Available at www.ons.gov.uk/ons/rel/vsob1/mortality-statistics--deaths-registered-in-england-and-wales--series-dr-/2012/sty-causes-of-death.html (accessed 20/3/14).

ONS (2014b) *Suicides in the United Kingdom, 2012 Registrations*. London: ONS.

Parsons, T. (1951) *The Social System*. London: Routledge & Kegan Paul.

Parsons, T. (1975) 'The sick role and the role of the physician reconsidered'. *Millbank Memorial Fund Quarterly* 53(3): 257–78.

Payne, S. (1998) 'Hit and miss': the success and failure of psychiatric services for women, in L. Doyal (ed.) *Women and Health Services: An Agenda for Change*. Buckingham: Open University Press, pp. 83–99.

Porter, S. (1992) 'The poverty of professionalisation: a critical analysis of strategies for the occupational advancement of nursing'. *Journal of Advanced Nursing* 17: 720–6.

Porter, S. (1999) *Social Theory and Nursing Practice*. Basingstoke: Macmillan – now Palgrave Macmillan.

Portes, A. (1998) 'Social capital: its origins and applications in modern sociology'. *Annual Review of Sociology* 24: 1–24.

Priest, N., Paradies, Y., Trenerry, B. et al. (2013) 'A systematic review of studies examining the relationship between reported racism and health and wellbeing for children and young people'. *Social Science and Medicine* 95: 115–27.

Putnam, R.D. (1995) 'Bowling alone: America's declining social capital'. *Journal of Democracy* 6(1): 65–78.

Radcliffe, E., Lowton, K. and Morgan, M. (2013) 'Co-construction of chronic illness narratives by older stroke survivors and their spouses'. *Sociology of Health and Illness* 36(7): 993–1007.

Roberts, I. and Power, C. (1996) 'Does the decline in child injury mortality vary by social class? A comparison of class specific mortality in 1981 and 1991'. *British Medical Journal* 313(7060): 784–6.

Robertson, S. (2006) '"Not living life in too much of an excess": lay men understanding health and well-being'. *Health* 10(2): 175–89.

Shaw, A. (2004) 'Discourses of risk in lay accounts of microbiological safety and BSE: a qualitative interview study'. *Health, Risk and Society* 6(2): 151–71.

Shaw, A., McMunn, A. and Field, J. (eds) (2000) *The Scottish Health Survey 1998*. London: TSO.

Shaw-Taylor, Y. (2002) 'Culturally and linguistically appropriate health care for racial or ethnic minorities: analysis of the US Office of Minority Health's recommended standards'. *Health Policy* 62: 211–21.

Stacey, M. (1988) *The Sociology of Health and Healing*. London: Unwin Hyman.

Townsend, P. and Davidson, N. (1982) *Inequalities in Health: The Black Report*. London: Penguin.

Türmen, T. (2003) 'Gender and HIV/AIDS'. *International Journal of Gynecology and Obstetrics* 82(3): 411–18.

Van Rossum, C., Shipley, M., van de Mheen, H. et al. (2000) 'Employment grade differences in cause specific mortality: a 25 year follow up of civil servants from the first Whitehall study'. *Journal of Epidemiology and Community Health* 54(3): 178–84.

Weich, S., Nazroo, J., Sproston, K. et al. (2004) 'Common mental disorders and ethnicity in England: the empiric study'. *Psychological Medicine* 34(8): 1543–51.

WHO (World Health Organization) (2008) *Closing the Gap in a Generation: Health Equity through Action on the Social Determinants of Health*. Final Report, Commission on Social Determinants of Health. Geneva: WHO.

WHO (2010) *Conceptual Framework for Action on Social Determinants of Health*. Geneva: WHO. Available at www.who.int/sdhconference/resources/ ConceptualframeworkforactiononSDH_eng.pdf (accessed 21/10/2011).

WHO (2014) *Global Health Observatory Data Repository: Life Expectancy by Country*. Available at http://apps.who.int/gho/data/node.main.688?lang=en (accessed 20/3/2014).

Wilkinson, R.G. (1996) *Unhealthy Societies: The Afflictions of Inequality*. London: Routledge.

Wilkinson, R.G. and Pickett, K. (2009) *The Spirit Level: Why More Equal Societies Almost Always Better*. London: Allen Lane.

Williams, G.H. (2003) 'The determinants of health: structure, context and agency'. *Sociology of Health and Illness* 25(3): 131–54.

Wilsnack, R.W., Kristianson, A.F., Wilsnack, S.C. and Crosby, R.D. (2006) 'Are US women drinking less (or more)? Historical and aging trends, 1981–2001'. *Journal of Studies on Alcohol* 67(3): 341–8.

Witz, A. (1992) *Professions and Patriarchy*. London: Routledge.

Zola, I. (1972) 'Medicine as an institution of social control'. *Sociological Review* 20(4): 487–504.

Geography and health

Overview	197
Introduction	197
Part 1 The contribution of geography to health studies	199
Linking places to health through the natural environment	200
Linking places to health through the built environment	206
Linking places to health through the sociocultural environment	210
Part 2 Theoretical and research approaches	213
Health mapping	214
Geographic information systems	216
Case study Obesity and the built environment	219
Summary	222
Questions for further discussion	222
Further reading	223
References	224

Learning outcomes

This chapter will enable readers to:

- Understand the role of the natural environment in the causation and control of disease
- Understand the role of the built environment in the causation and control of disease
- Appreciate how modern geospatial technology and techniques help to monitor, analyse and control disease
- Appreciate how human behaviour may change the environment, contributing to health problems

Overview

Think about where you are for a moment – your country, your city or town, where you work, the place you sleep; all the places where you spend different parts of your life, through various processes, affect your health. If you live in a poor, rural community in Nigeria, particularly if you spend time in and around local rivers, you might be at risk of contracting *onchocerciasis* (river blindness), caused by a parasitic nematode (roundworm), which can lead to blindness among victims as early as age 20. In Mexico City, you might occasionally experience extremely high levels of air pollution – so high that the city shuts down industry and restricts traffic for days at a time. On the other hand, Tokyo, an even larger city, has taken great measures to curb pollution over the past few decades, and the air quality is good by comparison. The environment can affect your health through social mechanisms, through how you are treated because of your identity – the way you and society view your race, gender and other social traits. Being a middle-income African woman in Costa Rica has different implications for health, healthcare and health-related behaviours than it does in South Africa or Scotland.

This chapter focuses on how the processes around locations affect health and how, by studying these processes, we can gain a more complete understanding of how places and spaces are linked to health. While a central tenet of geographic inquiry is recognition of the deep links between different facets of places, Part 1 is organized into sections by the key parts of environment examined by geographers: the natural, built and social environments. Part 2 discusses how maps – a basic part of the 'language' of the discipline – and modern geospatial technologies can contribute to studies of health. The chapter concludes with a case study of some of the ways that the recent obesity epidemic is profoundly related to places and the environment.

Introduction

The word 'geography' comes from the Greek roots *ge* (earth) and *graphein* (to write). Geography is the study the study of *places* and *spaces* and the processes that drive what happens in them. Space refers to *physical locations* and how they relate to one another. Work that considers how asthma incidence is related to the location of factories that emit sulphur dioxide is an example of a study chiefly concerned with space and *spatial relations*. Place refers to the constructed meaning given to spaces by culture and society. For example, research that examines how different health-related behaviours such as smoking are acceptable in some places and not others is chiefly concerned with place. The discipline has a long history of describing and characterizing geographical regions, but the primary focus of contemporary scholarship is exploring the processes that explain patterns and activities across the earth's surface.

Humans have described the earth with primitive maps for as long as they have conveyed language through writing (Utrilla et al., 2009). Thinking about where one is and one's environment may, in fact, be a fundamental component of human thought. Thus, it is perhaps unsurprising that space and place have played a role in the development of Western medicine since its inception. In his work *On Airs, Waters, and Places*, Hippocrates ([400 BCE] n.d.) wrote:

> Whoever wishes to investigate medicine properly, should proceed thus: ... when one comes into a city to which he is a stranger, he ought to consider ... the waters which the inhabitants use, whether they be marshy and soft, or hard, and running from elevated and rocky situations, and then if saltish and unfit for cooking; and the ground, whether it be naked and deficient in water, or wooded and well watered, and whether it lies in a hollow, confined situation, or is elevated and cold; and the mode in which the inhabitants live, and what are their pursuits, whether they are fond of drinking and eating to excess, and given to indolence, or are fond of exercise and labour, and not given to excess in eating and drinking.

The study of medicine and health in geography seeks to explore the powerful links between spaces, places and health. To understand what happens in a particular place or space, one must have some understanding of the **natural environment**, such as the climate, topography and geology, the **built environment**, such as buildings and transportation infrastructure, and the **social environment**, such as culture, power structures and wealth. Consequently, geographic studies of health, much like geographical study in its broader scope of inquiry, embrace holistic approaches to study; research that draws on a breadth of disciplines and perspectives.

As a result of this fundamentally holistic perspective, many of the distinctions in the topics discussed in this chapter are somewhat artificial. For example, while the distribution of mosquito vectors and their habitats are essential to understanding who gets malaria and where infection rates are high, the built environment, affecting, for example, how water is treated and how habitats are produced by human practices, and the sociocultural environment, such as people's ability and willingness to combat the vector (carrier) or take prophylactic measures against contracting the disease, are also important. While most research of health and disease is designed to address some narrow and focused facet of the environment, geographers are careful to recognize the holistic nature of health in their study. Consequently, many other approaches to the study of health are unified by the geographic study of spaces and places.

Part 1 The contribution of geography to health studies

example 6.1

The application of geography to the study of contemporary health issues

- The role of the natural environment in the causation and control of disease such as malaria
- Climate change and its impact on health through, for example, air quality or heat waves

- The role of the built environment in the causation and control of disease and in influencing health behaviours such as cycling
- The role of the social, cultural and political environments in the causation and control of disease
- Modern geospatial technology and techniques and their contribution to the monitoring, analysis and control of disease

While the deep roots of medical geography can be found among ancient Greek scholars, it emerged as a subdiscipline within geography in its modern sense in the nineteenth and twentieth centuries, perhaps beginning with John Snow's work to map cholera in 1854 (Griffith and Christakos, 2007). Since then, medical geography has evolved along with geography and scholarship more generally, sharing their shifts in paradigms and theoretical perspectives. The systematic study of medical geography as a named, formal subdiscipline of geography can be traced to the first 'Report of the Commission on Medical Geography of Health and Disease to the International Geographic Union' in 1952 (Meade and Emch, 2010).

Medical geography seeks to understand the spatial factors that influence the health of populations, similar to epidemiology (Chapter 3), which seeks to understand the patterning of disease.

connections

Much of the early work in the discipline was on disease ecology, the study of the physical environment and the conditions under which diseases flourish in the human population. The focus of this work was highly quantitative, dedicated to describing and explaining how human beings fit into the life cycle of particular disease pathogens. Similar to other disciplines discussed in this book, the study of medical geography eventually broke from traditional biomedical models and the doctrine of specific aetiology, which posits that there is a single, identifiable agent or pathogen that can cause a disease, and that, by extension, disease can be prevented by avoiding contact with the pathogenic entity. As geographers began to explore the broader relationships between health and space, many began to use an alternative name for the discipline, health geography, to signify that the study had moved 'beyond the driving metaphors of medicine and disease to embrace issues generated by emerging models of disease' (Kearns and Gesler, 1998, p. 2).

The acceptance of health geography perspectives signified a profound critique of the biomedical model, which excludes the social dimensions of health and fails to explain the many forms that health and illness can assume (King, 2010). The study of health and medical geography now includes substantive engagement with modern social theory to consider how culture, identity and power structures interact to affect health, across space and in different places.

connections	Chapter 5 looks at the social patterns of wealth, gender and ethnicity and how these impact on health.

Health and medical geography was forever changed by the emergence of modern geospatial technologies in the 1980s, specifically geographic information systems (GIS), which enable public health researchers and practitioners to map huge quantities of health data. Some of the functions facilitated by GIS include exposure assessment, disease surveillance, healthcare provision management, and spatial analysis of disease patterns, among others. Due in no small part to the emergences of these technologies and techniques, geographical perspectives have gained particular relevance in many health studies topics.

The study of geography in health embraces all these perspectives and approaches to encompass a broad variety of topics and themes, unified by the study of places and spaces, under the inclusive title of 'health and medical geography'. Because of geography's focus on places and the factors that constitute them, the discipline naturally assumes a global perspective, engendering the study with a strong international focus.

Linking places to health through the natural environment

Disease ecology and landscape epidemiology

In his seminal work, *The Ecology of Human Disease*, May (1958), physician and geographer, states that disease cannot arise without the convergence at a certain point in time and space of agent and host. The focus of his work was on the ecological conditions that come together to produce conditions under which diseases thrive. The disease ecology approach to the study of health views human beings as a single component in the life cycle of a disease pathogen. The life cycles of pathogens are often complex and can involve different hosts, or other living organisms the pathogen infects for part of its life cycle. The pathogen may travel between hosts through indirect transmission, via a non-living or living object in the environment. Often, disease vectors, such as mosquitoes or ticks, actively transport the pathogen. Some diseases may infect other animal reservoirs, making controlling the disease even more difficult. All the living organisms involved in the life cycles of disease interact with the biophysical environment in specific ways and are encouraged or deterred by environmental conditions (Figure 6.1).

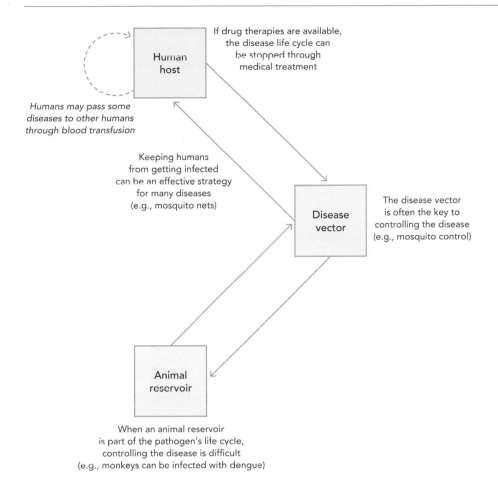

Figure 6.1 **The disease cycle**

Source: Adapted from Meade and Emch, 2010

Related to disease ecology, studies of landscape epidemiology consider the ways in which particular regions provide the conditions that enable disease in human population. Landscape epidemiology examines living and non-living factors of the natural environment. For instance, radon gas, which is emitted from certain types of rock and geological formations, can contribute to the risk of developing lung cancer. Radon gas is an important health problem in southwest England and the Rocky Mountains in western North America, for example, where particular care must be taken to ventilate buildings properly to avoid high levels of exposure to the gas.

The study of disease ecology and landscape epidemiology can enhance our understanding of spatial patterns in health. Once the ecological conditions and needs of the organisms in a disease are well understood, research in geography can then identify specific places that are at risk for disease outbreaks (Lleo et al., 2008), and inform methods for breaking the cycle. For example, hookworm is a parasitic nematode with a fairly simple life cycle that infects the digestive tracts of humans and is passed through faeces. In order to complete its life cycle, the eggs of the worm must be deposited on moist earth with a temperature of 15–25°C. They cannot survive if exposed to direct sunlight or if the acidity of the soil is too high (May, 1958). Thus, the geographical distribution of the disease is largely driven by these environmental factors. It is not prevalent in cold places, particularly in areas where there is significant freezing over winter, or in places with high-quality sanitation systems that prevent the eggs from ever contacting open soil.

Environmental change

Understanding the links between human health and the physical environment is especially important in the context of rapid **environmental change** resulting from human activity, such as urbanization, deforestation and pollution. These sorts of environmental change are closely tied to economic development, and have occurred at an alarmingly rapid pace over the past few centuries. Such rapid environmental change has the potential to fundamentally alter the established natural equilibria between humans and disease pathogens.

Humans and other mammals are at a grave disadvantage in the context of rapid environmental change because disease pathogens and vectors are able to adapt to new conditions far more rapidly. Human beings practise a 'K' reproductive strategy, which means that they produce relatively few offspring with a very high investment of time and energy in order to ensure survival. In contrast, disease pathogens are typically 'r' reproductive strategists, organisms with short life spans that produce a huge number of offspring (Walters, 2003). The 'r' strategy serves to ensure that at least some portion of the offspring will survive in the context of rapid change.

> **?** What changes to the natural environment caused by humans are responsible for infectious diseases?

In recent years, there have been numerous examples of emerging (and re-emerging) infectious diseases (EIDs) – diseases that may appear suddenly and with great virulence. Virtually all EIDs can be explained by human changes to the environment, such the construction of dams, the use of certain food production technologies, deforestation, or human travel or migration (Morse, 1995). Lyme disease is an example of a vector-borne EID. The disease is passed between organisms via tick vectors and requires mammal hosts, such as squirrels or deer, to complete its life cycle. As millions of acres of forest were removed to pave the way for growing cities and suburbs in the US, many of the local ecologies underwent ecosystem simplification, a rapid reduction in the diversity of species. The white-footed deer mouse is a critical species in the life cycle of Lyme disease. When the populations of the white-footed deer mice's natural predators dwindled precipitously as people built houses and settled in the area, the mice flourished. At the same time, human structures provided new, favourable habitats for the mice (hosts) and tick (vectors). The altered ecosystem has proved to be an ideal one for all the components of the Lyme disease cycle, while settlement patterns brought humans into contact with the tick vectors.

Other threats to human health have emerged as the consequence of agricultural practices. In the context of growing industrial agriculture, many producers discovered that they could save money by applying large quantities of antibiotics to livestock in order to prevent disease. In fact, far more antibiotics are currently administered to livestock than human beings. This practice has encouraged the emergence of antibiotic resistant disease – diseases that are highly virulent and resistant to human efforts to control them.

With the growing threat of climate change, the complex links between disease pathogens and the natural environment have become particularly obvious. The widespread – and sometimes seemingly subtle – changes to the environment may have profound impacts on human health through numerous mechanisms. Rising temperatures have enabled key disease vectors, such as mosquitoes, to expand their domain to new territory. Other problems, such as increased reproduction rates, and even the frequency of the vectors' interactions with humans, may also result from higher temperatures (Epstein, 2005). Climate change may affect air quality by altering the level of ozone in breathable air space or altering wind patterns to expose new populations to particulate matter (IPCC, 2007). In the context of warmer temperatures, people who are not accustomed to extremely high temperatures over extended periods of time, in places such as Paris or Chicago, are particularly vulnerable to heat stroke.

> **thinking about** What examples have you heard about the impact of global warming?

In summary, changes in the environment can affect human health by producing conditions to which we are not well adapted, while simultaneously giving disease pathogens an important survival advantage. As we continue to develop our understanding of the causes and consequences of climate change, keen attention to the complex and multifarious relationship between human health and the environment will become more critical than ever before.

example 6.2

Environmental change and dengue fever

Dengue fever is a virus that causes symptoms similar to flu, but can develop into a life-threatening form, known as 'severe dengue'.

The disease was originally endemic to particular regions in Africa, but spread out of the continent with colonialism and increased trade and human travel from the region. The primary vectors for the disease are the *Aedes aegypti* mosquito, the same species that is responsible for spreading malaria, and *Aedes albopictus*, a highly adaptable mosquito that can thrive in cooler environments (WHO, 2013a). The prevalence of dengue fever has increased thirtyfold over the past 50 years, and there have now been significant outbreaks in every WHO region outside Europe (Ranjit and Kissoon, 2011). By 2010, dengue was endemic in over 100 countries and over 2.5 billion people were at risk of contracting the disease (WHO, 2013a).

The reasons for the transformation of this disease from a regional endemic disease to a growing global pandemic can be explained largely through the processes of globalization, urbanization, and human changes to the environment, including climate change. International trade and migration were initially responsible for the disease's spread outside Africa and now that air travel has enabled individuals to travel halfway around the world within a day, there is a constant risk that the disease can spread to any region where the vectors are present.

Another key reason for the growth of the disease is the conditions produced by urbanization. Dengue is considered to be an urban disease because it thrives in the conditions found in urban settlements, which include a high concentration of susceptible human hosts and plenty of small pools of water. Breeding sites are in ample supply in urban settings, where there are ubiquitous discarded containers that fill with water, producing ideal mosquito breeding habitats. In fact, one study cites the proliferation of non-biodegradable packaging as an important factor behind the spread of the disease (Gubler, 1989). The WHO (2013a) recommends that prevention programmes focus on preventing egg-laying habitats for the mosquito by disposing of waste properly, covering outside water containers, and actively managing the local environment.

Climate change is expanding the range of habitats for the vector and disease. One of the critical limiting factors for the disease vector is freezing. Even *Aedes albopictus*, better adapted to cooler temperatures, is constrained by freezing during the winter months. As climate changes ushers in increased temperatures in all regions around the globe, it is only a matter of time before the disease will begin to spread along with warmer temperatures. Indeed, in 2013, there was an outbreak of dengue in the southern coast of Florida (National Public Radio, 2013) and there are growing concerns that it will spread to other places that are less equipped to combat the mosquito vectors.

Population and health

People are undeniably a part of disease ecosystems and many disease pathogens could not exist without a stable human population to infect. All the concepts discussed in this chapter are deeply linked to **demography**, the study of human population and the patterns of population growth. The relationship between human population and health is dynamic; human population and population structures affect health, and human health is, in turn, a driving force behind those structures.

Scholars have long expressed concerns about the implications of a growing human population on health. Thomas Malthus argued in his well-known work, *An Essay on the Principle of Population* (1798), that growth in human population will be limited by famine and disease, leading to the notion that the earth has a specific carrying capacity, a population beyond which the planet will no longer be able to sustain additional human life. Malthus also contributed to ideas about the relationship between economic prosperity and population size, arguing that population increases as a function of the food supply. Since Malthus's time, human beings have significantly expanded their ability to produce sustenance for life through improved agricultural technology and other means. The population of the earth is currently over 7 billion and the UN (2011) estimates that it will reach 8 billion by 2025.

The growth and development of human populations are closely tied to health and disease, described in the demographic transition model (Figure 6.2).

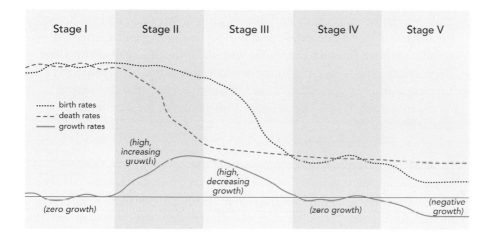

Figure 6.2 **The demographic transition model**

The model is divided into four distinct stages:

- *Stage 1:* In preindustrial society, overall mortality rates are very high. Without sanitation, clean water supplies or a formal healthcare system, infectious disease is a particularly grave problem. At the same time, fertility rates are also very high as families depend on a large number of children for economic and social subsistence.

- *Stage 2:* This is characterized by a precipitous drop in mortality rates as places industrialize. Many of the underlying causes for the high mortality rates improve; clean water and sanitation reduce the likelihood of infectious disease, and the benefits of economic growth reduce many traditional threats to health. At the same time, families continue to have large numbers of children, leading to rapid population growth. As a by-product of the processes of industrialization and economic growth, the burden of disease begins to shift from traditional risks of infectious disease, such as malaria and pneumonia, to modern risks, or diseases resulting from exposure to toxins, such as cancer. Industrialization eventually leads to postmodern risks, or 'lifestyle diseases', such as obesity and heart disease. The shift in the burden of disease is called the 'epidemiologic transition'.

connections   Chapter 3 discusses this shift in the burden of disease and the epidemiologic transition from infectious diseases to chronic diseases.

- *Stage 3:* The cost of having children increases with industrialization (with added education, medical and other costs), which discourages people from having too many children. Birth rates decline, to eventually bring overall growth rates into equilibrium once again.

- *Stage 4:* In industrial or postindustrial societies, birth and death rates exist in relative equilibrium and overall growth rates remain low. Some countries, such as Germany, Russia and Japan, have even experienced negative growth rates and are faced with the difficulties caused by a low dependency ratio – the ratio of the working population compared to the non-working population. Some have even argued that this period of negative growth may characterize a fifth stage of the demographic transition model.

?   What might be a criticism of this model of demographic transition?

One of the critiques of this model is that it oversimplifies the relations between economic development, population, fertility and health. As with any model, this approach to describing these relationships certainly involves substantial simplification of complex phenomena that, in reality, involve a large number of additional factors such as culture. For example, in some places, a deeply embedded tradition of having large families persists despite modernization, whereas in other places, such as China (Attané, 2002), stringent policies designed to curb rapid population growth have significantly reduced the growth rate.

Another critique of the model is that it was developed on the basis of historical European experiences with economic development and population. Nations in other parts of the world may not experience the same progression or may industrialize in a way that is distinct from the path assumed by Europe. In recent years, some countries, for example India, Mexico and Nigeria, have adopted Western lifestyles in their diets and exercise, resulting in increased rates of obesity, while they continue to struggle to overcome high rates of infectious disease (de Onis and Blössner, 2000). The rise of obesity and the health risks that come with it is almost a global phenomenon and many countries are beginning to experience a double burden of disease: high rates of infectious diseases and traditional health risks alongside modern-day health risks such as heart disease and cancer.

Linking places to health through the built environment

Health geographers often distinguish between the natural and built environments. Built environments are the components of the landscape that human beings have constructed, such as houses, roads, dams, schools and cars. Indeed, most of us now spend almost all our time in environments constructed by humans. The distinction between the natural and built environments is often ambiguous, however. Consider, for example, whether natural parks, places where human activity is limited to preserve the natural environment, are truly examples of nature, or a relatively 'natural' form of human construction?

thinking about How does the built environment where you live affect your health?

Urbanization

Throughout most of human history, the vast majority of people have lived in rural environments. With population growth and economic development, populations tend to aggregate in cities and towns, where modern lifestyles and economic opportunities – industry, education and other amenities of modern life – serve as strong pull factors. Urbanization comes with a host of environmental problems and challenges. As Europe urbanized, with increasing portions of its population moving to cities and towns, it was faced with overcrowding and overextended infrastructures, often leading to conditions that are ideal for disease. John Snow's well-known experience in nineteenth-century London, as he sought to determine the sources of a cholera outbreak, occurred precisely in this context (Johnson, 2006).

Chapter 3 describes some of the consequences of urbanization on human health and the nature of epidemiologic inquiry to determine the sources of   **connections** disease.

Starting in 2010, for the first time in human history, more than half of the world population lived in cities (WHO, 2013b). Many cities in low-income regions of the world are not able to accommodate rapid growth. As the industrializing regions of the world experience urbanization, health concerns are emerging that were familiar in Europe during the eighteenth and nineteenth centuries. An estimated 828 million people, roughly one-eighth of the world's population, currently reside in urban slums – areas in large cities where settlements have been improvised using scraps of available material (WHO, 2013c). Urban slums are a significant concern for human health and wellbeing, characterized by little or no access to safe water or sanitation. The WHO (2013c, p. 1) notes that urban slums are 'productive breeding grounds for tuberculosis, hepatitis, dengue, pneumonia, cholera, and diarrhoeal disease'.

Environmental exposures and environmental justice

Living in an urban environment comes with numerous health risks in the form of exposure to environmental toxins. Concentrations of industry in urban areas have introduced non-living agents of disease into the environment, posing a significant burden on human health (Pimentel et al., 2007). Exposures include common air pollutants, such as ozone, particulate matter, sulphur dioxide and lead, which result from daily activities in urban life such as energy production and transportation. Additionally, tens of thousands of synthetic chemicals are produced through industrial processes, of which we have little understanding of their health impacts. Novel synthetic chemicals are designed and produced much too quickly for their health effects to be carefully studied.

Determining the impacts of exposures to environmental pollutants is an extremely challenging research problem. While some environmental toxins have acute or immediate health impacts, most of the health burden is due to chronic or long-term exposures, meaning that decades may pass before the health impacts of an exposure are manifest in observable symptoms. Environmental exposures can be broadly characterized by what part of the environment they exist in – air, water or soil – as well as their route of exposure, or how they enter the human body.

> **?** How do studies in geography differ from epidemiology (Chapter 3) when considering the study of environmental exposures?

Studies in geography focus on the *patterns* and *processes* of exposure and *where* people are most at risk. All facets of the built and natural environments can be taken into account in this work, such as how the network of roads leads to exposures from vehicles or how wind and climate patterns affect where pollutants are transported.

Perhaps an even more interesting question is *why* environmental toxins occur where they do and how economic and social processes lead to the concentration of these toxins in certain locations, placing the health burden on particular groups of people.

> **connections**   Chapter 5 discusses inequalities in health and social determinants that shape health outcomes.

The study of environmental justice examines the social and political dimensions of exposure to health risks. Following roots in social organization, scholars and government organizations have begun to examine the ways that exposures are distributed across space, and many have found that race is the most significant factor explaining the locations of waste facility sites, providing evidence for environmental racism (Bullard, 1990).

example 6.3

Environmental justice

We must accept that there is a price to pay for living in an environment where, at least in rich countries, we can travel down the street or across town to obtain vegetables from another part of the world, we have access to a near-constant supply of power, and we enjoy modern products and technologies, such as computers and mobile phones. The production of these lifestyles inevitably leads to some degradation of the environment. Most forms of energy production, for example, require the release of toxic by-products or living with the risk of environmental disaster, such as nuclear meltdowns.

Everyone in society bears some health risk directly resulting from modern lifestyles. *Who* bears this risk and *how much* risk certain groups bear, however, are often not equal, which is the topic of environmental justice. The concept of environmental justice is rooted in the idea that certain groups in society, particular minority groups and the poor, bear an unequal burden of risk. The environmental justice movement began in the US in the early 1980s as an extension of the social justice activity. African American leaders began to organize in southern US states to protest the decision to locate new waste disposal sites in minority neighbourhoods. Since its origins, awareness of the concepts of environmental justice has expanded to include a variety of different geographical scales and contexts. For example, one study showed that poor and minority groups were more likely to be exposed to toxic release sites in Minneapolis, US (Sheppard et al., 1999), a matter of environmental injustice at the level of a city. The export of electronic waste, used in computer parts and other high technologies, from rich regions to poorer regions where they are recycled or disposed of, usually leading to significant impacts on the environment and health, can be viewed as an environmental justice issue at the global level.

Measuring environmental justice in cities can be tricky. Often, the available data are poor quality and it can be difficult to identify and map specific risks to health; it is often necessary, for example, to provide an incomplete estimate of environmental risk by mapping toxic release sites or high traffic roads. Information about the residents is usually aggregated to administrative units, such as census tracts or electoral districts,

which introduces limitations to analysis. In spite of these limitations, it is possible to use mapping techniques to make a compelling case for environmental justice. Raddatz and Mennis (2013), for example, use GIS to map toxic release sites, welfare recipients and immigrants in Hamburg, Germany. Using a variety of quantitative methods, they demonstrate that poor or minority neighbourhoods are more likely to be near to toxic release sites than wealthier neighbourhoods and other places with fewer immigrants.

There are several explanations for patterns of environmental injustice (Raddatz and Mennis, 2013):

- minorities and poor groups tend have less political power to control where facilities are sited
- the poor are often constrained by economic pressures and have less latitude in choosing where to live
- housing prices are likely to be lower in neighbourhoods with high exposures to environmental toxins
- poor and minority groups may experience discrimination in the housing market
- employment opportunities in industrial occupations, which are often assumed by immigrant groups and people with relatively low education, draw vulnerable groups to these high-risk areas.

In recent years, this field of inquiry has begun to examine equity with respect to environmental amenities, such as access to parks and green spaces, in addition to hazards. In the UK, for example, the most deprived communities are ten times less likely to live in the greenest areas, which are associated with increased longevity and reduced stress (Foresight, 2007). Since patterns of environmental justice are often deeply rooted in historical and political structures, addressing environmental injustice through policy will require much attention and careful research.

connections   Chapter 3 discusses lay epidemiology, whereby communities may collect data to make a case for the disproportionate or unusual impact of a phenomenon on health.

Linking places to health through the sociocultural environment

The concept of environmental justice provides an excellent example of the importance of integrating multiple facets of the environment into studies of health. While the patterns in exposure to environmental toxins are driven by human activities in and around the built environment, mapping those patterns does little to explain how they came to be. Decisions about where to build energy plants, waste sites, or factories occur in the context of the social, cultural and political environments of places. Individuals and institutions make decisions to locate factories and other entities that pose risks to health, ultimately producing the risk environment. Who is empowered to make these decisions is driven by the social and political context. Integrating the social, cultural and political components of environments is embraced by geographers because it enables scholars to consider 'the complex layerings of history, social structure, and built environment that converge in single places' (Kearns and Moon, 2002, p. 611).

Culture

Health geographers have focused their study of culture on how it relates to the natural environment through cultural ecology. May (1958, p. 30) wrote that 'culture influences disease in three main ways: by linking or separating the challenges of the environment and host; by changing the environment, and by changing the host population'.

In a classic example of cultural ecology, May (1958) describes a situation in Northern Vietnam to exemplify how the processes of culture and other characteristics of places come together to influence health. The hill dwellers from one region developed cultural practices that avoided some of the endemic risks to health. They wore shoes to avoid hookworm infection, designed houses to avoid contact with rats, and adopted a diet that prevented them from acquiring beriberi, which is caused by a nutritional deficiency of vitamin B1. When groups of plains dwellers moved into the region, bringing their native cultures with them, they experienced many of these health problems because their behaviours and practices were not adapted to the environment around their new homes.

connections   Chapter 7 discusses how the notion of what health is, what constitutes disease, and what behaviours are acceptable, are components of culture, which is often tied to particular regions and groups of people.

In recent years, geographers have begun to retheorize the very meaning of culture with respect to health. Notably, scholars have emphasized the relation between power and culture, with the recognition that the two are deeply linked. As Kearns and Gesler (1998, p. 13) wrote: 'culture should not be used as a source of explanation; rather it is something to be explained as it is continually being socially produced by people as they struggle to achieve power and meaning'.

Power

An important focus in the social sciences and health geography is the role of power, who controls decisions about health and the frequently subtle ways through which power can impact the lives of different groups of people. In discussions of power, there is often an implicit tension between the roles of individuals and the structures and constraints produced by society.

> Chapter 5 discusses sociological approaches to the study of the relationship between structure and agency.   **connections**

On the one hand, individuals possess the power to alter their own life course – people can decide whether they engage in risky behaviours, such as smoking or drug use. The role and power of individuals to drive their own behaviour is referred to as 'individual agency'. On the other hand, power structures are deeply linked to the processes that frame the social environments of particular places. Political economy approaches to health recognize the role of power structures to constrain (or enable) activities, often serving to produce high-risk environments that directly affect the health of particular groups or identities, a concept known as 'structural violence'. In discussing the extremely high rates of HIV/AIDS in Haiti, for example, Farmer (2001, p. 79) notes that: 'sickness is a result of structural violence: neither culture nor pure individual will is at fault; rather historically given (and often economically driven) processes and forces conspire to constrain individual agency'. Many women in Haiti are faced with dire economic situations that drive them into pressured sexual relations, where their power to engage in safe sexual practices is constrained by economic circumstances and notions of gender.

> Chapter 9 discusses the impact of patriarchal power structures on health outcomes.   **connections**

With geography's focus on human–environment interactions, political economy research is often framed in terms of how it affects human relationships with the environment, a field of inquiry known as 'political ecology'. The political ecology perspective views changes in the environment as a product of human decisions, which are in turn contextualized through political and economic power structures. Social, economic and natural systems are therefore linked in specific places to produce patterns in health. Political ecology can be applied to explain patterns of HIV/AIDS in South Africa, for instance, by drawing on historical power relations (King, 2010). Social and spatial patterns of the disease can be directly tied to interventions designed to intensify agricultural production by the South African government in the early twentieth century. The disease and the consequent impact of changes in adult mortality patterns in turn disrupt the way humans relate to the environment, as families in rural South Africa rely on natural resources – wood for fuel and construction, fruits and herbs, and medicinal plants. As King (2010, p. 49) explains: 'the reciprocal relationships between social and environmental systems merit greater scrutiny, therefore, to understand how human disease reworks demographic and livelihood patterns over time'.

Healthcare and healthcare delivery

The provision of healthcare is fundamental to understanding population patterns in health. Geographers are interested in examining healthcare systems to answer questions such as *how* and *why* it varies across space, where it is available, how social, cultural and political structures affect who has access to healthcare, and how healthcare delivery systems can be optimized across space to provide the most people with access to care.

---

example 6.4

Spatial access to healthcare

Access to healthcare has become an important issue worldwide as healthcare provision systems have only just been developed in some places, and are continually adapting to changing conditions in others. Geographers have employed advanced techniques using mapping and geographic information systems (GIS) to identify shortfalls in the healthcare system by identifying barriers to access or populations that are left out. Changes in the demographic makeup and distribution of a country, the disease profile, or the economic and political structures that govern healthcare can leave some populations underserved.

Much GIS work on analysing healthcare access estimates the service capacity of clinics and hospitals as well as the area they might potentially serve. Brabyn and Beere (2006) use maps of emergency hospitals, populations and the road network in New Zealand to estimate which populations, in which parts of the country, have poor access to emergency healthcare. They base their model on the notion that individuals should be able to reach an emergency healthcare service within an hour using the road network. Due to changes in the healthcare system, hospital closures and changes in the population distribution, they have determined that access has diminished in New Zealand and left some groups, such as the Māori, particularly vulnerable.

The study of healthcare systems is not limited to wealthy countries. In studies of Ghana (Masters et al., 2013) and Nigeria (Feikin et al., 2009), where transportation infrastructure is poor and many people have poor access to cars or public transport, distance is a key factor determining whether individuals are likely to utilize healthcare services when they need it. Geographic research on healthcare provision in low-income contexts can serve to:

- guide where new healthcare services should be located
- delineate where disease outbreaks are likely to occur so as to plan for healthcare provision
- provide evidence of areas in need in order to guide funders and assist them in working with healthcare providers (Brijnath et al., 2012).

Barriers to healthcare can assume a variety of forms, including economic, such as an inability to pay, cultural, such as language barriers for immigrant groups, or social, such as a distrust of the healthcare system. Geographers are especially interested in spatial or physical barriers, such as when there are not enough health facilities near enough to an area to meet the needs of the people who live there. Access to healthcare services is particularly relevant to people in poor, rural regions where resources are scarce (Kinman, 1999).

Chapter 8 outlines developments in health and social care policy. **connections**

Part 2 Theoretical and research approaches

example 6.5

Examples of research in the geography of health

Studies in the geography of health are extremely broad and encompass many topics, but are unified by a thematic focus on space and place:

- How migrating from one ecosystem to another can affect health outcomes (May, 1958)
- The ecological, environmental and demographic factors responsible for the emergence of infectious diseases (Morse, 1995; Ranjit and Kissoon, 2011)
- How climate change affects human health (Epstein, 2005)
- How population growth relates to environmental degradation, and how this affects human health (Pimentel et al., 2007)
- How the processes of globalization and structural changes to the international economic system have affected diets in low-income contexts (Hawkes, 2006)
- Food deserts and how they affect health (Pearson et al., 2005; Apparicio et al., 2007)
- The spatial factors relevant to who has access to healthcare (Brabyn and Gower, 2004; Masters et al., 2013)

A critical instrument in a geographer's toolbox is the map, a graphical representation of the earth's surface. Maps provide a special, spatial language through which geographers may communicate about, study and analyse places. As a biologist uses a microscope to examine processes and features that are too small to be seen by the naked eye, maps serve as a sort of 'macroscope', enabling people to visualize patterns across large areas that are similarly impossible to see with the naked eye. Consequently, geographers frequently utilize 'geospatial analysis', the methods and techniques of studying spatial patterns on the earth's surface. Maps are useful in health studies for communicating, exploring and analysing spatial patterns in health. A key argument throughout this chapter is that health is intimately tied to place, thus the analysis of spatial health information has offered a particularly fruitful perspective for health studies.

> **thinking about** What might a map tell you about the health of your neighbourhood?

Health mapping

The study of maps as a tool for communication has a long history that has involved a great deal of artistic and scientific accomplishment. Maps and spoken language have much in common; both text and maps are symbolic and condensed representations of reality. Maps have their own set of rules, or 'grammar', which, if ignored, may result in maps that are difficult or impossible to understand. Both language and maps, which are able convey a sense of authority to the reader, can be used in a way that can be intentionally or unintentionally misleading. Many geographers study cartography, or map-making, the art and science of communicating information through maps.

Many students of cartography begin by studying the map symbols, the language through which spatial information is conveyed. Health phenomena can be conveyed as:

- points: such as individual cases in an outbreak

- lines: to show the flow or travel of a disease pathogen or disease vector

- areas: as in a map that shows aggregated rates of a disease by a district or province.

Since all maps are hugely simplified abstractions or models of reality, all maps must, by their very definition, present only a tiny slice of reality in all its infinite complexity. Similar to telling a story about any subject, a map is a version of reality that is driven by the subjective preferences of the storyteller.

> **connections**   Chapter 3 includes the map produced by John Snow to examine the patterns of cholera infection in a London neighbourhood in 1854. By exploring the patterns of disease across space, it showed the clear link between cholera deaths and water pumps in the Soho area.

Following John Snow's work, the field of medical cartography grew slowly and steadily until experiencing sudden and transformative growth in recent decades. Organizations, such as the WHO and many national governments, collect and map a broad variety of health information. A common map used by health geographers is the 'choropleth' map, which comprises administrative units that are shaded to show the intensity of a disease rate or other facets of the social environment relevant to health, such as income. The UK's Office for National Statistics, for example, publishes choropleth maps of age-standardized mortality rates in England and Wales (ONS, 2013).

?   What do choropleth maps tell you about health?

When viewing the ONS choropleth maps, spatial patterns become immediately apparent: mortality rates are lowest in the central and southern portions of England, and relatively high in northern England and Wales, with a notable cluster of high rates around Liverpool. When health patterns are clearly visible on a map, physical and social environmental factors are likely to play some role.

Maps can also serve as an excellent tool for analysis and the production of new information or insights from health data. Figure 6.3 illustrates the global data on overweight in 2008, clearly showing on a map the differences across countries. An ecological study enables researchers to compare rates of different factors across aggregated aerial units, such as local authority districts. For example, if there is a correlation between districts with high rates of stomach cancer and certain dietary practices, such as high consumption of salty or smoked meats, the two factors might be related. In ecological studies, one must take caution not to commit the ecological fallacy, the assumption that an association at one scale, such as local authority districts, necessarily correlates to other scales, such as individuals.

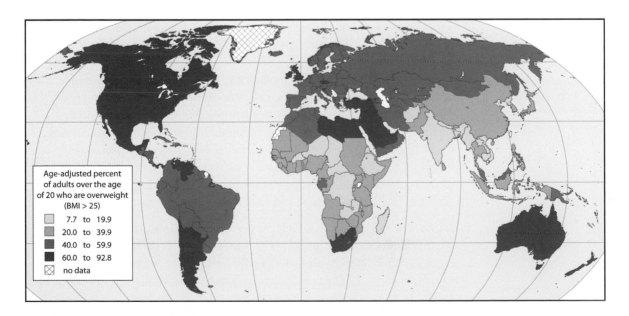

Figure 6.3 Prevalence of overweight, ages 20+, age standardized, both sexes, 2008
Source: WHO, 2013d

Spatial data, with information about location, require careful attention and great care must be taken in analysing and communicating spatial data. Since so much information is collected by administrative districts in health studies, health geographers must pay particular attention to the 'modifiable areal unit problem', the notion that the results of a study that uses aggregated data can change entirely if the borders are redrawn. Spatial epidemiology, also called 'geographical epidemiology', is the study of the methods and techniques for the analysis of spatial data. A key assumption in most parametric statistics is that events that are being analysed are statistically independent from one other, and that the outcome or status of one event is unrelated to other events. Events in space, however, are subjected to the phenomenon of spatial autocorrelation, which states that nearby observations are more alike than distant ones (Waller and Gotway, 2004) and may not be statistically independent.

Geographic information systems

Emerging alongside the advent of modern computer and database technologies over the past few decades, geographic information systems (GIS) have completely revolutionized the fields of mapping and geospatial analysis. A GIS can be defined as 'a computer system capable of capturing, storing, analyzing, and displaying geographically referenced information, that is, data referenced by location' (United States Geological Survey, 2007). In essence, a GIS is a computerized spatial database and map display system that enables spatial analysis. The use of GIS in studies of health continues to grow as the technology becomes more accessible and the availability of digital spatial data grows. A helpful way to think about GIS is to consider it in terms of its basic functions, that is, what it can do with spatial data:

1. *Data capture*: GIS can facilitate data capture, the collection or conversion of spatial data into a digital format. One of the greatest challenges of using GIS, particularly in studies of health, is finding appropriate and accurate data. There are multiple methods for performing data capture, including digitizing paper maps (manually converting written maps into digital form), using geographic positioning systems (GPS) to collect locations in the field, or using data from remote sensing, aircraft or satellites that scan the earth to provide up-to-date information.

2. *Queries of spatial data*: A GIS can perform queries of spatial data to identify features that satisfy specific criteria. For example, a district medical officer might want to identify the capacity for clinics to provide vaccinations for children in a city. Assuming that all the relevant data are available, they could use a query to identify the low-income, child-aged populations within a particular distance of the city's clinics to determine how many low-income people the clinics can serve.

3. *Modelling and analysis:* Most GIS can rapidly perform a large variety of calculations to describe how features relate to one another across space, such as the distance to the nearest hospital for individuals (see Brabyn and Gower, 2004). One of the most powerful analytical features of GIS is its ability to facilitate overlays of multiple sources (or 'layers') of spatial data. For instance, if one is interested in examining what built and natural features are associated with high malaria incidence across India, one might want to consider the locations of rivers, urban areas, precipitation and elevation, all of which can be combined and analysed in a single GIS. Through this kind of work, geographers have identified natural conditions and characteristics that are associated with malaria outbreaks, enabling links to be drawn between land use patterns and malaria (Pope et al., 2005).

To demonstrate the analytical and communicative power of GIS, Figure 6.4 presents a version of John Snow's classic map of cholera deaths around the Broad Street pump in Soho in 1854 that has been digitized into a GIS.

> **?** Compare this map with the conventional version reproduced in Chapter 3. How do they differ in their representation and what they can tell you?

In this map, Thiessen polygons were produced around each water pump, designating the area closest to each pump, and the number of cholera deaths was counted and reported for each polygon. This map clearly shows that the Broad Street pump polygon, the area within which the Broad Street pump was the closest source of water for the residents, had the highest number of cholera deaths.

4. *Display of data:* Most GIS have the ability to manipulate the display of data by changing what features are displayed and how they are symbolized. The rise of GIS has had a significant impact on the study of cartography, as they have expanded the formats and capabilities of maps. Data can now be presented as animated maps to show changes over time, which can highlight the spread or distribution of disease, while 3D visualization facilitates the display of a richer collection of spatial data in a more accessible way.

Key applications of GIS to studies of health

The capabilities of GIS have enabled a broad variety of application and advancement in the study and analysis of health. GIS has revolutionized the techniques for conducting exposure assessment of environmental toxins, such as air or water pollution. Consider, for instance, a study that seeks to examine exposure to air-borne environmental pollution from power plants (Dubnov et al., 2007). Since it is usually impractical or impossible to measure individual

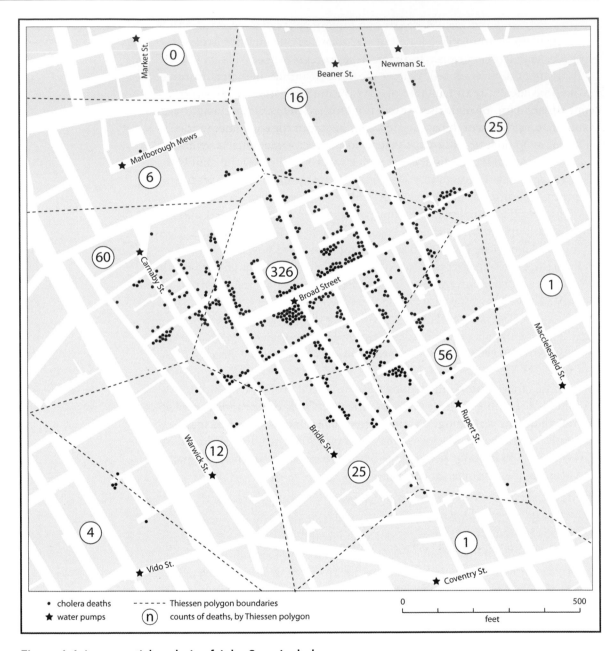

Figure 6.4 **A geospatial analysis of John Snow's cholera map**

exposures to specific pollutants, work must often rely on monitoring stations at a few points. GIS can serve to interpolate, or fill in, the spaces in between those measurements using sophisticated methods. The resulting model can be used to evaluate whether there is an association between exposures and a particular health outcome.

Another application of GIS is disease surveillance, systematic data collection designed to monitor signals that can indicate a new outbreak of disease or help direct interventions to tackle disease. There are now many disease surveillance systems online and available to the general public (see, for example, HealthMap, http://healthmap.org/en/index.php). Other scholarly work has identified 'hot spot' or high-risk areas, in order to target interventions (Srivastava et al., 2009). In combination with spatial epidemiological methods, GIS can be used to identify disease clusters, areas that experience a relatively high rate of a particular disease or health outcome. This work should be approached with great care and thought, as it is not uncommon for disease clusters to appear on a map on casual viewing. Clusters are often little more than statistical phantoms that occur randomly, which may lead to unfounded public alarm. Careful statistical analysis can determine how likely the cluster is to appear by chance alone.

Finally, GIS has broad applications in the provision and planning of healthcare services, both for research and application, which include mapping healthcare services, evaluating access to services, and analysing patterns of utilization (Cromley and McLafferty, 2012). Scholars have used GIS as a tool to evaluate the impact of healthcare utilization in poor regions (Feikin et al., 2009) and structural change in healthcare systems (Brabyn and Beere, 2006), and for determining access to prenatal healthcare among particular immigrant groups (McLafferty and Grady, 2005).

While these examples illustrate some of the key lines of research using GIS in recent years, the technology continues to evolve. Open-source and internet-based GIS has expanded its use beyond specialized and highly trained technicians, potentially enabling greater access to the technology and use of spatial data. However, users must always bear in mind that there is potential for the tool to be misused, as the products of GIS can be no better than the data geospatial analysis is based on. The future of GIS as a facilitator of the study of health will depend on a continued interest in medical and health geography and its exploration of the links between human health and their environments.

case study obesity and the built environment

As geographers Pearce and Witten (2010, p. 4) write about obesity:

the rising epidemic reflects profound changes that have been accompanied by rapid and widespread changes to the environment ... to understand the worldwide rise in obesity prevalence, it is necessary to consider a whole host of environmental factors.

Many geographers have focused their study of nutrition environments on obesogenic environments at the scale of cities and neighbourhoods, including access to healthy food and opportunities for exercise.

Research has investigated the existence and distribution of 'food deserts', areas in cities where affordable, nutritious food is difficult to obtain. In these areas, where residents often live in poverty and have poor access to transportation, fruit and vegetables are difficult to find, whereas cheap, processed foods exist in abundance. Since the concept began to be investigated in the mid-1980s and eventually appeared in official British government documents a decade later (Cummins and Macintyre, 2002), the link between built environments and access to healthy nutrition has been heavily investigated. A great deal of research has used GIS to evaluate which areas of cities are food deserts. Because transportation is a critical component of physical access, measures of accessibility often analyse the transportation network in order to evaluate the walking or driving distance to sources of healthy food for residents.

What objective factors can we map to designate which parts of a city are in a food desert? One basic problem in this research has been how to define a food desert, as there are no widely accepted set of criteria. The US Department of Agriculture (2013) defines a food desert as:

> urban neighborhoods and rural towns without ready access to fresh, healthy, and affordable food. Instead of supermarkets and grocery stores, these communities may have no food access or are served only by fast food restaurants and convenience stores that offer few healthy, affordable food options.

In the UK, the term has been used to highlight poverty, social exclusion as well as unsupportive local food environments.

In a study to identify food deserts in Montreal, Aparricio et al. (2007) 'geocode', that is, convert text information to locations on a map, addresses of supermarkets into a GIS and then estimate food accessibility by calculating:

- the distance to the nearest supermarket
- the number of supermarkets within 1,000 metres

- the average distance to supermarkets belonging to different companies.

These measures are intended to provide an estimate of physical access and access to a diversity of foods and products. The criteria for what constitutes a food desert vary considerably, and should take into account the local cultural, social and economic context. While living three kilometres from a grocery store in the suburbs of Canada might not be a significant barrier if nearly everyone in the area has access to personal transport such as a car, that distance might be a huge problem in other contexts, such as an urban slum in Brazil.

Research on the relationship between food deserts and local residents' income and health status has burgeoned over the past decade. While there is good evidence that food is more expensive for low-income residents of cities in developed countries, such as the UK (Cummins and Macintyre, 2002), the causal link between BMI and access to food is mixed.

This research, and indeed any research that attempts to establish a causal link between environments and health, faces difficult methodological challenges. For instance, it is possible that sociocultural attitudes towards food are a primary cause for poor diet (Pearson et al., 2005), and those attitudes may be associated with income and food deserts, resulting in a problem of scientific confounding. Other local environments, such as where one works, may also play an important role (Story et al., 2008), ultimately distorting results in studies that are based on residence. Finally, much of this work is data driven, meaning that study conditions and parameters are defined by what data are available, rather than by what theory suggests or what the authors truly wish to examine (Thornton and Kavanaugh, 2010). Despite the existence of a vast body of scholarly work on this topic, much additional work is needed in order to guide city planners and policy-makers to the best policies and approaches to the problem.

One of the other causes in the recent worldwide rise in obesity prevalence rates is a decrease in the amount of time children spend in physical activity. In response to this problem, cities around the world have invested heavily in providing children with safe spaces where they can engage in healthy playtime behaviour and develop physical activity habits. Despite the huge body of research that seeks to improve our understanding of the link between the built environment and health, evidence-based research on specific design practices that can be implemented to encourage healthy behaviour in school spaces has only recently begun. For example, some work demonstrates that newly constructed or renovated spaces are associated with higher rates of vigorous physical activity among children in schools and parks (Anthamatten et al., 2011; Colabianchi et al., 2011).

More recently, scholars have begun to examine children's behaviour *within* these spaces in order to determine specific guidelines for designers. This work strives to address key questions to provide those guidelines:

- Does constructed playground equipment encourage children to be more active during school break times?
- How important are open spaces for children's activity; for example, is it important to include fields where children can play organized games or is constructed play equipment more important?
- Are there observable differences between the genders?

In work that can be described as 'behaviour mapping' or the study of the 'microgeographies of play', scholars have begun mapping children's behaviour within school grounds in order to understand how this behaviour relates to the design features of activity spaces. Fjortoft et al. (2010) monitored 14-year-old children in schools in Norway. Children were asked to carry a GPS, which enabled the authors to track children's movement over time, as well as heart monitors, to estimate the intensity of their activity. The authors found that students engaged in the most intense activity in handball courts, which suggests that such facilities are important components of activity spaces in Norway.

The US city of Denver implemented a city-wide programme to renovate playgrounds in all the schools in the city. Researchers used the opportunity to evaluate which parts of the playground were particularly effective at attracting children and encouraging them to engage in intense physical activity. They found that design features did relate to children's activity in a modest capacity. Boys were more likely to engage in vigorous activity in spaces without playground equipment, and girls were more likely to spend time in zones with equipment (Anthamatten et al., 2014a). In a related study, the authors determined that parts of the playground with high densities of constructed playground equipment were associated with a slightly higher rate of vigorous activity (Anthamatten et al., 2014b). Future work, with more nuanced analysis, may serve to provide specific guidelines for designing healthy activity spaces for children.

Summary

- This chapter has shown that where you are and how you relate to spaces and places is a critical factor to health

- The geography of health approaches topics in a broad and integrative way

- To understand how particular places affect health, it is critical to consider not only the physical ecology of a place, such as climate, flora and fauna, but also the social ecology – the ways that cultural norms, economic structure and political forces come together to construct places and drive what happens in different spaces

- Geographic information systems (GIS), remote sensing and online mapping have greatly enhanced our ability to explore and analyse health data in ways that would have been inconceivable 20 years ago

- Due in no small part to these advances in geospatial and mapping technology, public health scholars have become increasingly aware of the critical role of location in driving health

- By viewing and analysing health data, it is easy to see that there are clear spatial patterns in health and that *where you are* matters

- As the planet struggles with the global problems of the twenty-first century, ushered in by climate change, globalization and population growth, geography will continue to play a critical role in our understanding of the drivers of human health

Questions for further discussion

1. Think about the places you live and work in. How do these places protect or harm your health? Try to produce examples that draw from the natural, built and social environments.

2. What kind of disease vectors can thrive in the ecosystem in which you live? How could environmental change, and climate change specifically, alter the health risk environment?

3. Do you think your neighbourhood is an example of an obesogenic or a leptogenic (slimming) environment? Provide examples of the components in your environment that encourage or discourage obesity.

4. Think about culture, identity and power in different places as they relate to health. How can these components of the social environment serve to harm an individual's health?

Further reading

Anthamatten, P. and Hazen, H. (2011) *An Introduction to the Geography of Health*. New York: Routledge.
Introductory text to the study of the geography of health, intended to accompany undergraduate courses and designed to provide an overview of theories, methods and techniques. Introduces readers to key themes in health geography research on natural, built and social environments, and concludes with an overview of geospatial techniques and concepts. The final chapter examines disease eradication as an exercise in applying the holistic perspectives offered by study in geography.

Cromley, E.K. and McLafferty, S. (2012) *GIS and Public Health* (2nd edn). New York: Guilford Press.
As GIS has gained an increasingly critical role in the study of health, interest in GIS has broadened to include scholars and researchers in a variety of public health studies. Written for the broader public health community, provides an overview of spatial data, GIS and geospatial applications and techniques across a variety of health topics.

Curtis, S. (2004) *Health and Inequality: Geographical Perspectives*. London: Sage.
Useful analysis of how geographical perspectives can be used to understand the problems of health inequalities.

Kearns, R.A. and Gesler, W.M. (1998) *Putting Health into Place: Landscape, Identity, and Well-being*. Syracuse, NY: Syracuse University Press.
Served as a key work in the transformation of 'medical geography' to include 'geographies of health', more broadly cast to incorporate social and cultural theory to the study of health and places. Draws on worldwide research to illustrate the relevance and potential of the geography of health in three thematic parts: therapeutic landscapes, identity, difference and health, and place, policy and wellbeing.

Meade, M.S. and Michael, E. (2010) *Medical Geography* (3rd edn). New York: Guilford Press.
First published in 1988, now a staple among graduate students of the geography of health. Rich coverage of the quantitative methods within the field, including key topics relevant to medical geography, such as newly emerging diseases, natural environmental process, and healthcare delivery and access.

Pearce, J. and Witten, K. (eds) (2010) *Geographies of Obesity: Environmental Understandings of the Obesity Epidemic*. Farnham: Ashgate.
Edited book with contributions from top researchers on obesity, with in-depth coverage of the key foci of geographic research on the obesity epidemic. Divided into sections that examine food environments, physical activity environments, policy responses and research challenges.

Shaw, M., Dorling, D. and Mitchell, R. (2002) *Health, Place and Society*. London: Pearson Education.
Combines medical sociology with geography; explores how environmental and social factors determine the geography of health, particularly the degenerative diseases of the Western world. Compares examples from Europe, America and the former Soviet Union/communist bloc with British case studies. Dorling has written extensively and much of his work is published on his personal website www.dannydorling.org.

Waller, L.A. and Gotway, C.A. (2004) *Applied Spatial Statistics for Public Health Data*. Hoboken, NJ: John Wiley and Sons.
Seminal book in spatial epidemiology provides an in-depth overview of the analysis of spatial exposure and health data. As the first part provides an introduction to statistical methods that form the foundation for the rest of the text, readers should have some proficiency and comfort with quantitative methods.

References

Anthamatten, P., Brink, L., Lampe, S. et al. (2011) 'An assessment of schoolyard renovation strategies to encourage children's physical activity'. *International Journal of Behavioral Nutrition and Physical Activity* 8(27): 1–9.

Anthamatten, P., Brink, L., Kingston, B. et al. (2014a) 'An assessment of schoolyard features and behavior patterns in children's utilization and physical activity'. *Journal of Physical Activity and Health* 11(3).

Anthamatten, P., Fiene, E., Kutchman, E. et al. (2014b) 'A microgeographic analysis of physical activity behavior within elementary school grounds'. *American Journal of Health Promotion* 11(3).

Apparicio, P., Cloutier, M. and Shearmur, R. (2007) 'The case of Montreal's missing food deserts: evaluation of accessibility to food supermarkets'. *International Journal of Health Geographics* 6(4): 1–13.

Attané, I. (2002) 'China's family planning policy: an overview of its past and future'. *Studies in Family Planning* 33(1): 103–13.

Brabyn, L. and Beere, P. (2006) 'Population access to hospital emergency departments and the impacts of health reform in New Zealand'. *Health Informatics Journal* 12(3): 227–37.

Brabyn, L. and Gower, P. (2004) 'Comparing three GIS techniques for modelling geographical access to general practitioners'. *Cartographica* 39(2): 41–9.

Brijnath, B., Ansariadi, and de Souza, D.K. (2012) 'Four ways geographic information systems can help to enhance health service planning and delivery for infectious diseases in low-income countries'. *Journal of Health Care for the Poor and Underserved* 23(4): 1410–20.

Bullard, R. (1990) 'Ecological inequities and the new south: black-communities under siege'. *Journal of Ethnic Studies* 17(4): 101–15.

Colabianchi, N., Maslow, A. and Swayampakala, K. (2011) 'Features and amenities of school playgrounds: a direct observation study of utilization and physical activity levels outside of school time'. *International Journal of Behavioral Nutrition and Physical Activity* 14(8): 32.

Cromley, E.K. and McLafferty, S. (2012) *GIS and Public Health*. New York: Guilford Press.

Cummins, S. and Macintyre, S. (2002) 'A systematic study of an urban foodscape: the price and availability of food in Greater Glasgow'. *Urban Studies* 39(11): 2115–30.

De Onis, M. and Blössner, M. (2000) 'Prevalence and trends of overweight among preschool children in developing countries'. *American Journal of Clinical Nutrition* 72(4): 1032–9.

Dubnov, J., Barchana, M., Rishpon, S. et al. (2007) 'Estimating the effect of air pollution from a coal-fired power station on the development of children's pulmonary function'. *Environmental Research* 103(1): 87–98.

Epstein, P.R. (2005) 'Climate change and human health'. *New England Journal of Medicine* 353(14): 1433–6.

Farmer, P. (2001) *Infections and Inequalities: The Modern Plagues*. Berkeley, CA: University of California Press.

Feikin, D.R., Nguyen, L.M., Adazu, K. et al. (2009) 'The impact of distance of residence from a peripheral health facility on pediatric health utilisation in rural western Kenya'. *Tropical Medicine and International Health* 14(1): 54–61.

Fjortoft, I., Lofman, O. and Thoren, K. (2010) 'Schoolyard physical activity in 14-year-old adolescents assessed by mobile GPS and heart rate monitoring analysed by GIS'. *Scandinavian Journal of Public Health* 38(5): 28–37.

Foresight (2007) *Tackling Obesities: Future Choices – Project Report* (2nd edn). London: Government Office for Science.

Griffith, D. and Christakos, G. (2007) 'Medical geography as a science of interdisciplinary knowledge synthesis under conditions of uncertainty'. *Stochastic Environmental Research and Risk Assessment* 21(5): 459–60.

Gubler, D. (1989) '*Aedes aegypti* and *Aedes aegypti*-borne disease control in the 1990s: top down or bottom up'. *American Journal of Tropical Medicine and Hygiene* 40(6): 571–8.

Hawkes, C. (2006) 'Uneven dietary development: linking the policies and processes of globalization with the nutrition transition, obesity and diet-related chronic diseases'. *Globalization and Health* 2(4). Available at www.ncbi.nlm.nih.gov/pmc/articles/PMC1440852/ (accessed 2/10/2014).

Hippocrates ([400 BCE] n.d.) *On Airs, Waters, and Places*, trans. Francis Adams. Available at http://classics.mit.edu/Hippocrates/airwatpl.html (accessed 7/10/2013).

Hossain, P., Kawar, B. and Nahas, M.E. (2007) 'Obesity and diabetes in the developing world: a growing challenge'. *New England Journal of Medicine* 356(3): 213–15.

IPCC (International Panel on Climate Change) (2007) Climate change 2007: impacts, adaptation, and vulnerability, in M. Parry, O. Canziani, J., Palutikof et al. (eds) *Contribution of Working Group II to the Third Assessment Report of the Intergovernmental Panel on Climate Change*. Cambridge: Cambridge University Press, p. 30.

Johnson, S. (2006) *The Ghost Map: The Story of London's Most Terrifying Epidemic and How it Changed Science, Cities, and the Modern World*. New York: Riverhead Books.

Kearns, R. and Gesler, W. (1998) *Putting Health into Place: Landscape, Identity, and Well-Being*. Syracuse, NY: Syracuse University Press.

Kearns, R. and Moon, G. (2002) 'From medical to health geography: novelty, place and theory after a decade of change'. *Progress in Human Geography* 26(5): 605–25.

King, B. (2010) 'Political ecologies of health'. *Progress in Human Geography* 34(1): 38–55.

Kinman, E. (1999) 'Evaluating health service equity at a primary care clinic in Chilimarca, Bolivia'. *Social Science and Medicine* 49(5): 663–78.

Lleo, M., Lafaye, M. and Guell, A. (2008) 'Application of space technologies to the surveillance and modelling of waterborne diseases'. *Current Opinion in Biotechnology* 19(3): 307–12.

McLafferty, S. and Grady, S. (2005) 'Immigration and geographic access to prenatal clinics in Brooklyn, NY: a geographic information systems analysis'. *American Journal of Public Health* 95(4): 638–40.

Malthus, T.R. (1798) *An Essay on the Principle of Population*. Available at www.esp.org/books/malthus/population/malthus.pdf (accessed 30/1/2014).

Masters, S., Burstein, R., Amofah, G. et al. (2013) 'Travel time to maternity care and its effect on utilization in rural Ghana: a multilevel analysis'. *Social Science and Medicine* 93: 147–54.

May, J.M. (1958) *The Ecology of Human Disease*. New York: MD Publications.

Meade, M. and Emch, M. (2010) *Medical Geography*. New York: Guilford Press.

Morse, S. (1995) 'Factors in the emergence of infectious-diseases'. *Emerging Infectious Diseases* 1(1): 7–15.

National Public Radio (2013) Florida officials swat at mosquitoes with dengue fever. Available at www.npr.org/blogs/health/2013/09/12/221791874/florida-officials-take-swat-at-mosquitoes-with-dengue-fever (accessed 10/11/2013).

ONS (Office for National Statistics) (2013) *Age-standardised Mortality Rates: Persons*. Available at www.neighbourhood.statistics.gov.uk/HTMLDocs/dvc171/map.html (accessed 29/1/2014).

Pearce, J. and Witten, K. (2010) *Geographies of Obesity: Environmental Understandings of the Obesity Epidemic*. Farnham: Ashgate.

Pearson, T., Russell, J., Campbell, M.J. and Barker, M.E. (2005) 'Do "food deserts" influence fruit and vegetable consumption?: A cross-sectional study'. *Appetite* 45: 195–7.

Pimentel, D., Cooperstein, S., Randell, H. et al. (2007) 'Ecology of increasing diseases: population growth and environmental degradation'. *Human Ecology* 35: 653–68.

Pope, K., Masuoka, P., Rejmankova, E. et al. (2005) 'Mosquito habitats, land use, and malaria risk in Belize from satellite imagery'. *Ecological Applications* 15(4): 1223–32.

Raddatz, L. and Mennis, J. (2013) 'Environmental justice in Hamburg, Germany'. *Professional Geographer* 65(3): 495–511.

Ranjit, S. and Kissoon, N. (2011) 'Dengue hemorrhagic fever and shock syndromes'. *Pediatric Critical Care Medicine* 12(1): 90–100.

Sheppard, E., Leitner, H., McMaster, R. and Tian, H. (1999) 'GIS-based measures of environmental equity: Exploring their sensitivity and significance'. *Journal of Exposure Analysis and Environmental Epidemiology* 9(1): 18–28.

Srivastava, A., Nagpal, B., Joshi, P. et al. (2009) 'Identification of malaria hot spots for focused intervention in tribal state of India: a GIS based approach'. *International Journal of Health Geographics* 8: 30.

Story, M., Kaphingst, K., Robinson-O'Brien, R. and Glanz, K. (2008) 'Creating healthy food and eating environments: policy and environmental approaches'. *Annual Review of Public Health* 29: 253–72.

Thornton, L. and Kavanaugh, A. (2010) Understanding the local food environment and obesity, in J. Pearce and K. Witten (eds) *Geographies of Obesity: Environmental Understandings of the Obesity Epidemic*. Farnham: Ashgate, pp. 79–111.

UN (United Nations) (2011) *World Population Prospects: The 2010 Revision*. vol. 1: *Comprehensive Tables*, Department of Economic and Social Affairs, Population Division. Available at http://esa.un.org/wpp/Documentation/pdf/WPP2010_Volume-I_Comprehensive-Tables.pdf (accessed 14/11/2013).

United States Department of Agriculture (2013) Food Deserts. Available at http://apps.ams.usda.gov/fooddeserts/foodDeserts.aspx (accessed 07/11/2013).

United States Geological Survey (2007) Geographic Information Systems. Available at http://egsc.usgs.gov/isb//pubs/gis_poster/ (accessed 23/3/2014).

Utrilla, P., Mazo, C., Sopena, M. et al. (2009) 'A palaeolithic map from 13,660 calBP: engraved stone blocks from the Late Magdalenian in Abauntz Cave (Navarra, Spain)'. *Journal of Human Evolution* 57(2): 99–111.

Waller, L. and Gotway, C. (2004) *Applied Spatial Statistics for Public Health Data*. Hoboken, NJ: John Wiley & Sons.

Walters, M. (2003) *Six Modern Plagues and How we are Causing Them*. Washington: Island Press/Shearwater Books.

WHO (World Health Organization) (2013a) Dengue and severe dengue. Available at www.who.int/mediacentre/factsheets/fs117/en/, accessed 21/10/2013.

WHO (2013b) Urban population growth. Available at www.who.int/gho/urban_health/situation_trends/urban_population_growth_text/en/ (accessed 28/9/2013).

WHO (2013c) Slum residence. Available at www.who.int/gho/urban_health/determinants/slum_residence_text/en/ (accessed 28/9/2013).

WHO (2013d) Global Health Observatory map gallery. Available at http://gamapserver.who.int/mapLibrary/Files/Maps/Global_Overweight_BothSexes_2008.png (accessed 10/10/2013).

Winson, A. (2004) 'Bringing political economy into the debate on the obesity epidemic'. *Agriculture and Human Values* 21(4): 299–312.

Yang, W., Kelly, T. and He, J. (2007) 'Genetic epidemiology of obesity'. *Epidemiologic Reviews* 29: 49–61.

7

Cultural studies and anthropology

Overview   229

Introduction   229

Part 1 The contribution of cultural studies and anthropology
to health studies   230
Cultural practices in relation to health   233
Health and illness across cultures   235
Lay knowledge and beliefs   240
Representations of health   243

Part 2 Theoretical and research approaches   248
Ethnography   251
Discourse and conversation analysis   253
Semiotics   255

Case study Breastfeeding and infant feeding across cultures   256
Summary   258
Questions for further discussion   259
Further reading   259
References   259

Learning outcomes

This chapter will enable readers to:

- Understand what is meant by culture and how it can be applied to health
- Gain an overview of the discipline and development of cultural studies and anthropology, including its theoretical and research approaches
- Reflect on the insights that cultural studies and anthropology can give to our understanding of health, illness and healthcare

Overview

Health and illness are commonly defined in biological terms but can also be seen as being shaped by **culture** – a system of shared meanings, experiences and practices. Culture is reflected in the customs and areas of knowledge of social life, including religion, ethnicity, diet and dress. Cultural studies is a relatively new field that adopts a multidisciplinary approach to the study of culture, drawing on insights from anthropology, sociology, communication studies, literature and the visual arts, among others. Social anthropology is the study of aspects of society from a cross-cultural perspective and medical anthropology explores the cultural dimensions of health, sickness and death. Part 1 explores the relationship between medical discourses and ethnic beliefs, customs and traditions relating to health and lay knowledge and beliefs regarding health and illness. These illustrate the complexity and diversity of cultural concepts of health and illness. Official and unofficial representations of health in the media are compared and contrasted. Part 2 discusses the contribution of different methodological approaches, including ethnography, discourse analysis and semiotics, to cultural studies. The chapter concludes with a case study exploring the cultural significance of different forms of infant feeding.

Introduction

Individual health is shaped by the context in which we live and how we make sense of the world. Cultures are the systems of shared meanings, **representations** and practices that comprise the whole of social life. Thus, cultural manifestations may be found in religious beliefs, ethnic identity, diet, dress, leisure, codes of behaviour and systems of knowledge. Culture is the way in which we make sense of the world:

> To some extent, culture can be seen as an inherited 'lens', through which the individual perceives and understands the world … and learns how to live within it. Growing up within any society is a form of enculturation, whereby the individual slowly acquires the cultural 'lens' of that society. (Helman, 2007, p. 2)

Every object, action and person is assigned a meaning by us as we try to interpret our encounters and fit them into a unifying framework. The study of culture is thus the study of signification: we examine and deconstruct what certain cultural practices or objects signify. Certain ideas and representations can become dominant in society, particularly if they are disseminated through the mass media. It would, however, be far too simplistic to portray cultural ideals as being unanimously held: culture should not be understood as a homogeneous entity.

Part 1 The contribution of cultural studies and anthropology to health studies

example 7.1

The application of cultural studies and anthropology to contemporary health issues

- Help-seeking behaviour and the use of cure practices

- The interaction of new biotechnologies with traditional beliefs and practices
- Stigma and health
- The use of communication technologies including mobile phones to promote health
- How people adapt to changed bodies or circumstances as a result of illness

Cultural studies is a relatively new discipline. However, the study of culture is also the principal focus of anthropology, which has a much longer history. In the past, anthropology tended to be associated with nineteenth-century colonialism and a somewhat voyeuristic focus on other cultures. As Russell and Edgar (1998, p. 3) describe, it was traditionally 'the study of "exotic" peoples in "other" places'. Contemporary anthropology is a much more wide-ranging and reflexive discipline, which studies culture in many settings, from the unusual to the familiar. While the general meaning of anthropology is the study of humanity, it has several specialisms. In particular, medical anthropology has made an important contribution to understandings of health. The main focus of medical anthropology is seeking to explain people's ideas and behaviour in relation to health by examining the influence of their culture. It does so by exploring the relationship between the biological and the social. However, ideas about health and illness are inevitably linked to wider cultural beliefs and influences. As such, the anthropological approach is holistic. It also stresses understanding cultures from within, that is, studying them in their own terms as opposed to measuring them against a different cultural standard.

If culture shapes how we interpret the world, then health and illness are part of this process of finding meaning. Adopting this approach to health makes certain issues of interest:

- who is classed as healthy and who is ill

- how we feel and describe symptoms

- how illness is treated

- whether an illness is seen as stigmatizing

- how we seek help and from whom.

These forms of knowledge may be hierarchical. One way of understanding health and illness may be considered less legitimate within one society than another. For example, laypeople's ideas of what counts as healthy eating may have less authority than the views of health professionals, who have taken on the beliefs of a distinctive culture of learning and practice in the course of their medical training. Culture can thus be seen as linked to power. This is also evident in the fact that laypeople's ideas, across a range of cultures within a society, are likely to reflect dominant ideas to some extent. Cultural ideas of specific groups seldom constitute a wholly separate system, but take elements of the dominant culture and interweave them with alternate beliefs. An example of this could be someone who combines the use of complementary medicine with mainstream treatments. Wiese et al. (2010) report that mainstream medical practice has been forced to adopt an attitude of 'grudging acceptance' towards complementary medicine, given its growing popularity. Dominant ideas of health and health-care are that they are scientific and primarily rooted in biological fact; medicine and healthcare have tended not to be seen as culturally determined. Research into the health and cultural beliefs of ethnic minority groups has represented minority cultures as faulty for supporting health practices, such as the use of ghee for cooking, that are not in keeping with Western norms (Ahmad, 1996).

Culture embraces the whole of our social life and systems of knowledge, including knowledge relating to health and healthcare. Information on health comes to us via numerous sources apart from the medical profession, such as our families and friends, literature, the media, self-help groups and the internet. Health is not only a property of our bodies, but also an item of **consumption**. Many products, from sportswear and slimming aids to organic foods and water filters, are marketed as 'healthy' or 'healthier'. These products not only reflect our current conceptions of health, but also help create new beliefs and ideas. Our health, illnesses and lifestyles cannot be divorced from the culture within which we live. Culture is also important in defining ourselves, our bodies and our identities.

In contrast to Marxist perspectives, which state that culture is produced from economic structures, some theorists argue that culture should be seen more as autonomous and dynamic. **Structuralists** such as de Saussure (1960) and Lévi-Strauss (1970) focus on the ways in which meaning is socially created, especially through language. From de Saussure's perspective, different languages share the essential quality of ordering the world into interrelated categories. Thus, language orders our conceptual understanding of the world. Lévi-Strauss applied this idea of conceptual structure to all cultural practices, such as kinship networks, cooking and myths, as described by Fiske (2011, p. 116):

> All cultures make sense of the world, and while the meanings that they make of it may be specific to them, the ways by which they make those meanings are not; they are universal. Meanings are culture-specific, but the ways of making them are universal to all human beings.

For Lévi-Strauss, the fundamental contribution of language was the construction of binary oppositions: the division of the world into two categories that are mutually dependent on one another for their meaning, for example hot and cold. Health and disease can also be understood as binary oppositions. Concepts that defy being placed into oppositional categories, possessing characteristics that blur the boundary, are termed 'anomalous categories'. When these categories are seen as being too disturbing to established social knowledge, they become the subject of taboos. Thus, Lévi-Strauss argued that homosexuality was seen as taboo because it undermined gender identity. The category in which someone is placed, such as mentally ill/physically ill or able bodied/disabled, may have profound consequences for how people perceive themselves and how they are treated. Transitions between one category and another, such as deciding when someone is officially well, are also socially significant and culturally specific (Helman, 2007). An example of tensions surrounding such categories comes in Moscowitz et al.'s (2013) work on illness appraisals following HIV diagnosis. Before the development of effective antiretroviral treatments, receiving such a diagnosis was effectively being classed as terminally ill. Now HIV can be seen as a manageable chronic condition. However, this does not automatically mean that people appraise their illness positively. The authors identify considerable variations in response, emphasizing that healthcare practitioners should avoid assumptions about reactions to diagnosis in order to tailor support appropriately.

Postmodernists argue that, in our postindustrial world, identities and ideas proliferate to create a pluralistic society. Pluralism means that there is a variety of subcultures and groups, each of which is valid. **Postmodernism** rejects the grand narratives of perspectives such as Marxism that seek to explain society by reference to a unifying underlying set of ideas (Doyle, 1995). The modernist concept of linear progress is dismissed, as is the search for an ultimate objective truth such as economic determinism. Within a postmodern world, traditional sources of solidarity and **identity** become dislocated. As family and working structures fragment, we are left without easy certainties. Geographic or social class location, for example, will not be sufficient to give us a central, lifelong identity. In this context, the **body** can act as a source of identity, giving a stability that we lack from other sources. The pursuit of a certain look, level of fitness or lifestyle can all be ways for us to define ourselves; they are not simply reflections of whether we are ill or healthy (see, for example, Kelly and Millward, 2013).

connections   Chapter 5 also discusses structuralist and postmodern perspectives on society and social roles. It explains contemporary critiques in sociology, including the focus on embodiment and the meanings attached to our corporeal selves.

Postmodernity is characterized by a plurality of discourses. An extreme form of this view is very relativist, and any boundaries between high and low, good or bad, are rejected. No forms of knowledge or belief are superior, they are simply different. So, a doctor's knowledge of a medical condition is not intrinsically more valid than a layperson's, and biomedicine is not more grounded in 'reality' than homeopathy. All knowledge and practice must be understood within discourse and culture: there is no external or absolute reality that can be known. There are also less extreme forms of postmodernist perspectives, for example the acknowledgement that there are incontrovertible biological aspects of health and illness, but that these are mediated and made meaningful through social processes.

Cultural practices in relation to health

Contemporary concerns are particularly focused on the relationship between lifestyles and health, and lifestyles derive – at least in part – from cultural beliefs. In order to understand why individuals eat certain foods, take exercise or drink too much, we need to see these activities as everyday cultural practices and look at their meanings.

Usually, people are not consciously aware of carrying out cultural practices. Activities and behaviour simply feel normal or 'common sense'. While many everyday activities have a bearing on health, individuals may not interpret them in this way or have thoughts of health uppermost in their minds. As Bury (2005, p. 8) notes: 'Health risks vie with the routine nature of daily life, with its own pressures and pleasures, constraints and potentialities.' Putting extra blankets on a baby may not be just to stop the baby getting cold, but because it is an outward show of our caring, and loving parenting is an important cultural value. However, this practice may put babies at higher risk of sudden infant death syndrome, and runs counter to official advice (NHS Choices, 2013). Practices such as sunbathing or using tanning equipment are carried out because of a cultural preference for tanned skin, although this may have damaging implications for health in the form of promoting melanoma.

Cultural practices can be deeply embedded in social groups and are a vital part of the expression of identity, therefore they can also be highly resistant to change. Health promotion activities, either at the individual or collective level, are unlikely to be successful if they simply exhort people to live more healthily and fail to engage with the meanings behind cultural practices. For example, the food choices that people make are often circumscribed not only by material factors such as cost and accessibility, but also by ideas of tradition or emotional significance. Friedman (2012) flags up that 'fat-shaming' discourses, in the name of a fight against global obesity, serve as a form of oppression and moral regulation.

example 7.2

Food as culture

According to Caplan (1997, p. 3):

> Food is never 'just food' and its significance can never be purely nutritional.

Furthermore, it is intimately bound up with social relations, including those of power, of inclusion and exclusion, as well as cultural ideas about classification (including food and non-food, the edible and the inedible), the human body and the meaning of health.

One of the most powerful ways in which food is intertwined with culture is through the family. The rise in family diversity, brought about by factors such as a higher divorce rate, cohabitation, lone parenthood and same-sex relationships, has led many to decry the demise of the 'traditional' nuclear, patriarchal family. This social anxiety is exemplified in the concern that the family meal, when the whole family sits down to eat together, is under threat. The supposed downfall of this ritual has been linked to a rise in the consumption of unhealthy food. Murcott (1997) argues that the notion that families always ate together in the past is an idealized one: upper-class families, for example, tended to separate adults and children, so that children would eat either in the nursery or at boarding schools away from home. Murcott traces concerns about the decline in the family meal to the earlier part of the twentieth century, arguing that this is a recurrent metaphor for the state of the family.

The shared meal has come to signify the ideal family. Symbolic meals, such as Sunday dinner, acquire great importance. The roles family members take within this meal communicate their position. In the UK, the husband traditionally carves the meat, displaying his authority and role as provider. The woman is placed in the subject position of wife and mother by cooking a meal, while the children are placed as dependants, the grateful recipients of their parents' care. This family ideal remains the dominant model, although it faces continual challenges from the growth in family diversity. Recent studies continue to support this model of eating. Larson et al. (2013) argue that shared mealtimes promote better nutrition among adolescents, while McIntosh et al. (2010) emphasize mothers' roles and motivations in encouraging children to participate in family dinners.

Food has traditionally been used as a marker of cultural identity: 'Simple equations such as "we eat meat, they don't" … affirm, in shared patterns of consumption and shared notions of edibility, our difference from others' (James, 1997). James (2004) studied the food choices of African Americans, a group who are at a particularly high risk of conditions such as obesity and diabetes. Aspects of poor diet among this group include consuming foods high in fat, calories and sodium, while eating insufficient quantities of fruit, vegetables and high-fibre foods (DHHS, 2000, in James, 2004). However, these choices are not simply made in wilful disregard of healthy eating messages; food is an essential part of a cultural identity. In the case of African Americans, diet reflects the history of a group shaped from slavery and segregation. Food is also a large part of family gatherings, where providing or asking for 'healthy' food as opposed to more traditional food could be seen as rude. James (2004, p. 357) illustrates this with a quote from one of her participants:

> I tried to tell my dad that if we have beans and rice, we don't need to eat meat because the beans already have the protein. He didn't like that and I still had to get up and fix him some meat.

Participants in James's study felt that relinquishing their customary foods was also relinquishing their cultural heritage and acquiescing to the dominant culture. There was thus considerable reluctance to give up food choices, coupled with difficulties such as the expense of healthier alternatives.

Notions of what comprises British food can be seen as ways of identifying and placing oneself in the world, just as we may categorize ourselves as members of communities or workplaces. However, just as some of these traditional sources of identity begin to break down into multiple possibilities, so British food has become subject to tremendous diversity. James (2004) points out that a new trend is occurring in British eating habits, namely 'food Creolization', in which hybrid dishes evolve. However, class differences in the type of food eaten persist, with the middle and upper classes tending to shun Creolization in favour of authentic cooking, either British or foreign. Similarly, the British preoccupation with food as an easily prepared necessity continues. The recent popularity of cooking programmes, competitions and celebrity chefs highlights that food preparation is a cultural activity.

Food is intimately related to identity and social relations rather than purely nutrition. Strategies to promote healthier diets are therefore directly attempting to refashion cultural practices. Success is more likely if the context of these practices is understood and acknowledged than if they are denied. Adapting a diet to maximize its positive elements and minimize negative ones is more likely to result in change rather than pursuing a prescriptive and culturally insensitive approach. Stead et al. (2011) found that young people saw food choices as a way of signifying their identity; healthy choices were in conflict with the types of food they felt would help them fit in with their peer group.

> **thinking about** How important are family eating patterns in determining children's food choices? What was your experience?

Health and illness across cultures

One of the clearest ways of demonstrating the importance of the relationship between health, illness and culture is to examine variations in beliefs across groups. The dominance of biomedicine within Western societies tends to suggest that health and illness are natural, universal phenomena and the body simply a biological entity. Yet understandings can vary both across and within cultures and societies. Health and illness are culturally specific concepts and experiences, so must be understood from *within* cultures.

> Chapter 1 is illustrative of a biomedical and mechanistic approach to the study of health that also adopts the Cartesian dualism paradigm or the separation between the mind and the body of an individual. Chapter 2 discusses how this is a modern development and that, historically, health was perceived holistically.
>
> **connections**

There are many cultures within the boundaries of a wider society; these may gain their cultural identity from a number of factors, such as class, region, gender or ethnicity. Ethnicity has most commonly been associated with cultural beliefs and practices but it is not the only basis for the identification of a cultural grouping.

> Chapter 5 discusses the ways in which ethnicity and race have been used to classify populations and examines the reasons why ethnicity is strongly associated with poor health status and access to health services.
>
> **connections**

The relationships between ethnicity and culture are seldom straightforward or simplistic:

● Members of an ethnic group will not necessarily share a single culture

- Not all members will adhere strictly to specific cultural or religious beliefs, for example some Muslims drink alcohol

- Cultural beliefs may not necessarily be the overriding factor in decisions and understandings about health

- What a person believes may not always dictate what they do in practice.

> **?** Ahmad (1996, p. 215) argues that culture needs to be treated as a set of 'flexible guidelines' that influence behaviour rather than as something that determines actions and outlook. Why might this be the case and what are the implications for professional practice?

There are numerous ways in which ethnicity may influence belief and practice in relation to health and illness. For example, different ethnic groups may have different forms of self-care activity and use different remedies if ill. A variety of herbal or other forms of traditional remedies may be used, either in conjunction with Western medicine or instead of it. The treatment of illness is often dependent on assumptions about its causes. Very different explanatory models may be used, linking illness to a variety of internal, external or social factors. Many cultures would attribute forms of illness not to disease agents, but to the evil eye, in various manifestations. In Italy, for example, amulets may be worn to combat the evil eye (Spector, 2012). Illness attributable to such forces, including witchcraft or voodoo, may be avoided by certain forms of behaviour, such as taking care not to antagonize practitioners.

Illnesses may not be defined and understood in the same way as Western conceptualizations that are rooted in biology. Kaur (1996, in Dein, 2006) notes that there are several languages that do not contain a word for cancer. Cancer may be classified as another kind of illness or as separate illnesses depending on their site of occurrence.

---

example 7.3

Cultural perceptions of mental health

Mental illnesses are conceptualized differently across cultures. Pote and Orrell (2002) have explored perceptions in relation to schizophrenia, a diagnosis that is frequently open to dispute and contestation. They asked their sample, taken from 13 broad categories of ethnicity, to rate different symptoms in terms of how indicative they were of mental illness. Significant differences were that hallucinatory behaviour and suspiciousness were less likely to be seen as signs of being mentally ill by Bangladeshis, whereas African-Caribbeans were less likely to see unusual thought content in these terms. Ethnicity emerged as the most significant predictor of these differences between perceptions, but other factors such as religion, education, sex and contact with people with mental health problems were also influential.

Reactions to illness or disability may also vary in terms of fatalism or emotional response. Katbamna et al.'s (2000) research involving people from British South Asian communities identified similarities and differences in attitudes to disability between the communities and in relation to white groups. For example, while stigmatizing disability is widespread, they found that female carers who were Pakistani Muslim or Gujarati Hindu were most likely to feel that they were being blamed for producing a disabled child. A common preoccupation was that disclosing disability would negatively affect marriage prospects, particularly in the case of arranged marriages. Hindus and Sikhs were more likely to perceive disability as 'karma' (destiny) and hence struggle with the notion of being punished. Caring responsibilities were even more heavily gendered than among most white ethnic groups in Britain. Scior et al. (2010) found that attitudes towards people with intellectual disabilities were less favourable among a Hong Kong Chinese sample group than among a white British sample.

Medical practitioners therefore need to be sensitive to the various ways in which health and illness are interpreted by different ethnic groups, without separating culture from the wider social framework.

example 7.4

Meanings of hypertension

Morgan (1996) carried out a study largely in response to concerns expressed by a GP relating to difficulties he experienced in communicating information about hypertension and its treatment regimen to his African-Caribbean patients, a group with a higher than average incidence of the condition.

Morgan (1996) found that African-Caribbean patients had a greater tendency not to take prescribed medication, often preferring to use familiar herbal remedies. This group found the commonness of this condition among family and friends to be a reassuring indication of normality, rather than seeing a high incidence as being illustrative of elevated risk. Among both groups, there was a relatively low level of awareness that hypertension and high blood pressure were one and the same thing. Several respondents understood hypertension to be a nervous condition relating to stress. This reiterates the fact that different groups may understand diseases differently. Medical discourse provides forms of knowledge and language that are not universally shared by lay groups.

One factor that did vary between ethnic groups was that African-Caribbeans were more likely to identify strokes as a dangerous outcome, whereas white males highlighted heart conditions. Each group thus correctly identified the risk to which it was most likely to be exposed. African-Caribbeans, however, tended to take a more fatalistic approach, which appeared to increase acceptance and reduce anxiety. Thus, whereas Morgan (1996) identifies some differences in perception relating to hypertension between white and African-Caribbean people, she also draws out a number of similarities that characterize lay understanding as opposed to medical interpretation.

However, it is also important not to overstate cultural differences. Schuster et al. (2011) studied the way ethnic groups within the Netherlands employed metaphors to make sense of their experiences of hypertension. Although there were differences between groups, these were outnumbered by similarities, indicating that certain cultural metaphors, such as the body as a machine, override ethnic difference.

Many studies of health and culture have sought to explain 'bad' health and health behaviours in a simplistic manner as a result of culture. What cultural studies can contribute to this debate is a challenge to such notions, highlighting the interplay between culture, resistance, power and inequality within society.

The role of traditional healers illustrates what can be a negative response by a biomedical healthcare system to aspects of traditional cultures (Spector, 2012). Traditional healing includes many different approaches. For example, Catholics associate different saints with different ailments, such as St Vitus (epilepsy), or may undertake pilgrimages to holy sites such as Lourdes to pray for healing. The phrase 'traditional healer' is commonly used to describe someone who seeks to heal the sick using methods and a belief system outside Western biomedicine. Healers may have different origins. They may be religious figures, have undergone special training or be regarded as wise women, for example. They may be purely secular technicians skilled in a particular aspect of care, like childbirth, or they may draw on sacred knowledge. Often, their approach is characterized as much by a different relationship with the person seeking help as by the belief system under which they practise (Spector, 2012). This is indicated in Table 7.1, which compares the role of a medical professional in the US to that of a traditional healer.

Table 7.1 **A comparison of a traditional homeopathic healer versus a modern allopathic physician**

Healer	Physician
Maintains informal, friendly, affective relationship with the entire family	Businesslike, formal relationship; deals only with the patient
Comes to the house day or night	Patient must go to the physician's office or clinic, and only during the day; may have to wait for hours to be seen; home visits are rarely, if ever, made
For diagnosis, consults with head of house, creates a mood of awe, talks to all family members, has social rapport, builds expectation of cure; is not authoritarian	Rest of family usually ignored, deals solely with the ill person and may deal only with the sick part of the person; authoritarian manner creates fear
Generally less expensive than the physician	More expensive than the healer
Has ties to the 'world of the sacred', has rapport with the symbolic, spiritual, creative or holy force	Secular, pays little attention to the religious beliefs or meaning of a given illness
Shares the patient's worldview – speaks the same language, lives in the same neighbourhood, or in some similar socioeconomic conditions; may know the same people; understands the patient's lifestyle	Generally does not share the patient's worldview – may not speak the same language, live in the same neighbourhood, or understand the socioeconomic conditions; may not understand the patient's lifestyle

Chapter 1 describes the features of biomedicine and its scientific processes of investigation in contrast to those forms of care that do not separate mind from body.

connections

These properties of traditional healers can also be seen in societies where there is little access to Western-style healthcare. In sub-Saharan Africa, for example, the majority of the rural population are excluded from healthcare provision due to travel, costs and lack of services. In these circumstances, the role of healers is crucial.

example 7.5

Traditional healers and people with epilepsy

In Zambia, epilepsy is a highly stigmatizing condition that can undermine social networks and employability, leading to great disadvantage. Traditional healers are usually the main source of care. A notable feature of their involvement is that they focus on the individual and social circumstances of the person with epilepsy, contextualizing the disease, and providing causal explanations. Taking a detailed personal and medical history is a central part of their approach, and underscores the fact that they share a conceptual and social framework with the person consulting them. Baskind and Birbeck (2005) found that there is a high correlation between healers' accounts of the symptoms of epilepsy and those recognized by modern medicine. However, there is divergence over causality. Traditional healers see witchcraft as the underlying cause of epilepsy, although this may operate alongside other factors. Treatment involves providing an antidote, often using ingredients thought to have been used in the original witchcraft. There is also a role for 'immunizing' family members, as

the seizures are thought to be contagious via bodily fluids. If treatment fails, the person with epilepsy might be referred to other more powerful healers, or to hospitals, which are seen as able to mobilize specific treatments effectively. Treatment may be ineffective or dangerous, and fees can be expensive. Nevertheless, there can be significant benefits:

If a healer's treatment allows the family members of a PWE [person with epilepsy] no longer to fear contagion, perhaps the family is more willing to assist the PWE when they experience seizures … In addition, after a first seizure, some individuals worry constantly about the possibility of another seizure. Many will never have a second seizure, or the next seizure will not occur for months or years. Perhaps the TH's [traditional healer] ritual treatment alleviates this worry and allows the person to return to the social fold as 'normal'. At times, the THs seem to function as the community's moral conscience – pointing out broken taboos and violated norms. (Baskind and Birbeck, 2005, p. 1125)

? Should traditional healers be included in the management and treatment of conditions such as HIV/AIDS?

Traditional healers can retain a powerful role in contemporary healthcare, either because there is no readily accessible alternative or they offer a personalized service compatible with the patient's conceptual framework. Medical professionals need to acknowledge the role they play in different societies, as they may well be involved in shared care.

Lay knowledge and beliefs

There are three sectors of knowledge and belief about health (Kleinman, 1980):

1. The professional sector refers to orthodox Western medicine

2. The alternative sector refers to beliefs about health that stem from other medical traditions, such as folk medicine or complementary therapies

3. The lay sector represents the general public or patients, notably someone who is not a professional.

There has often been a tendency to devalue lay understandings as being an inaccurate version of medical expertise.

> **thinking about** Think about someone you know with a long-standing condition. Do you think they have expert knowledge about it?

In recent years, people with long-standing conditions or disabilities have come to be seen as experts on their experiences, in a way that medical professionals, lacking personal knowledge, can never hope to emulate. The terms 'lay knowledge' and 'lay expert' have been used to denote authority. However, Prior (2003) claims that it is misleading to use the idea of the lay expert. He argues that laypeople may have a highly developed awareness of living with and managing illness, but they lack the technical medical knowledge acquired through professional education and training. Nevertheless, there is an increased emphasis on harnessing lay experiences within orthodox medicine; this is one way in which a blurring of the boundaries between the different sectors identified by Kleinman (1980) is occurring.

> **connections** Chapter 3 discusses the emergence of a 'lay epidemiology', in which the information collected by members of the public has been used to profile diseases or conditions.

Evidence of the recognition now afforded to lay understandings is provided in initiatives such as the expert patient programme (DH, 2001). This approach seeks to encourage self-management programmes among patients who experience chronic, long-term conditions. It recognizes that living with conditions such as rheumatoid arthritis, diabetes or epilepsy involves the development of day-to-day strategies to cope with issues such as pain, fatigue and poor sleep. The illness may also have adverse consequences, such as disruption to employment prospects or an impact on other family members. In the absence of a cure, often the best approach is developing coping strategies to mini-mize problems associated with the illness. This may entail identifying effective ways of dealing with diet, exercise, energy levels or social situations. A recent meta-synthesis of studies examining self-management within chronic illness identified three key processes: focusing on illness needs, activating resources, and living with a chronic illness (Schulman-Green et al., 2012).

Approaches such as the expert patient programme seek to capitalize on the growth of lay self-help groups. Kelleher (1994) identifies various ways in which such groups operate, from being focused on members to heightening public awareness, fundraising and repositioning specific medical conditions or social groups higher on the political agenda. Self-help groups also vary in their relationship to medical professionals: some operate hand in hand, others occupy a complementary role, and others are more directly challenging. One recurring feature of self-help groups is their emphasis on the emotional experience of illness, which is often ignored by medical professionals, who focus purely on clinical factors. This represents differing interpretations of the *meaning* of illness.

> **thinking about** Have you been part of a self-help group? What support did you hope it would provide?

There has been extensive research into lay constructions of health and illness. Blaxter's (1990) study found five common concepts of health:

1. *Health as not-ill:* health as the absence of symptoms or medical input. This concept meant that some people with ongoing conditions were still able to define themselves as healthy. It was more commonly used by people in good health than those in bad health.

2. *Health as physical fitness:* usually associated with having energy and being fit. This concept was most used by younger men.

3. *Health as social relationships:* associated with maintaining one's social role and network; it was used more frequently by women than men.

4. *Health as function:* being able to carry out tasks and activities. It was a concept often employed by older people of both sexes.

5. *Health as psychosocial wellbeing:* health as a mental state of wellbeing. While it was the commonest definition, it was less used by young men and most used by those from higher occupational groups.

What is evident from these concepts is that their use is shaped, although not dictated, by membership of different social groups stratified by a range of factors. Thus, whether someone considers themselves to be healthy, and what this idea of healthy means, is variable.

connections   Chapter 4 explores the attributions people have for their illness and the ways in which these are explored in psychology.

Medical professionals and laypeople may therefore:

- define health differently

- have different causal explanations for illness

- have different understandings of risk

- have different priorities when controlling illness, perhaps not rating medical compliance as foremost over social obligations or employment (Kelleher, 1994).

---

example 7.6

The menopause and hormone replacement therapy: understandings of risk

Women's attitudes to risk are shaped by a number of factors, including:

- personal experiences and histories
- core beliefs about illness
- the construct of being a woman
- ideas about concepts such as fatalism and control.

According to Walter and Britten (2002, p. 584):

Risks were given meaning by placing knowledge, context and presentation against personal experience and core beliefs. The patient's perspective thus varies markedly from the medical perspective which views risk in terms of numerical descriptions.

Medical assessments of risks in relation to treatments like hormone replacement therapy need to be communicated to patients in ways that are meaningful. For example, risks could be related to other familiar processes such as antenatal care or the use of contraceptives. Risk assessment in antenatal care is often individualized; for example, a woman will be given her own risk of having a child with Down syndrome. Walter and Britten's (2002) study suggests general risk information is less easy for people to relate to. They recommend that medical practitioners ask patients about their attitudes to and experiences of risk, as well as about their symptoms. This would enable them to personalize and communicate information more effectively.

---

connections   Chapter 5 discusses the ways in which patients experience pain, showing that its physiological cause may be mediated by psychological elements such as anxiety or distraction.

The communication of pain between patient and medical professional is not a simple exchange of information. It is mediated by many factors, including the cultural repertoire of understandings available to each, the explanatory models used, the expectations of how they think the other party is behaving or interpreting behaviour, and personal responses to pain. There can be differences in reactions to and expressions of pain, emotion or stoicism across different ethnic groups (Davidhizar and Giger, 2004).

example 7.7

Accounts of pain

While many aspects of illness can be observed or measured, this is not always the case. Even aspects that can be rendered visible to the medical gaze require interpretation. In addition, there are symptoms and experiences associated with illness that cannot easily be quantified by an observer and medical practitioners rely on patients' accounts. One example of this is pain. It is possible to observe physical trauma that would be assumed to cause pain, such as injuries, but some episodes of pain may be unexplained. This means that practitioners may judge a person's pain on several levels:

- as part of a diagnostic process
- in terms of whether it seems a plausible reflection of their physical condition
- whether it is being expressed at a level they consider reasonable in view of their expectations.

One important issue that shapes the communication of pain is the fact that pain can be perceived in moral terms; to express too much pain, particularly if it does not match a medical professional's assessment of symptoms, can lead to assumptions of malingering, deceit or exaggeration. May et al. (1999) discuss attitudes surrounding chronic lower back pain (CLBP), a widely experienced condition that is often difficult to attribute to a specific observable cause. This has led to suspicion regarding the integrity of patients complaining of CLBP. The authors discuss

various historical shifts in perceptions, from the construction of 'railway spine' in the nineteenth century (when it was assumed that damage to the back was claimed in order to receive compensation from railway companies), to the notion of hysteria, which was linked to, among others, Freud's theories, and established the idea that back pain could be a neurotic and somatic symptom rather than a physical problem. May et al. comment that a divide began to be constructed between 'real', that is, organic, pain and 'untrustworthy' pain that could not as easily be explained. This divide has continued to be reflected in contemporary attitudes to CLBP, as demonstrated by this extract (May et al., 1999, p. 530):

- The patient expresses symptoms of pain and fatigue; these are formulated in terms of biomechanical degeneration or exhaustion of functional performance and are undoubtedly *real* experiences. The patient interprets these within a strict 'biomedical' model of organic cause and expects the clinician to act upon this basis.
- The clinician investigates potential organic cause, discounts the presence of sinister pathological signs and interprets expressed symptoms in the context of a psychosocial model. The patient understands this as casting doubt upon the *reality* of embodied experiences and is demoralized and dissatisfied. Both parties are ultimately pessimistic about the extent to which the other is 'willing' to hear their interpretation of expressed symptoms.

Representations of health

One of the most important arenas in which we can observe the cultural properties of health is that of the media, where messages on health are formulated, interpreted and exchanged. The mass media helps us to make sense of the world by shaping our commonsense, cultural ideas and interpretation of the world. Russell and Edgar state (1998, p. 4): 'Representations, linguistically and symbolically codified, are seen as creating social reality rather than just reflecting it.'

Ideas about health are conveyed through two channels, which are not discrete but overlap:

- official channels, the sphere of public health and health information
- non-official channels, discourses concerning health within popular culture.

Public health and health information

Public health and health information includes the concepts of health and illness contained within policy documents, public health initiatives, health promotion initiatives and publicity campaigns by charities. In many ways, public health campaigns resemble advertising: they are designed to sell us an idea of good health and the means of achieving it. Change4Life is a recent example of an extensive health promotion campaign designed to encourage a healthier diet and more exercise (DH, 2009).

? Why is it more difficult to 'sell' health in a public information campaign than to advertise a commercial product?

The differences between selling health in a public information campaign and advertising a commercial product are summarized in Table 7.2.

Table 7.2 **A comparison between a public information campaign and advertising a commercial product**

Public information campaign	Commercial marketing of a product
The aim is to effect fundamental behavioural changes among a large section of the population	The aim is to effect a small change in behaviour, such as brand-switching, among a section of the market
The budget is likely to be limited	The budget may be considerable
Market research is likely to be limited	Market research is likely to be detailed
It may be perceived as unethical to oversell potential gains from following advice	Exaggerated claims may be made, albeit within legal standards
The rewards for acquiescence may not be immediate	The rewards of consumption are perceived as being immediate

Health and popular culture

Health issues appear in popular culture in different ways, including:

- press reports, which may be based on official government pronouncements
- medical advisory columns
- television dramas.

The media act as gatekeepers of the public's awareness, reporting material that is deemed to be most interesting, most important or likely to increase circulation or viewing figures. Oinas (1998) presents an analysis of how medical advisory columns promote a medicalized construction of menstruation. The most common response to queries from teenage girls, most of which required no specialist expertise to answer, was advice to visit a doctor, either to have a problem solved or for a general check-up. The message conveyed is thus that of an expert monopoly on the body. Magazines act as a bridge between the medical profession and those initially reluctant to consult them.

Health issues are a favourite subject of dramas, documentaries, films and soap operas. *Casualty* and *Holby City*, for example, are popular TV programmes, interweaving the lives of medical staff with incidents of illness, accident and death. Much attention has been paid to how the health messages in these programmes are consumed by their viewers. Some analyses have shown that doctors are routinely portrayed in heroic ways, whereas nurses are usually nurturing or sexy (Karpf, 1988; Turow, 1989). In contrast, Bury and Gabe (1994) argue that whereas the massive growth in media representations of health and medicine strengthens their influence over consumers, the portrayals increasingly reflect shifting and contested power relations. Eisenman et al. (2005) report that viewers may passively absorb useful medical information, such as knowledge of resuscitation techniques.

Health and illness have also been powerful subject matter within literature. In recent years, there has been an upsurge in what has been dubbed 'confessional writing', in which authors explore and detail their encounters with illness, including terminal illness (for example Moore, 1996; Picardie, 1998; Diamond, 1999). Wurtzel (1996) draws on her experience of depression and its treatment to present the use of antidepressant medication as a cultural phenomenon. Some see these books as a symbol of self-indulgence, while others cite them as a powerful evocation of subjects previously treated as taboo.

> **thinking about** How do you regard literature or films of people's encounters with serious illness or death – gratuitous or insightful?

In recent years, the internet has become an increasingly significant forum for the exchange of ideas and representations of health. Online information often crosses the boundary of official and unofficial channels, as the two types may exist side by side, with some users uncertain about the differences. The internet can be used as a way for individuals and groups to challenge media representations. Access to the internet is not governed or filtered in the same way as conventional media – anyone can post any form of health information. Some, principally in the medical profession, have been disturbed by this, arguing that the public may access misleading information (Abbott, 2000). Others see the challenge to the medical profession's stranglehold on knowledge and expertise as a positive development.

---

example 7.8

HIV/AIDS and the internet

Gillett (2003) carried out a study on media activism and internet use by people with HIV/AIDS, and identified the following themes:

- Websites maintained by people living with HIV/AIDS strongly affirm the role of lay knowledge
- Many sites had autobiographies intended to inspire and inform others in a similar situation
- People with HIV/AIDS shared their experiences of treatments and symptoms
- Self-promotion was a common theme
- Individuals publicized their own activities or projects

- A less prevalent theme was that of dissent. Individuals challenged what were seen as perceived orthodoxies from within or outside the medical establishment on topics such as specific medications or the causes of HIV/AIDS.

In the main, these sites sought to give a voice to their individual producers' experiences without being formally affiliated to media activism. In this way, they escape the institutionalization that has occurred in relation to much earlier activism. Gillett's (2003) research illustrates the profound need people have to describe, share and represent their illness experiences as part of their identity.

A different perspective comes from Seale (2005), who argues that the old and new media are converging. Established media institutions now have a consolidated internet presence where they provide links to mainstream health resources. This means that internet users, far from experiencing a democratizing of knowledge, are increasingly directed to resources that replicate the dominant discourses of the old media. In part, this is because most popular (non-medical) search engines flag up mainstream sites.

thinking about What characterizes discourses about breast cancer in the media?

Women with breast cancer are portrayed as being on intense emotional journeys, in which cancer transforms their lives and the lives of those around them. Prostate cancer, on the other hand, is less reported; imagery tends to show men as more isolated, with a focus on fighting illness. Such representations clearly reinforce stereotypical views of men and women, while reinforcing dominant expectations of how they should behave and attach meaning to their illnesses. Seale's (2005) study of internet sites revealed similar trends. For example, a breast cancer site had a high number of photos representing women with breast cancer, often shown with family or friends, or doing activities such as trying on wigs. A prostate cancer site, by contrast, featured far less photos of men. Those that were shown were usually of people connected with the site in some way, such as fundraisers, rather than being representations of men with prostate cancer. Pictures were more often based on medical or technical diagrams, using mechanical imagery. Thus, the assumption that the internet may prove a vehicle for challenging discourses of illness experience seems not to hold true in this case. This is also reflected in regular controversies surrounding the publication on Facebook of images of women after breast cancer surgery. Many have been removed or attracted disapproval.

This view is affirmed by Nettleton et al. (2005), who argue that people's internet use is linked to specific conditions and complements more traditional sources, such as medical professionals, rather than representing an alternative perspective. Their research indicates that people who use internet health sites are aware of the potential for risk in terms of the trustworthiness of information. However, they tended to see this as a general risk and one to which they themselves would not fall prey. Nettleton et al. (2005) see the convergence of information as representing a form of third way between the idea of the internet as liberating people from the constraints of medical discourse and the idea that it conveys damaging and incorrect messages.

Reporting of diseases in the media tends to draw on a familiar stock of metaphors and imagery. Often these involve military language, in which diseases are characterized as invaders, while people with illnesses are portrayed as battling them bravely. Another common image is that of plague.

example 7.9

SARS in the media

An example of a disease that received a high degree of coverage in the media is severe acute respiratory syndrome (SARS). SARS attracted widespread attention and reporting in 2003 after the World Health Organization sent out an international alert. Most cases were in China, although a number of other locations were affected. In the UK, newspaper coverage tended to vary between portraying the disease as a major threat or dismissing fears as an alarmist panic. The focus was strongly on any perceived threat to the UK. Two sets of metaphors were used: 'SARS as killer', with its brutal properties represented in terms like 'hit' and 'attack'; and 'control', represented in terms like 'contain' and 'tackle', and institutional and bureaucratic responses (Wallis and Nerlich, 2005, p. 2632). The lack of war metaphors contrasts with reporting in countries where the threat was more immediate, where they continued to feature heavily. War metaphors failed to gain ground in UK reporting as no sole country could be identified as the prime site, the threat was distant, so the main aim was to avoid panic, and there was no clear expectation of victory. In addition, the fact that the UK was involved in a war in Iraq may have made militaristic metaphors less palatable.

Eichelberger (2007) identified a high level of blame and stigma directed at the community of New York's Chinatown in 2003, despite the fact that there were no reported cases of SARS there. Media speculation on the likelihood of an epidemic led to a drop in tourism and business in Chinatown. Eichelberger (2007) argues that there was a high degree of 'othering' in the media coverage: 'China was defined as a diseased threat to the modern healthy world.' The remedy was for China to effect cultural change. Reportage in the US was heavily racialized, with frequent images of Asians wearing face masks, portraying them as a source of infection. Eichelberger notes that in the May 2003 edition of *Time* magazine, the only photos of Asians were included in the context of SARS stories.

In China where the majority of cases occurred, Zhang (2006) outlines how media coverage ranged from restrictive, in the early days of SARS cases, to overwhelming, when the number of cases rose dramatically. He notes that this has been credited with having a permanent impact on the nature of the media in China, which has traditionally been secretive and subject to strong central control. In relation to TV coverage, Zhang argues that while the frequency of reports increased, the content still reflected the continuing political status quo rather than signifying any wholesale shift in dominant discourses. The key current affairs programme in China concentrated on praising government officials for their handling of the situation. This contrasted with the alarmist tone of reporting in other countries far less affected by the disease, as in the media's use of 'killer' metaphors in the UK. The language used in the Chinese media was more moderate, and drew on military imagery to invoke feelings of solidarity and heroic struggle.

The differences in the representation of SARS show that even when dealing with a contagious disease that has the potential to cross boundaries swiftly, the meaning of the disease is still demonstrably a cultural product. As such, it is fluid and open to different interpretation in different contexts. Reporting of the disease was shaped by a number of factors:

- the previous cultural repertoire of disease imagery
- the political and international context
- ideas of blame or compassion for people with the disease
- the perceived level of risk
- a managerial approach to global problems.

Part 2 Theoretical and research approaches

example 7.10

Examples of research in cultures and health

- How different diseases and illnesses (breast cancer, AIDS) are portrayed in popular culture
- The relationship of cultural beliefs and practices in connection with health and illness, for example in maternity and childbirth
- How health and wellbeing are socially and culturally constituted in comparative and transnational contexts
- The practice of medicine and the process of healing for the individual and community
- The cultural meaning and significance of certain health-related behaviours, for example smoking and excessive drinking
- How the experiences and perceptions of the body, self, or notion of the individual or person influence the illness experience

The study of culture is interdisciplinary and draws on a vast framework of knowledge and approaches, including sociology, media studies, philosophy, literature, anthropology and the visual arts. Its outlook is, above all, that of a *critical* perspective. Cultural studies challenges the boundaries, status and concerns of many more rigidly defined fields of study. Thus, cultural studies can perhaps best be thought of as a 'cross-disciplinary and anti-disciplinary field as well as an intellectual movement' (Alasuutari et al., 1998). In some ways, it is most easily characterized by its preoccupations, which centre on culture and meaning, and the complex power relations that shape them.

Many writers make a different claim for the origins of cultural studies. It has been variously traced back to Victorian observers such as Charles Booth and Henry Mayhew, early US sociologists (Jenks, 1993), or, less traditionally, to the work in the 1970s of the Kamiriithu Community Education and Cultural Centre in Kenya (Wright, 1998). However, most accounts of the development of cultural studies (Hall, 1980) cite the influence of three seminal figures and their works: Raymond Williams' *Culture and Society* (1961), E.P. Thompson's *The Making of the English Working Class* ([1963] 1978) and Richard Hoggart's *The Uses of Literacy* (1958). These authors, while divergent in their approaches and concerns, were notable for identifying and celebrating working-class culture. Hoggart became the first director of the Birmingham Centre for Contemporary Cultural Studies (founded in 1964), often credited as the academic grouping that consolidated the identity of cultural studies and provided the impetus for growth and expansion within universities across the world.

In theoretical terms, the key concept articulated by these authors was that culture began to be seen as a social feature that could not be reduced solely to a materialist base. This signalled a theoretical shift away from classical Marxism, which saw the whole of social life, and hence culture, as a product of the economic structure, designed to maintain and legitimate the status quo. It is here that the concept of ideology becomes central. From the classical Marxist perspective, ideological beliefs are often false: they serve to obscure the realization that society ultimately works in the best interests of the dominant classes.

Chapters 1, 3 and 6 explore disease aetiology and discuss models of disease causation. Culture is one of the factors to be considered alongside genetics, environment and others.	**connections**

Anthropology is the study of all aspects of society from a cross-cultural perspective. Historically, it was concerned with other 'exotic' cultures and was much criticized as the 'handmaiden' of colonialism. Contemporary anthropology is concerned with all cultures, while medical anthropology explores the social and cultural dimensions of health, ill health and medicine. Increasingly, it has focused on a critique of hegemonic power structures such as biomedicine as a potentially oppressive structure.

> **?** In what ways are people hailed or reaffirmed as patients within the healthcare system?

Doctor–patient relationships serve to reinforce the power of the medical professional over the layperson. The use of professional titles, coupled with the use of symbolic clothing such as white coats, serves to confirm the power of the expert. Thus, while this form of ideological practice and perpetuation is more subtle than Marx's concept of oppression, it still involves the collusion of all subjects in ideological dominance. Marxist analyses of the social structure remain a strong, if contested, influence within cultural studies. Few, however, now subscribe to the idea that all the features, beliefs and ideologies of a society are determined by its mode of production or economic organization. This shift away from reductionism is, in part, derived from the influence of the work of writers such as Althusser and Gramsci.

Althusser (1971) theorized that ideologies and cultures could be seen as having relative autonomy from the economic superstructure, and that all classes participated in the promotion and processes of ideology, rather than the dominant class imposing beliefs on others. In a classic text, Turner (1992) states that cultural studies draws on Althusser's view that key 'ideological state apparatuses', for example the family, the education system and religion, are every bit as significant as economic conditions. One of the most pervasive mechanisms of ideology is that of 'interpellation', also referred to as 'hailing'. This refers to the fact that we are continuously placed in our subject positions, such as mothers, older people or patients, by the way in which we are addressed within different forms of communication.

Gramsci (1971) suggests that for ideologies to become dominant (or hegemonic), they must continually struggle to reassert themselves through winning the consent of individuals and institutions. When a system of beliefs becomes dominant, this is often achieved by such a high degree of consent that the beliefs become naturalized. The most powerful set of ideas are those which deny their ideological quality by portraying themselves as natural and 'true'. Thus, the biomedical model of health could be described as hegemonic, in that it has become so firmly established that we see it as objective and rooted in the natural realm of biology.

Across a range of disciplines that explore the interface of culture and health, a variety of approaches that could be termed 'social constructionist' have taken hold, reflecting the influence of postmodernism discussed earlier in this chapter. Social constructionism (or social constructivism, as it sometimes called) looks at ways in which our understanding of the world is shaped within specific societies. At one extreme, there are 'strong' versions of social constructionism that are very relativistic. At this end of the spectrum, nothing has any objective reality, not even the physical world; everything must be understood as a social construction. At the other end of the spectrum, 'weak' approaches acknowledge a physical, material reality but see social issues as being constructed. Between these two extremes, many writers take an approach that acknowledges the biological and the social. This recognizes objective phenomena, but states that they are only given meaning through social processes. As Blaxter (2004) notes, this means that processes such as disease, pathogens and pain are acknowledged, but the way they are responded to and conceptualized is socially constructed. Blaxter (2004, p. 28) states: 'What counts as disease or abnormality is not "given" in the same sense as biological fact is given. It depends on cultural norms and culturally shared rules of interpretation.'

Given the eclectic, multidisciplinary nature of cultural studies, it inevitably makes use of a wide range of methodologies that originate in a range of different academic fields. Alasuutari (1995, p. 2) states that: 'Cultural studies methodology has often been described by the concept of *bricolage*: one is pragmatic and strategic in choosing and applying different methods and practices.' In theory, then, all methodologies are appropriate for use. However, given the emphasis that cultural studies places on meaning, it tends, maybe unsurprisingly, to focus primarily on qualitative approaches. These approaches can perhaps best be conceived as forming a broad spectrum, ranging from those focusing on people as the direct source of information to those that study texts.

Methods that centre on people may include or combine different forms of observational studies, types of direct questioning, such as semi-structured interviewing, or less formal means, such as the use of narratives or life histories. At the other end of the spectrum, there is the direct study of cultural artefacts or texts. A *text* is any cultural product – TV, films, newspapers, broadcasts, adverts, pictures or architecture – that can be analysed for the meanings it contains. Along the spectrum lie a variety of methodologies that incorporate a range of techniques.

Ethnography

The use of ethnography in cultural studies derives principally from anthropology. It stems from the fieldwork tradition in which researchers immerse themselves in the group or community being studied in order to understand its culture from within. Many methods may be employed in the search for understanding, including interviewing, observation and informal conversations. Data may be noted in a number of ways, such as tape-recordings, but the principal method of collection is the use of the researcher's notes and observations recorded in a fieldwork diary. One of the aims of ethnography is often termed 'thick description', following Geertz's influential work (1973).

Two issues immediately become apparent with this method of research. First, there is an ethical question. Observation may be overt or covert. The latter approach seeks to avoid 'contaminating' findings, which may occur if the research subjects know they are being observed. This method can, however, be characterized as exploitative. Given the time-consuming nature of an extended period of fieldwork, there is also the danger that the findings may, in practice, be based on sketchy or sporadic observations, a tendency characterized by Murdock (1997) as 'thin descriptions'.

Second, however fully the researchers immerse themselves within the group, there will inevitably be an element of subjective interpretation. In attempting to understand any culture and its practices, researchers' interpretations will be shaped by their own cultural location. Many critiques of an earlier, more confident and authoritative ethnography have come from feminist writers who have challenged the notion of the traditional research hierarchy by which subjects become objectified (Atkinson and Coffey, 1995). Feminist researchers have been at the forefront of the cultural studies' goal of enabling the voice of marginalized groups to be heard; ethnography can be a valuable method in this cause.

---

example 7.11

Ethnography and concepts of health among the Cree in Quebec

Adelson's (1998) study of health beliefs among the Cree of Whapmagoostui in northern Quebec clearly illustrates the fact that concepts of health must be understood as cultural. She characterizes her research as participant observation, including interviews with over 20% of the adults in the community, which took place over a two-year period. Adelson found that there was no direct translation of the term 'health'; the term used by the Cree translates most closely as 'being alive well'. This concept is closely bound to the Cree's specific sociocultural context (Adelson, 1998):

> 'being alive well' is defined through local beliefs and practices, simultaneously incorporating references to an idealized past and consolidating issues of cultural identity. 'Being alive well' is inseparable from community, history, identity, and ultimately resistance.

The history of the Cree village studied is one of contact with prospectors, hunters and traders. As for many indigenous people exposed to outside groups, this contact altered the traditional way of life and introduced new diseases. The community was transformed by contact, modernization and cultural exchange. In 1989, the community was mobilized by its opposition to a proposal by the Quebec provincial government to initiate a hydroelectric project that would have had an immense impact on the local environment. Although successful in their opposition, they face continual challenges in the face of sovereignty disputes. The specific history and conditions of the Cree form a vital context in understanding concepts of health.

The concept of 'being alive well' is distinct from Western biomedical constructions of health and is not rooted in physiology. It is possible to be unwell in the Western sense of the word, yet still to be in a state of 'being alive well'. 'Being alive well' relates more to a way of life associated with practices such as carrying out physical activity, keeping warm and eating traditional Cree foods, which reflects the people's strong relationship with the land and its preservation. The vigour of the land and the Cree themselves is associated with an idealized past that existed before the 'white man' came. The customs and conditions introduced by the 'white man' are seen as weakening the sense in which the Cree can 'be alive well'. This study illustrates the ways in which groups can be studied by ethnographic methods in order to bring cultural practices and beliefs alive. In this example, health is a product of sociocultural conditions and a marker of cultural identity.

Discourse and conversation analysis

Broadly speaking, a **discourse** is a series of terms, values, symbols and words that gather about a topic or group. Discourses are permeated and shaped by cultural and ideological connotations. In the linguistic sense, discourse analysis involves analysing patterns and structures of talk in order to reveal the forms and constraints of social interaction. Within this broad approach, the term 'conversation analysis' is often used more narrowly to describe a specific methodology for analysing how language shapes the discussion of two or more parties.

Conversation analysis permits us to go beyond an examination of the content of a conversation or interview in order to examine how both parties interact and construct their subject positions. Any conversation can be analysed for the incidence of patterned regularities of speech that allow the participants to position themselves in relation to one another. For example, we can examine how men and women talk to one another, how couples structure a narrative when they are relating an event, and how medical consultations establish the relative social positions of doctor and patient. A crucial element of this approach is that it is only the conversation that is subjected to analysis: all other forms of context or background must be excluded. Thus, for the purposes of analysis, transcriptions of conversations follow detailed rules. All speech must be reproduced verbatim, pauses timed to within a tenth of a second, and the points at which interruptions and responses occur precisely noted.

At the heart of conversation analysis is the recognition that conversations tend to follow certain rules. At a basic level, this comprises turn-taking, that is, the way in which participants negotiate the order of utterances. One important feature is that of pairs of utterances, for example question–answer, invitation–acceptance/refusal. Subverting these implicit rules may result in a call for justification or explanation (Alasuutari, 1995). There can, however, be a significant difference between the types of conversation. An everyday discussion may have different properties from 'institutional talk' such as meetings or layperson–expert interactions. Conversation analysis, then, reveals how structures of power within society operate through the formal, if often unacknowledged, rules of speech engagement. While conversation analysis is a rigorous approach with a carefully detailed focus, it is also possible to combine its insights with knowledge of broader cultural patterns and relationships.

Ten Have (1991) argues that such talk is asymmetrical and reflects a hierarchical organization of speech interaction. This is in part the result of inherent power imbalances between the layperson and medical expert. In addition, the talk itself actively produces asymmetry. First, the patient's, rather than the doctor's, problems are the focus. Second, the carrying out of the tasks of the encounter (complaint presentation, examination, diagnosis and treatment) is dominated by the doctor. Ten Have discusses a number of ways in which this asymmetry becomes manifest in talk. For example, how doctors elicit information frames patients' replies, and is often designed to produce brief answers. Patients are not encouraged simply to narrate an account of their illness. Doctors also display control by questioning without context or justification: they are not required to explain the reasoning behind their questions. Doctors' noncommittal replies reveal nothing of their reaction to responses. Thus, ten Have states that asymmetry is produced by doctors' role as initiators and their control of the information they divulge.

An interesting example of discourse analysis, a broader approach than conversation analysis, is found in Blumenreich and Siegel's (2006) study of the imagery used in children's books about HIV/AIDS. They examine the way in which children's understandings become shaped by dominant discourses. One text is shown to reproduce messages of social stigma, even though its explicit aim appears to be to generate understanding for HIV-positive children. The child with HIV is depicted as naturally an outcast, for whom sympathy is required as befitting his victim status. The child's mother, who is shown as a drug user, does not receive much compassion. The author makes frequent use of war metaphors in discussing how the AIDS virus operates. In their analysis, Blumenreich and Siegel (2006) found that common themes were a tendency to use outdated information, a neglect of new treatments that help people live with HIV, a lack of ethnic diversity among characters, and the use of stereotypical views of people with HIV/AIDS.

Blumenreich and Siegel (2006) identify three principal discourses:

1. *A public service discourse:* has a health education approach and deals with themes of transmission and appropriate behaviour. **Risk groups** are portrayed as threats to the general population, who are somehow different. When members of the general population become infected, they are seen as innocent victims, with the unspoken inference that others are 'guilty' victims. The main aim of this discourse appears to be to reassure the general population.

2. *Medical discourse:* much medical scientific writing about AIDS uses war metaphors. Typical terminology is about 'fighting off invaders', 'defences' and 'enemies'. Children's texts draw heavily on this imagery, which again sets up divisions between good and bad, normal and abnormal.

3. *Secrecy:* characters often discuss secrets associated with diagnosis, or the fact that they have to lie about situations, or piece together facts by themselves rather than being told information directly. This secrecy is often echoed in plots that conceal characters' sexuality or personal circumstances.

Countering these discourses, however, were some texts that sought to convey oppositional discourses. A limited number show children who are HIV positive being healthy or misbehaving like other children. Sometimes, HIV-positive children are shown as being good friends and having something to offer rather than just people who require kindness. Only a couple of books include direct treatment of the topic of death, although texts featuring children's own discussions of living with HIV/AIDS show that this is an issue uppermost in their minds.

Most of the books Blumenreich and Siegel (2006) studied engage with common cultural concerns about HIV and AIDS. In doing so, their intent is often to reassure and inform children, helping them deal with difficult situations. However, in the process, they draw on dominant imagery and reinforce constructions of disease, which shapes children's understandings. In Althusser's language, children interpellate these images and messages and take them on as their own.

Semiotics

Semiotics (or semiology) focuses on the study of *signs* contained within texts. Signs comprise two components:

- signifiers – sounds, words or images

- the signified – the concepts represented by signifiers.

Thus, a photograph of someone with a stethoscope around their neck (the signifier) would suggest the concept of medical power (the signified). Meaning emerges from the relationship between the signifier and the signified.

> **?** Consider well-known adverts such as those for Marlboro cigarettes. The Marlboro man was depicted as a cowboy riding a horse in 'Marlboro country'. What is signified by this image?

The Marlboro man brings forth ideas of the Wild West, freedom, masculinity and independence. These images successfully made consumers and potential consumers perceive Marlboro to be a man's cigarette. By contrast, cigarettes such as Kim or Silk Cut, aimed at female consumers, emphasized the 'lightness' or mildness of the cigarette.

When we are part of a culture, we learn and internalize complex and shifting patterns of associations, which can be termed 'codes'. Thus, we develop a way of making sense of the world in which we learn to read off meanings and associations from signs within everyday life. This is not necessarily something we carry out consciously: the process may become instinctive and automatic. However, as these relationships and associations are dynamic and changing, not everyone will work with the same system of codes or understand codes in the same way. This can lead to what has been termed 'aberrant coding': a mismatch of meaning between those who produce cultural artefacts and those who receive them. Thus, a public health message, for example, may fail because its makers use terms or images that do not conjure up the same pattern of associations in the minds of its target group.

case study breastfeeding and infant feeding across cultures

The prevalence of childhood overweight and obesity worldwide has greatly increased over the past few decades. There is some evidence that a risk of obesity is influenced by exposures early in life. Among other factors, breastfeeding has been proposed as a potential protective factor against overweight (Arenz et al., 2004; Beyerlein and von Kries, 2011). Breastfeeding is therefore seen as a central strategy in addressing childhood obesity.

The ability to breastfeed is in many respects universal, although there will always be women who find it difficult or impossible. However, the meaning and value afforded to breastfeeding, its duration, the way in which difficulties are perceived and responded to, and the transition to weaning are all subject to tremendous cultural variation. Currently, the dominant wisdom regarding breastfeeding in the West is that it is demonstrably best for babies. Despite this evidence, considerable disparities in rates of breastfeeding exist between cultures. Attitudes towards breastfeeding among mothers, families and potential support networks, the general public, medical professionals and policy-makers all contribute to the cultural milieu in which breastfeeding either does or does not take place.

One way to identify how breastfeeding is mediated by cultural factors is to explore changes in practices over time. Formula milk, a heavily modified version of cow's milk that is safe for babies to drink, is a comparatively recent invention. Its introduction opened up a new range of possibilities for infant nutrition, as well as associated shifts in discourse surrounding the desirability of breastfeeding. Prior to this, although many of the concerns of breastfeeding, such as insufficient milk, were familiar, dilemmas, values and strategies often differed. Fildes (1986) has conducted extensive research on the history of infant feeding and identifies a wealth of associated practices. For example, in ancient India, newborn babies would be given a mix of ghee and honey until the mother's milk came in some three to four days later. She states that colostrum is still commonly regarded as a harmful or taboo substance in certain developing societies, in spite of current medical evidence suggesting it is a vital source of antibodies and proteins for the newborn baby. In their study of neonatal care in Pakistan, Fikree et al. (2005) identified 'risky traditional newborn care practices', such as giving babies honey, water or tea as their first feed.

Such practices are not confined to developing countries. Bentley et al.'s (1999) study of young African American mothers from low-income backgrounds found that semi-solids, such as cereals, were introduced as early as within the first two weeks. Introducing solids too early has been associated with allergies and obesity (Skinner, 1997, in Bentley et al., 1999). The babies' grandmothers often played a valued and key role in childcare, so their views on infant feeding became part of the cultural common sense on which the young mothers drew. Therefore, grandmothers' advice was often followed, even when it conflicted with that of health professionals. There was a strong sense that milk alone was inadequate and babies who were seen as small or who cried or woke up frequently needed solids. Babies' behaviour was also frequently interpreted as signs that they were 'greedy'. Giving solids was a way of responding positively to a hungry baby, and was constructed as a sign of good parenting. This study shows the importance of engaging with the social context when attempting to promote breastfeeding, in this case understanding why solids would be given and realizing that the mother is not the only significant carer.

In a different setting, Aubel et al. (2004) found that engaging grandmothers in a community health programme had a significant impact on raising awareness of optimal feeding practices. In Senegal, although breastfeeding is widespread, it is often supplemented by other foods and fluids rather than being exclusive, and it is not always immediate. In Aubel et al.'s study, involving grandmothers in education sessions increased their knowledge of nutrition, raised self-esteem and increased the respect shown for them within households and the wider community.

Throughout history, an inability to breastfeed is well documented. In the past, however, the recommended strategy was to use a wet nurse – another lactating woman who could nurse the baby instead of its mother. This practice ensures that a baby benefits from breast milk. Elements of this practice are still witnessed today when women donate excess milk to milk banks. In some periods and cultures, wet nurses could be of high standing. At other times, they were poor and seen as either exploited or as potentially dangerous and exploitative themselves.

Entwined with ideas about wet nurses and breastfeeding are concerns about the concept of motherhood and how women should behave. Fildes (1986) discusses the views of Roman philosophers such as Pliny and Tacitus, who stressed the importance of maternal breastfeeding for nutrition and attachment. They also noted a class element, deploring the fact that poor women fed their own children while richer mothers employed wet nurses. Fildes highlights a contrast with medical writers of the time, who were keener that the most suitable person would breastfeed. This would not necessarily be the mother, especially if she were ill or became pregnant, as this was seen to spoil her milk and potentially damage the child. Nevertheless, debates about breastfeeding versus wet nursing continued in many societies, echoing contemporary debates concerning breastfeeding versus formula feeding. In relation to Europe in the late sixteenth and seventeenth century, Fildes (1986, p. 100) notes that:

Wet nursing was an ancient, deeply-ingrained and widely-accepted social custom, and wealthy mothers who decided to nurse their own babies were sufficiently exceptional to attract comment (often adverse) both from close friends and from the wider social circle.

Women's objections to breastfeeding largely centred on the fear of losing their looks or becoming ill. Breastfeeding was thought to make women look older, produce sagging breasts, and inhibit the range of fashionable clothing that could be worn. There is documentation of women enduring considerable damage to their breasts from feeding. Repeated cuts became infected, scar tissue resulted and sometimes children chewed through nipples. Here, we see a dilemma for women – whether to conform to the role of good mother or the role of attractive, desirable woman.

The breast can be seen as a complex signifier. Its biological function is to provide breast milk to nurture a baby. However, this cannot be separated from the social value we attach to the process and the woman who nurses. The breast is a signifier not just of motherhood, but also sexuality and feminine identity. Promoting the advantages of breastfeeding currently takes place in a cultural context that sees breasts as primarily sexualized rather than nurturing. Because of these connotations, exposing the breast can also be seen as indecent, which can impose restrictions on mothers being able to feed in public places.

Among women who are keen to breastfeed, the inability to do so can provoke intense feelings of shame and grief. However, even successful feeding can be tremendously stressful. Flacking et al.'s (2007) study of mothers of premature infants in Sweden found that establishing a secure bond was sometimes difficult due to the need for their babies to receive specialist care, which often entailed physical separation, and the intense emotions and exhaustion associated with anxiety for their babies' wellbeing. Mothers felt under tremendous pressure to breastfeed, as its nutritional value was critical for their vulnerable babies. Sweden has a strong culture of breastfeeding, which is seen as a marker of good mothering. Being able to breastfeed was a vital aspect of these women's role of good mother. Unhappy experiences of breastfeeding or failing to find the experience enjoyable created feelings of anxiety in mothers about the nature of their bond with their child. Women who bottle-fed expressed feelings of shame about doing so in public.

In order to promote breastfeeding among mothers, health professionals have to understand the specific cultural factors that contribute to women's decisions. These can be variable. Scavenius et al. (2007) studied breastfeeding in Brazil, and found that an extremely high intention to breastfeed among pregnant women translated into a much lower rate of continuing breastfeeding – 29% at six months compared to rates of between 50–63% in other Latin American countries. In poorer countries, the protective effect of breastfeeding is even more important, so the public health goal of exclusive breastfeeding for at least six months is crucial. As 98% of newborn deaths occur in developing countries, care practices are key to survival (WHO, 1996). Scavenius et al. (2007) traced the discrepancy between intent and breastfeeding practice in Brazil to features of the social context in recent years, including the promotion of formula milk via the US development programme in the 1970s, which contrasts with the strong health promotion emphasis on breastfeeding. They draw on van Esterik's (1988, in Scavenius et al., 2007) distinction between breast milk as 'product' and breastfeeding as 'process' to characterize Brazil's cultural understanding. Cultures that focus on breast milk as a product are more likely to have beliefs about the quality or supply of milk, use supplements and cease exclusive breastfeeding comparatively early. Cultures that see breastfeeding as a process perceive it as a complex social activity and have ways to facilitate this pattern of interaction between mother and child, including overcoming difficulties. This results in longer exclusive breastfeeding. Scavenius et al. (2007) argue that their research demonstrates an important interaction between the biological and the social. In biological terms, milk is stimulated by frequent suckling. However, the frequency of suckling is linked to social factors, such as the value attached to mothers' breastfeeding, its acceptability in public, whether other roles such as employment constrain mothers, or the way in which identity is intertwined with nursing. In the UK, it became illegal under the Equality Act 2010 to treat a breastfeeding woman unfavourably. However, this has not led to breastfeeding becoming an unproblematic activity.

Summary

- All cultures have systems of health beliefs to explain what causes illness, how it can be cured or treated, and who should be involved in the process

- This chapter has explored the ways in which popular Western culture constructs illness as 'battles' and patients as 'survivors' or 'victims', reflecting the dominance of natural science explanations for illness

- The ethnographic methods used in anthropology enable a focus on human relations and the meanings other communities give to health and illness

- Cultural competence is a key area of health and social care practice. This means appreciating and living with difference

Questions for further discussion

1. The term 'cultural competence' is widely used to describe organizations that recognize and address issues of diversity. What elements would you expect to be included?

2. Why should health professionals understand the cultural context of health decisions?

3. What does the widespread use of products such as organic foods, farmers' markets and water filters indicate about our cultural attitudes to food and health?

4. Consider how a product such as alcohol is marketed. What type of analysis would you use to investigate this?

Further reading

Alasuutari, P. (1995) *Researching Culture: Qualitative Method and Cultural Studies*. London: Sage. Useful, comprehensive account of various methodologies.

Dein, S. (2006) *Culture and Cancer Care: Anthropological Insights on Oncology*. Maidenhead: Open University Press.
Thoughtful, comprehensive comparative text, focusing on a range of cultural issues in relation to cancer.

Helman, C. (2007) *Culture, Health and Illness* (5th edn). Oxford: Butterworth Heinemann. Clear account from the perspective of medical anthropology, which has a longer tradition of analysing health as a cultural phenomenon.

Turner, G. (2003) *British Cultural Studies: An Introduction* (3rd edn). London: Routledge. Accessible overview of the discipline and development of cultural studies. Explores language, semiotics, Marxism and ideology, individualism, subjectivity and discourse.

Turner, G. (2012) *What's Become of Cultural Studies?* London: Sage. Explores whether cultural studies still has relevance.

Some journals explicitly address issues of culture in relation to health, for example *Culture, Health and Sexuality, Ethnicity and Health* and *Sociology of Health and Illness*.

References

Abbott, V.P. (2000) 'Web page quality: Can we measure it and what do we find? A report of exploratory findings'. *Journal of Public Health Medicine* 22(2): 191–7.

Adelson, N. (1998) 'Health beliefs and the politics of Cree well-being'. *Health* 2(1): 5–22.

Ahmad, W.I.U. (1996) The trouble with culture, in D. Kelleher and S. Hillier (eds) *Researching Cultural Differences in Health*. London: Routledge, pp. 190–219.

Alasuutari, P. (1995) *Researching Culture: Qualitative Method and Cultural Studies*. London: Sage.

Alasuutari, P., Gray, A. and Hermes, J. (1998) 'Editorial'. *European Journal of Cultural Studies*, 1(1): 5–11.

Althusser, L. (1971) *Lenin and Philosophy and other Essays*, trans. B. Brewster. New York: Monthly Review Press.

Arenz, S., Rückerl, R., Koletzko, B. and von Kries, R. (2004) Breast-feeding and childhood obesity: a systematic review. *International Journal of Obesity* 28(10): 1247–56.

Atkinson, P. and Coffey, A. (1995) Realism and its discontents: on the crisis of cultural representation in ethnographic texts, in B. Adam and S. Allan (eds) *Theorizing Culture: An Interdisciplinary Critique after Postmodernism*. London: UCL Press, pp. 41–57.

Aubel, J., Toure, I. and Diagne, M. (2004) 'Senegalese grandmothers promote improved maternal and child nutrition practices: the guardians of tradition are not averse to change'. *Social Science & Medicine* 59(5): 945–59.

Baskind, R. and Birbeck, G. (2005) 'Epilepsy care in Zambia: a study of traditional healers'. *Epilepsia* 46(7): 1121–6.

Bentley, M., Gavin, L., Black, M.M. and Teti, L. (1999) 'Infant feeding practices of low-income, African-American, adolescent mothers: an ecological, multigenerational perspective'. *Social Science & Medicine*, 49: 1085–100.

Beyerlein, A. and von Kries, R. (2011) 'Breastfeeding and body composition in children: Will there ever be conclusive empirical evidence for a protective effect against overweight?' *American Journal of Clinical Nutrition* 94(6 Suppl): 1772S–5S.

Blaxter, M. (1990) *Health and Lifestyles*. London: Routledge.

Blaxter, M. (2004) *Health*. Cambridge: Polity.

Blumenreich, M. and Siegel, M. (2006) 'Innocent victims, fighter cells, and white uncles: a discourse analysis of children's books about AIDS'. *Children's Literature in Education* 37(1): 81–110.

Bury, M. (2005) *Health and Illness*. Cambridge: Polity.

Bury, M. and Gabe, J. (1994) Television and medicine: medical dominance or trial by media?, in J. Gabe, D. Kelleher and G. Williams (eds) *Challenging Medicine*. London: Routledge, pp. 65–83.

Caplan, P. (1997) Approaches to food, health and identity, in P. Caplan (ed.) *Food, Health and Identity*. London: Routledge, pp. 1–31.

Davidhizar, R. and Giger, J.N. (2004) 'A review of the literature on care of clients in pain who are culturally divers'. *International Nursing Review* 51(1): 47–55.

Dein, S. (2006) *Culture and Cancer Care: Anthropological Insights on Oncology*. Maidenhead: Open University Press.

De Saussure, F. (1960) *Course in General Linguistics*, trans. W. Baskin. London: Peter Owen.

DH (Department of Health) (2001) *The Expert Patient: A New Approach to Chronic Disease Management for the 21st Century*. London: TSO.

DH (2009) *Change4Life Principles and Guidelines for Promotion*. London: TSO.

Diamond, J. (1999) *Because Cowards Get Cancer Too*. London: Vermillion.

Doyle, B. (1995) Changing the culture of cultural studies, in B. Adam and S. Allan (eds) *Theorizing Culture: An Interdisciplinary Critique after Postmodernism*. London: UCL Press, pp. 174–85.

Eichelberger, L. (2007) 'SARS and New York's Chinatown: the politics of risk and blame during an epidemic of fear'. *Social Science & Medicine* 41(7): 957–68.

Eisenman, A., Rutestski, V., Zohar, Z. and Stolero, J. (2005) 'Subconscious passive learning of CPR techniques through television medical drama'. *Australasian Journal of Paramedicine*, 3(3). Available at http://ro.ecu.edu.au/jephc/vol3/iss3/3 (accessed 1/9/2014).

Fikree, F.F., Ali, T.S., Druocher, J.M. and Rahbar, M.H. (2005) 'Newborn care practices in low socioeconomic settlements of Karachi, Pakistan'. *Social Science & Medicine* 60(5): 911–21.

Fildes, V. (1986) *Breasts, Bottles and Babies: A History of Infant Feeding*. Edinburgh: Edinburgh University Press.

Fiske, J. (2011) *Introduction to Communication Studies* (3rd edn). London: Routledge.

Flacking, R., Ewald, U. and Starrin, B. (2007) '"I wanted to do a good job": experiences of "becoming a mother" and breastfeeding in mothers of very preterm infants after discharge from a neonatal unit'. *Social Science & Medicine* 64(12): 2405–16.

Friedman, M. (2012) 'Fat is a social work issue: fat bodies, moral regulation, and the history of social work'. *Intersectionalities* 1: 35–69.

Geertz, C. (1973) *The Interpretation of Cultures: Selected Essays*. New York: Basic Books.

Gillett, J. (2003) 'Media activism and internet use by people with HIV/AIDS'. *Sociology of Health & Illness* 25(6): 608–24.

Gramsci, A. (1971) *Selections from Prison Notebooks*. London: Lawrence & Wishart.

Hall, S. (1980) 'Cultural studies: two paradigms'. *Media, Culture & Society* 2: 57–72.

Helman, C. (2000) *Culture, Health and Illness* (4th edn). Oxford: Butterworth Heinemann.

Hoggart, R. (1958) *The Uses of Literacy*. London: Penguin.

James, A. (1997) How British is British food?, in P. Caplan (ed.) *Food, Health and Identity*. London: Routledge, pp. 71–86.

James, D.J. (2004) 'Factors influencing food choices, dietary intake, and nutrition-related attitudes among African Americans: application of a culturally sensitive model'. *Ethnicity & Health* 9(4): 349–67.

Jenks, C. (1993) *Culture*. London: Routledge.

Karpf, A. (1988) *Doctoring the Media: The Reporting of Health and Medicine*. London: Routledge.

Katbamna, S., Bhakta, P. and Parker, G. (2000) Perceptions of disability and care-giving relationships in South Asian communities, in W.I.U. Ahmad (ed.)

Ethnicity, Disability and Chronic Illness. Buckingham: Open University Press, pp. 12–27.

Kelleher, D. (1994) Self-help groups and their relationship to medicine, in J. Gabe, D. Kelleher and G. Williams (eds) *Challenging Medicine*. London: Routledge, pp. 104–17.

Kelly, M. and Millward, L. (2013) Identity and illness, in D. Kelleher and G. Leavey (eds) *Identity and Health*. London: Routledge, pp. 1–19.

Kleinman, A. (1980) *Patients and Healers in the Context of Culture: An Exploration of the Borderland between Anthropology, Medicine and Psychiatry*. Berkley, CA: University of California Press.

Larson, N., Fulkerson, J., Story, M. and Neumark-Sztainer, D. (2013) 'Shared meals among young adults are associated with better diet quality and predicted by family meal patterns during adolescence'. *Public Health Nutrition* 16(5): 883–93.

Lévi-Strauss, C. (1970) *The Raw and the Cooked: Introduction to a Science of Mythology*, vol. 1. London: Jonathan Cape.

McIntosh, W.A., Kubena, K.S., Tolle, G. et al. (2010) 'Mothers and meals: the effects of mothers' meal planning and shopping motivations on children's participation in family meals'. *Appetite* 55(3): 623–8.

May, C., Doyle, H. and Chew-Graham, C. (1999) 'Medical knowledge and the intractable patient: the case of chronic low back pain'. *Social Science & Medicine* 48(4): 523–34.

Moore, O. (1996) *PWA: Looking AIDS in the Face*. Basingstoke: Macmillan – now Palgrave Macmillan.

Morgan, M. (1996) The meanings of high blood pressure among Afro-Caribbean and white patients, in D. Kelleher and S. Hillier (eds) *Researching Cultural Differences in Health*. London: Routledge, pp. 11–37.

Moscowitz, J.T., Wrubel, J., Hult, J.R. et al. (2013) 'Illness appraisals and depression in the first year after HIV diagnosis'. *PLoS One* 8(10): e78904.

Murcott, A. (1997) Family meals: a thing of the past?, in P. Caplan (ed.) *Food, Health and Identity*. London: Routledge, pp. 32–49.

Murdock, G. (1997) Thin descriptions: questions of method in cultural analysis, in J. McGuigan (ed.) *Cultural Methodologies*. London: Sage, pp. 178–92.

Nettleton, S., Burrows, R. and O'Malley, L. (2005) 'The mundane realities of the everyday lay use of the internet for health, and their consequences for media convergence'. *Sociology of Health & Illness* 27(7): 972–92.

NHS Choices (2013) Reducing your baby's risk of cot death. Available at www.nhs.uk/conditions/pregnancy-and-baby/pages/reducing-risk-cot-death.aspx (accessed 4/9/2014).

Oinas, E. (1998) 'Medicalisation by whom? Accounts of menstruation conveyed by young women and medical experts in medical advisory columns'. *Sociology of Health & Illness*, 20(1): 52–70.

Picardie, R. (1998) *Before I Say Goodbye*. London: Penguin Books.

Pote, H.L. and Orrell, M.W. (2002) 'Perceptions of schizophrenia in multi-cultural Britain'. *Ethnicity & Health* 7(1): 7–20.

Prior, L. (2003) 'Belief, knowledge and expertise: the emergence of the lay expert in medical sociology'. *Sociology of Health & Illness* 25(3): 41–57.

Russell, A. and Edgar, I.R. (1998) Research and practice in the anthropology of welfare, in I.R. Edgar and A. Russell (eds) *The Anthropology of Welfare*. London: Routledge.

Scavenius, M., van Hulsel, L., Meijer, J. et al. (2007) 'In practice, the theory is different: a processual analysis of breastfeeding in northeast Brazil'. *Social Science & Medicine* 64: 676–88.

Schulman-Green, D., Jaser, S., Martin, F. et al. (2012) 'Processes of self-management in chronic illness'. *Journal of Nurse Scholarship* 44(2): 136–44.

Schuster, J., Beune, E. and Stronks, K. (2011) 'Metaphorical construction of hypertension among three ethnic groups in the Netherlands'. *Ethnicity & Health* 16(6): 583–600.

Scior, K., Kan, K., McLoughlin, A. and Sheridan, J. (2010) 'Public attitudes towards people with intellectual disabilities: a cross-cultural study'. *Intellectual and Developmental Disabilities* 48(4): 278–89.

Seale, C. (2005) 'New directions for critical internet health studies: representing cancer experience on the web'. *Sociology of Health & Illness* 27(4): 515–40.

Spector, R. (2012) *Cultural Diversity in Health and Illness* (8th edn). Upper Saddle River, NJ: Pearson Prentice Hall.

Stead, M., McDermott, L., MacKintosh, A.M. and Adamson, A. (2011) 'Why healthy eating is bad for young people's health: identity, belonging and food'. *Social Science & Medicine* 72: 1131–9.

Ten Have, P. (1991) Talk and institution: a reconsideration of the 'asymmetry' of doctor–patient interaction, in D. Boden and D.H. Zimmerman (eds) *Talk and Social Structure*. Cambridge: Polity, pp. 138–63.

Thompson, E.P. ([1963] 1978) *The Making of the English Working Class*. London: Penguin.

Turner, B. (1992) *Regulating Bodies: Essays in Medical Sociology*. London: Routledge.

Turow, J. (1989) *Playing Doctor: Television Storytelling and Medical Power*. New York: Oxford University Press.

Wallis, P. and Nerlich, B. (2005) 'Disease metaphors in new epidemics: the UK media framing of the 2003 SARS epidemic'. *Social Science & Medicine* 60(11): 2629–39.

Walter, F.M. and Britten, N. (2003) 'Patients' understandings of risk: a qualitative study of decision-making about the menopause and hormone replacement therapy in general practice'. *Family Practice* 19(6): 579–86.

WHO (World Health Organization) (1996) *Perinatal Mortality: A Listing of Available Information*, FRH/MSM, 96.7. Geneva: WHO.

Wiese, M., Oster, C. and Pincombe, J. (2010) 'Understanding the emerging relationship between complementary medicine and mainstream health care: a review of the literature'. *Health* 14(3): 326–42.

Williams, R. (1961) *Culture and Society 1780–1950*. Harmondsworth: Penguin.

Wright, H.K. (1998) 'Dare we de-centre Birmingham?: Troubling the "origin" and trajectories of cultural studies'. *European Journal of Cultural Studies* 1(1): 33–56.

Wurtzel, E. (1996) *Prozac Nation*. London: Quartet Books.

Zhang, X. (2006) 'Reading between the headlines: SARS, *Focus* and TV current affairs programmes in China'. *Media, Culture & Society* 28(5): 715–37.

CLARE BAMBRA, KATHERINE SMITH and LYNNE KENNEDY

Politics and health

chapter

8

Overview	266
Introduction	266
Part 1 The contribution of political science to health studies	267
The political and the non-political	268
The political nature of health	270
Part 2 Theoretical and research approaches	274
Conservatism	275
Liberalism (and neoliberalism)	276
Socialism and social democracy	278
Nationalism (and fascism)	280
Feminism	281
Environmentalism	283
Case study The politics of 'fat'	284
Summary	287
Questions for further discussion	288
Further reading	288
References	289

Learning outcomes

This chapter will enable readers to:

- Compare competing definitions of politics and variants of political science
- Understand the political nature of health
- Examine the influence of politics and political ideology on health
- Assess the emerging contribution of politics to health studies

Overview

The discipline of politics examines the debates, ideas and institutions that surround community organization and collective decision-making about resources. In this chapter, the contribution of politics to health studies is examined. Part 1 considers how politics is defined and how this underpins the various strands of political science. It examines some of the key concepts of political study: power, ideology, democracy, government and the state. It also explores what contribution politics has and can make to health studies. Part 2 considers some of the theoretical and research approaches within political science. It looks at political ideologies, how they offer competing definitions of politics, varied views of the social and political world, and divergent views on health and health improvement. A case study explores how recent changes in many contemporary societies, associated in particular with neoliberal economic policies, have led to a greater emphasis on freedom through choice. Individuals are called on to take a greater role in self-care and risk management in relation to their bodies. At the same time, the development of large multinational companies has given rise to a system of production whereby their size and dominance have provided them with an ability to structure the food market.

Introduction

In broad terms, politics is about **community** organization, how people choose to live together, and collective decision-making about resources or, as Laswell (1936) has claimed, 'who gets what, when, how'. A variety of competing definitions have been utilized over time and by different political **ideologies**, and it has been suggested that the definition of politics is in itself a political act (Leftwich, 1984). Following Heywood (2007), a broad fourfold classification is possible:

1. *Politics as government:* The word 'politics' is derived from *polis*, the Greek for city-state. Traditionally, politics has been associated with the art of government and the activities of the state, and its academic study focuses on the personnel and machinery of government, excluding the many arenas in which political activities take place in civil society.

2. *Politics as public life:* Politics is primarily concerned with the conduct and management of community affairs through the institutions of the state (the courts, police, the NHS), excluding the political activity of families, personal relationships and so on.

3. *Politics as conflict resolution:* Politics is concerned with the expression and resolution of conflicts through compromise, conciliation, negotiation and other strategies. Politics is thus seen as a process privileging debate and discussion.

4. *Politics as power:* Politics is the process through which the production, distribution and use of scarce resources is determined in all areas of social existence, including personal relationships.

This classification shows a large variation in the conceptualization of politics; for example, the first concept is very narrow and the last is very broad. The first concept, the most prevalent definition within mainstream political discourse, places restrictive boundaries around what politics is – the activities of governments, elites and state agencies – and therefore also restricts who is political and who can engage in politics, that is, the members of governments, state agencies and other elite organizations. It is a 'top-down' approach that essentially separates politics from the community. By contrast, the last definition offers a much more encompassing view of politics: politics, effectively, is everything, from personal power struggles upwards. In between, lie definitions that encompass the politics of voluntary collective activities and public debate.

While politics may be seen as concerned with compromise and conciliatory activity, for many it is the exercise of power and how legitimacy for the exercise of that power is achieved. Authority is one means, alongside wealth, strength or violence, of exercising power. Politics is thus a term that can be used to describe any 'power-structured relationship or arrangement whereby one group of persons is controlled by another' (Millett, 1969). This is a 'bottom-up' approach, which suggests that any and every issue is political and, likewise, anyone and everyone can engage in a political act.

> **thinking about** Why are there calls to take the politics out of health?

These competing definitions of politics have also permeated the contemporary discipline of political science (the study of politics), where the different academic approaches similarly operate divergent conceptualizations about what should be studied (Stoker, 2010).

Part 1 The contribution of political science to health studies

example 8.1

The application of politics to contemporary health issues

- The impact of social and welfare policies on health including the rise in food banks in England
- Private versus public healthcare systems
- Regulation, individualism and the role of the state in controlling unhealthy products, for example alcohol, ultra-processed food, sugary drinks and tobacco
- Globalization and trade and its impact on health

The concepts and methods of political science have a clear potential to contribute to the study of health. However, to date (aside from specific discussions about healthcare), health has not been widely considered as a political entity within academic debates or, more importantly, broader societal ones. In this part, we examine some of the reasons behind this, and then discuss more recent arguments, which suggest that health is political and, therefore, that political science has much to offer our understanding of health.

The political and the non-political

The marginalization of the politics of health is unlikely to have a simple solution because the treatment of health as apolitical (that is, not political) is almost certainly the result of a complex interaction of a number of different factors.

Health equals healthcare

Health is often reduced and misrepresented as healthcare or, in the UK, as the NHS. Consequently, the *politics of health* becomes significantly misconstrued as the *politics of healthcare* (Freeman, 2000), and, more specifically, as the politics of the NHS. For example, the majority of popular political discussions about health concern issues such as NHS funding and organization, NHS service delivery and efficiency, or the demographic pressures on the future provision of healthcare. The same applies in most other high-income (developed) countries.

connections   Chapters 9 and 10 study health as ways in which care is organized and delivered.

The limited, one-dimensional nature of this political discourse surrounding health can be traced back to two ideological issues: the definition of health and the definition of politics (Carpenter, 1980). The definition of health that has conventionally been operationalized under Western capitalism has two interrelated aspects to it: health is considered as the absence of disease (a biomedical definition) and as a commodity (an economic definition). Both definitions focus on individuals, as opposed to society: health is seen as a product of individual factors such as genetic heritage or lifestyle choices, and as a commodity that individuals can access either via the market or, in the UK's case, the health system (Scott-Samuel, 1979). In this sense, health is an individualized commodity produced and delivered by the market or the health service. Inequalities in the distribution of health are therefore a result either of the failings of individuals through, for example, their lifestyle choices, or the way in which healthcare products are produced, distributed and delivered.

connections   Chapter 11 claims that health is produced and that the study of economics enables a society to decide how much and to whom scarce resources should be allocated in relation to healthcare. It discusses the advantages and limitations of using the market to allocate resources such as healthcare.

It is important to note that this limiting, one-dimensional view of health is common across the political spectrum, with left-wing versus right-wing health debates usually focusing on the role of the NHS.

Health and concepts of politics

Earlier, we outlined four broad definitions of politics and suggested that the first one, politics as the art of government and the activities of the state, was the most prevalent within current political discourse. The **hegemony** of this conceptualization of politics influences which aspects of health are considered to be political. Especially in countries like the UK where the state's role is significant, healthcare is an immediate subject for political discussion as it involves differences over funding and delivery. While such differences may be partly resolved through negotiation and conciliation, there has been recourse to the economic marketplace and rational decision-making. The establishment of the NHS in 1948 as a service free at the point of delivery might have been expected to be a fair and acceptable mechanism for delivering healthcare. Yet, the allocation of treatment and care has come to be determined by market mechanisms, which has caused dissatisfaction and conflict.

Calls to replace politics with managerialism especially in relation to healthcare emerged in the 1970s. Using available information to conduct detailed option appraisals might be expected to be a rational form of decision-making. Instead, this process also caused dissatisfaction because professional judgement was thought to be sacrificed to managerial expertise and the interests of the community were thought to play too little a role.

Chapter 10 discusses the factors influencing the structure of the NHS and what has driven its various reorganizations and shows how the welfare state reflects the degree to which societies take care of their citizens. The welfare state and labour market policies have an effect on income and social inequalities in the population.

connections

example 8.2

Politics and the NHS

When the NHS was launched by Aneurin Bevan, then minister of health, on 5 July 1948, it was based on three core principles:

- that it meet the needs of everyone
- that it be free at the point of delivery
- that it be based on clinical need, not ability to pay.

The Labour Party's election manifesto in 1997 warned that only Labour could 'save the NHS'. By 2005, a resolution at its party conference attacked the Labour government's moves towards fragmenting the NHS and embedding a marketized system of public services with a growing role for the private sector. The main driver of healthcare has become 'choice'. For example, personalized budgets allow people living with long-term conditions to determine how they wish welfare payments to be spent, but there are fewer claimants and the assessment of eligibility is carried out by an independent company, challenging the notion of universal provision. Patients are seen as consumers and in order for them to exercise choice, there must be sufficient and reliable information, which healthcare services must collect. Targets include a four-hour waiting time in A&E departments that is consistently 'breached', incurring financial penalties. Alongside the shift to patient power is the growing role for the healthcare professional, particularly GPs who run clinical commissioning groups purchasing services. Such local services (including diagnostics, such as blood tests and X-rays, mental health services, GP services and out-of-hours care, community health and pharmacy services) are increasingly put out to tender and won by private companies. These changes led to the formation in 2005 of an active campaign group – Keep Our NHS Public (www.keepournhspublic.com).

Health and political science

To date, health has not been seriously studied within political science nor, for that matter, has politics within health. This has compounded its exclusion from the political realm. Health, to a political scientist (in common with more widely held views) often means only one thing: healthcare and, usually (in the UK), the NHS. Some political scientists will argue that they do study health as a political entity but what is usually under analysis is the politics of health*care*.

Understanding why this has happened requires us to consider the various schools of thought within political science and their corresponding definitions of the political, as discussed in the introduction. These schools of thought have not been equally successful in political science and the discipline is dominated, especially in the US, by the behavouralist, institutionalist and rational choice strands. To adherents of these schools, politics – and therefore political science – is concerned with the processes, conditions and institutions of mainstream politics and government. As the politics of healthcare revolves around the politics of institutions, systems, funding and elite interactions, it fits the priorities of these mainstream schools of political science. Health, in its broader sense, therefore tends to be thought of as apolitical and of academic concern only to disciplines such as sociology, public health or medicine.

| connections | Chapter 5 examines two strands of concerns about health: inequalities and the ways in which groups and societies perceive and experience health. |

The political nature of health

That health outcomes are determined in high-income countries as much by the circumstances in which people live as by access to health services has long been recognized. The impact of globalization on health is extensive, from the financial crisis and introduction of austerity measures that impact on the poor, to transnational corporations and their production and retail of health-damaging products, such as tobacco, alcohol, ultra-processed foods and weapons, as well as their support for trade agreements that encourage, for example, the migration of health workers, which deprives poor countries of resources (Horton and Lo, 2014). Yet, political scientists have taken little interest in health, and it is not until relatively recently that a body of work has emerged overtly arguing that health is itself a political issue (see, for example, Navarro, 2004; Borrell et al., 2007), and should therefore be examined using political science perspectives (Bambra et al., 2005, 2007). For example, applying a political science lens draws attention to why and how policy decisions about tobacco are made. Although evidence about the harms caused by tobacco has been widely acknowledged from the 1950s onwards, it has only been in the past 20 years or so that many countries, including the UK, have taken extensive policy action to regulate the tobacco industry and its products – via very high rates of taxation, bans on tobacco advertising, restrictions on smoking in public places, and action to limit the ability of the tobacco industry to influence policy debates. To understand why such a delay occurred between evidence and action, and why extensive policy reforms were subsequently introduced, it is necessary to explore the interests and actors involved in tobacco debates and examine how the competing 'sides' of this debate have each worked to frame evidence and arguments with a view to attracting public and political support (see Smith, 2013).

Bambra et al. (2005, p. 187) have argued that 'health, like almost all other aspects of human life, *is* political in numerous ways'. They identify four key aspects of the political nature of health: unequal distribution, health determinants, organization, and citizenship. Ultimately, health is political because power is exercised over it. The health of a population is not entirely under the control of individual citizens but is under the control of the wider political relations of society. Changing society is only achievable through politics and political struggle.

The ways in which inequalities in health became an issue on the political agenda are discussed in Chapters 5 and 9.　**connections**

Unequal distribution

Evidence that the most powerful determinants of health in modern populations are to be found in social, economic and cultural circumstances comes from a wide range of sources and is also acknowledged by governments (Commission on Social Determinants of Health, 2008). Yet, differences in health experiences between areas and social groups (socioeconomic, education, ethnic and gender) remain. How these inequalities in health are approached by society is highly political and ideological. Are health inequalities to be accepted as 'natural' and inevitable results of individual differences in respect of genetics and the silent hand of the economic market, or are they an abhorrence that needs to be tackled by a modern state and a humane society? Underpinning these different approaches to health inequalities are not only divergent views of what is scientifically or economically possible, but also differing political and ideological opinions of what is desirable. This is reflected in the terminology used to describe such inequity: in the US, the term 'disparity' is used, reflecting a mere difference in health outcomes. Similarly, in the UK, the Conservative government of the 1980s adopted the term 'variations'. Neither term encapsulates the injustice implicit in the term 'inequality' or 'inequity'.

Health determinants

While genetic research is helping us to better understand why some people are predisposed to experience certain diseases, and other causes of ill health are becoming better understood, it is evident that environmental triggers are, in most cases, even more important and that the major determinants of health or ill health are inextricably linked to the social environment (Marmot et al., 2010). In this way, factors such as housing, education, income and employment – indeed many of the issues that dominate political life – are all important determinants of health and wellbeing. The importance of these factors, which are beyond the realm of the health sector, also help demonstrate why non-healthcare policies are of such importance to health. As Marmot et al. (2010, p. 4) state in the most recent review of health inequalities in England: 'This link between social conditions and health is not a footnote to the "real" concerns with health – healthcare and unhealthy behaviours – it should become the main focus.'

connections	Chapter 5 gives a detailed description of the social determinants of health.

Organization

Health is political because any purposeful activity to enhance health needs 'the organised efforts of society' (Secretary of State for Social Services, 1988) or the engagement of 'the social machinery' (Winslow, 1920): both require political involvement and political actions. Population health can only be improved through the *organized* activities of communities and societies. In most countries, the organization of society is the role of the state and its agencies. The state, under any of the four definitions of politics outlined earlier, is a (and more usually, *the*) subject of politics. Furthermore, it is not only who or what has the power to organize society, but also how that organizational power is processed and operated that makes it political.

Health and citizenship

Health is political because the right to 'a standard of living adequate for health and well-being' (UN, 1948, Article 25) is, or should be, an aspect of citizenship and human rights. Citizenship is 'a status bestowed on those who are full members of a community. All who possess the status are equal with respect to the rights and duties with which the status is endowed' (Marshall, 1963).

Following Marshall, it is possible to identify three types of citizenship rights: civil, political and social. While the right to health includes the right to healthcare, it goes beyond healthcare to encompass the underlying determinants of health, such as safe drinking water, adequate sanitation and access to health-related information and a standard of living adequate for health and wellbeing.

example 8.3

Health and human rights

Article 25 of the UN Universal Declaration of Human Rights of 1948 states that:

(1) Everyone has the right to a standard of living adequate for the health and wellbeing of himself and of his family, including food, clothing, housing and medical care and necessary social services, and the right to security in the event of unemployment, sickness, disability, widowhood, old age or other lack of livelihood in circumstances beyond his control.

(2) Motherhood and childhood are entitled to special care and assistance. All children, whether born in or out of wedlock, shall enjoy the same social protection.

In the UK, the welfare state ensured that certain health services and a certain standard of living became a right of citizenship. However, the extent to which health is a right of citizenship is a continued and constant source of political struggle. In the US, the Patient Protection and Affordable Care Act of 2010 attempted to extend health insurance to 45 million Americans previously without access to healthcare, and even in the UK's NHS, access to healthcare is rationed through high charges for drug prescriptions (at least in England – Northern Ireland, Scotland and Wales do not apply prescription charges), dentistry and optometry services.

Thus, to maintain that politics and health can remain separate is incoherent since many of the determinants of health are themselves politically determined, because the technical agenda of medicine is set by political forces and the provision of healthcare involves the distribution of scarce resources.

example 8.4

Politics in medical publications

According to Barr et al. (2004), many medical journals have rightly never subscribed to this distinction between political and technical, trying instead to widen their readership's perspective on health. The *BMJ*'s stated aim is to publish 'papers commenting on the clinical, scientific, social, political, and economic factors affecting health'. Similarly, the *Journal of the American Medical Association* recognizes a 'responsibility to improve the total human condition' and 'inform readers about non-clinical aspects of medicine and public health, including the political'. Thomas Wakley, surgeon, MP and 'medico-political polemicist', founded *The Lancet* in 1823, with the aim of introducing a 'radical slant' to the 'corrupt medical establishment'.

This approach does present some difficulties. One problem is that political bias may creep into a profession that requires objectivity. Maintaining high standards of evidence can guard against such subjectivity. Yet, the current evidence is that many high-impact general medical journals ignore major medico-political issues altogether. Since September 2001, neither the *New England Journal of Medicine*, nor the *Annals of Internal Medicine*, has published any article containing the word 'Afghanistan' or 'Iraq'. The suppression of important health issues is even more worrying than the threat of subjective bias, which can be countered as all social research is political.

Part 2 Theoretical and research approaches

example 8.5

Examples of research in politics and health

- The impact of social and welfare policies on health and social inequalities, for example Institute of Health Equity, www.instituteofhealthequity.org
- Policy-making and health systems and equity of healthcare, for example the European Observatory on Health Systems and Policies, www.euro.who.int/__data/assets/pdf_file/0007/164383/e96159.pdf
- Labour markets and the relationships between work, worklessness and health inequalities, for example Bambra, 2011
- The social determinants of health, for example WHO Collaborating Centre for Policy Research on Social Determinants of Health, www.liv.ac.uk/psychology-health-and-society/research/who
- Understanding corporate influences on health and the policies impacting on health, for example Smith et al., 2010; Corporations & Health Watch, http://corporationsandhealth.org

The nature of politics as an academic discipline is much debated, some seeing it as branch of philosophy or history and others as a science. Aristotle (384–322 BC), the Greek philosopher, claimed politics was the 'master science', in that all we do in life, in society, in arts and in science is influenced by politics. His classification of the constitutions of the Greek city-states was systematic and rigorous. Many social scientists have since tried to build a body of political theory using scientific methods of **empirical** observation. Karl Marx, for example, sought to uncover the scientific laws driving historical development. However, in the latter half of the twentieth century, the main academic strand of political science was behaviouralism, reflecting a view that only that which could be observed and quantified should be studied, leading to a focus on voting behaviour and electoral systems. The modern discipline of politics combines many approaches and focuses:

- Political theory examines theories of institutions, forms of government and systems of representation

- Political philosophy looks for answers to more philosophical questions concerning freedom, justice, equality and rights

- Comparative government tries to generalize about political power and systems from the analysis of groups of countries, international relations being the study of how countries relate through war and diplomacy

- Political ideology is concerned with ideas about the ways states should be organized.

In addition, politics includes many subdisciplines examining the role of the state in the economic system (political economy), the formation of political attitudes, the exercise of power in society, and the policy-making processes of government.

> Several chapters examine political concepts and theories. Chapter 2 provides a summary of a Marxist approach to the study of history. Chapter 9 describes a systems model of the political process.   **connections**

In this part, we focus on political ideologies and how these have informed health policy and approaches to health. An **ideology** is a system of interrelated ideas and concepts that reflect and promote the political, economic and cultural values and interests of a particular societal group (Bambra et al., 2007). Ideologies, like societal groups, are therefore often conflicting, and the dominance of one particular ideology within a society largely reflects the power of the group it represents (hegemony). Ideology can be used to manipulate the interests of the many in favour of the power and privileges of the few (Ledwith, 2001). So, for example, liberal democratic ideology, with its emphasis on the individual, the market and the neutral state, can be seen as a reflection of the power of business interests within capitalist society (Bambra et al., 2005). A hegemonic (that is, universally prevailing) ideology is usually one that has successfully incorporated and cemented a number of different elements from other competing ideologies and thereby fuses the interests of diverse societal groups and classes (Gramsci, 1971). There is emerging evidence that ideology plays a key role in determining mortality and population health (Navarro, 2004).

?   What are the key characteristics of dominant ideologies?

Conservatism

The literal interpretation of conservatism is to 'conserve', that is, maintain what has been tried and tested, rather than seek radical change. Part of maintaining the traditional order of things includes a belief that human talent varies naturally and, consequently, that attempts to 'level' things out (in the way many socialists advocate) are artificial and destined to fail. The existence of a social hierarchy is not only viewed as inevitable but also desirable as it is thought to promote innovation and success, and allows the majority to benefit from the leadership of particularly talented individuals. Rich people tend to be thought of as creators of prosperity rather than plunderers of the poor (a view that contrasts with socialist and communist ideas about wealth). Hence, conservatism differs from many other political ideologies in its vindication of inequality (Heywood, 2012).

Conservative preferences for maintaining tradition are associated with preserving the dominance of particular groups (e.g. wealthy white men) or a religion (e.g. Christianity) or culture (e.g. 'Britishness'). Taken to an extreme, these preferences may be linked to xenophobia, nationalism and racism. More often, these preferences are associated with a morality emphasizing the importance of self-discipline, decency, the 'nuclear family unit', and a respect for the rule of law.

As well as a tendency towards tradition, other features of conservatism include a view of society as a collection of self-interested individuals, a belief underlying Margaret Thatcher's infamous claim that 'there's no such thing as society, only individuals and families'. Of particular importance to health, conservatives tend to see the role of the state as minimal, with a preference for limited (if any) welfare provision. While some conservatives favour a society in which the privileged classes provide basic welfare (e.g. housing) to the 'deserving poor', there is agreement that too much provision by the state removes incentives from the poor to improve themselves, creating a dependency culture and a permanent underclass of what Thatcher called 'moral cripples'. The only exception to conservative preferences for minimal government intervention in society tends to be around law and order, where significant state intervention is often viewed as essential to maintain the smooth running of society.

Despite the association between conservatism and tradition, some strands of conservatism have involved advocating for radical change. For example, although the New Right movement of the 1980s (strongly associated with Thatcherism in the UK and Reaganism in the US) employed a traditionally conservative moral rhetoric, the drive towards the free market and competitive individualism (see Friedman and Friedman, 1980) took its inspiration from liberal thinking (Dearlove and Saunders, 2000). Such ideas, when applied to health and healthcare, resulted in widespread restructuring and privatization of the welfare state in the 1980s, with negative impacts on health and inequalities (Scott-Samuel et al., 2014).

Liberalism (and neoliberalism)

At its heart, liberalism is essentially an economic approach but, like all economic doctrines, it has far-reaching political and social repercussions. With its focus on freedom and choice, liberalism emphasizes the importance of individual rights over those of social groups. Classical liberals believe that a free market guarantees social justice, allowing all those with talent and a willingness to work to succeed. The flip side of this presumption is that poor social circumstances are explained by liberals in rather social Darwinian terms, as a result of individual weakness and/or laziness (Heywood, 2012). This genre of liberalism was popular in the eighteenth and nineteenth centuries, when its proponents advocated minimal state intervention in the economy and the importance of the 'invisible hand of the market' and free trade. Popular discontent with the social consequences of this approach (including extensive material deprivation such as that of the Great Depression in the 1930s) resulted in the emergence of strong political opposition (from communism, socialism and social democracy) and put pressure on liberals to adapt. Out of this situation, 'modern liberalism' emerged, which conceded that state intervention to reduce the excesses of market economics and mitigate its negative effects was desirable. In postwar Britain, this resulted in the emergence of Keynesian welfare capitalism.

The crisis of welfare in the late 1970s led to the re-emergence of classical liberal ideas, especially in relation to economics, exemplified by the approaches of the Thatcher and Reagan governments. This form of liberal thinking, which resurrected market economics, is known as **neoliberalism** (neo meaning new). Under the neoliberal governance of Thatcher in Britain, state intervention was scaled back and public expenditure cut, the economy was deregulated and state-owned companies were privatized. Once again, the primacy of the individual came to the fore, with a corresponding rise in the emphasis placed on traditional morality and responsibility. Politically, neoliberalism is associated in particular with the US but economic **globalization** means that it has increasingly become perceived as hegemonic, to the extent that some commentators argue there is now no alternative (Fukuyama, 1989).

| Chapter 9 discusses the changes in welfare provision in England since 1948 and how these reflect the prevailing ideology. | **connections** |

Neoliberalism has been criticized for:

- its negative impact on health

- increased inequalities in wealth, which many health researchers believe are directly related to health inequalities (Marmot et al., 2010)

- an erosion of social cohesion, which is also thought to be important for health (Wilkinson and Pickett, 2010)

- the dismantling of the welfare state, reducing the 'safety net' available to people living on low incomes and exacerbating poverty in some groups (UCL Institute of Health Equity, 2012).

Other critiques of neoliberal policy in relation to health focus on the individualistic nature of the ideology. Authors such as Galvin (2002) claim that neoliberal governments have deliberately emphasized the importance of avoiding 'risky behaviours' in such a way that individuals are positioned as responsible for their own health status. This, Galvin (2002, p. 119) argues, leads to assertions about individual culpability for those living with chronic diseases: 'for if we can *choose* to be healthy by acting in accordance with the lessons given us by epidemiology and behavioural research, then surely we are culpable if we do become ill'. In achieving public consensus that risky behaviours (such as excessive consumption of alcohol, lack of exercise and poor diet) cause chronic disease, governments are able to shift responsibility for health improvement away from themselves and onto individuals, thereby allowing the kind of minimal state intervention advocated by liberalism.

In a critique of the 2001 Report of the Commission on Macroeconomics and Health (the Sachs Report), Katz (2004) compares a neoliberal approach to health with a social justice perspective, in which health is seen as a right and human necessity (Table 8.1).

Table 8.1 **Neoliberal and social justice approaches to health**

Neoliberal approach to health	Social justice/human rights approach to health
Underlying assumptions	*Alternative assumptions*
Economic growth, within a globalized 'free' market, is the aim	Fair distribution and sustainable use of resources is the aim
Health is what you get from a health service	Health is what you get from meeting basic needs
International aid, with conditionalities to enforce certain policies, is the only way to finance health	Sovereign and solvent states must provide for their people's basic needs without outside interference
Democracy is alive and well in the developed world and is the model for the developing world	Democracy is in crisis everywhere; self-determination of nation states and a rules-based system of international governance are required
Key features	*Key features*
Addresses symptoms, short term	Addresses root causes, long term
Promotes 'magic medical bullets'	Promotes the meeting of basic needs
Promotes interventions delivered through health services	Promotes public works to free people from miserable living conditions
Identifies charity and international aid as the only sources of funds for health	Identifies redistribution and economic justice as sources of funds for health
Maintains the status quo of extreme concentrations of wealth and power	Demands a fair and rational international economic order
Focuses on individual behaviour and tends to blame victims	Focuses on structural poverty and violence and tends to blame 'the system'

Socialism and social democracy

According to Heywood (2012), socialism is the broadest of political ideologies, containing a variety of perspectives from revolutionary communists to reformist social democrats. The meaning of socialism is therefore not fixed and differs by place and time. Originally, socialism was associated with the Marxist/communist tradition, and used to describe material equality (common ownership of the productive wealth and a classless society) in contrast to the purely political equality (right to vote and be represented) of capitalism (Heywood, 2012). The social democratic parties of Western Europe were originally based within the Marxist tradition but by the early twentieth century, a split occurred: the communist parties continued to advocate revolution and the overhaul of capitalism, while the social democrats supported the reform of capitalism and proposed a parliamentary road to socialism. The social democrats were therefore no longer committed to the abolition of capitalism but to reforming it on moral grounds (in the UK particularly, social democratic ideology was strongly influenced by the utopian socialism of Robert Owen and William Morris). In the immediate postwar period, this entailed using increased state intervention, such as the public ownership of key parts of the economy and the establishment of the welfare state, to mitigate the effects of capitalism and thereby achieve needs-based social justice (Heywood, 2012). However, there is little agreement among social democrats about how much state intervention is required in the economy and this has been notable in the policy differences between countries (compare, for example, the UK and Sweden). The most recent evolution of social democracy – the Third Way (associated with Blairism in the UK) (Giddens, 2002) – has seen the abandonment of previous commitments to public ownership and a dilution in views of the extent to which capitalism is seen to require reform (Giddens, 1998). This, alongside the collapse of socialism in the Eastern bloc, has led to speculation as to whether socialism is dead.

---

example 8.6

Socialist approaches to improving the health of populations

A comparison of the level of population health among 29 developed countries over the period 1945–80 (Navarro and Shi, 2001) demonstrates that population health fared best in countries that had social democratic governments in rule for most of this time. In this period, these countries (Sweden, Finland, Norway, Denmark and Austria) all had extensive welfare states, funded by relatively high taxation, which allowed higher expenditure on social security (health, education and family support services) than in countries under other types of governance. This suggests that the socialist values of

equality, redistribution of wealth and a strong welfare state are beneficial for health, which makes sense in light of a recent and growing consensus on the importance of social determinants of health. Evidence from regions of India (Kerala) and northeast Italy, where significant improvements in population health outcomes (reduced health inequalities and associated population health improvement) have also occurred under socialist governance (Navarro and Shi, 2001), adds support to those who argue that socialist programmes are most compatible with healthy populations. Even Cuba, which is governed by a non-elected socialist government, demonstrates impressive health outcomes, with life expectancy rates that are on a par with developed countries that spend twenty times as much on health

(Veeken, 1995). The poorest health outcomes of all the countries Navarro and Shi looked at were in Spain, Greece and Portugal, all of which had undergone significant periods of fascist rule in the period of study. This suggests, at the very least, that extreme incarnations of nationalism are likely to be damaging to health. The authors claim that the causes of poor health outcomes in these ex-fascist countries are likely to result from a combination of regressive fiscal policies, that is, policies that tend to favour the wealthy without benefiting the poor, underdeveloped welfare states, and the general repressive nature of such regimes.

? What might account for the purported better health outcomes in social democratic/socialist countries?

The key to these health improvements may lie in a more egalitarian society, as Wilkinson (2005; Wilkinson and Pickett, 2010) would suggest, or in better government responses to material deprivation. Whatever the cause of reduced health inequalities and improved population health in these countries might be, the dominance of governments of a socialist persuasion demonstrates the importance of political ideology for health.

Nationalism (and fascism)

Unlike other political ideologies discussed in this section, nationalism does not describe an interrelated set of values and is probably better thought of as a belief, rather than an ideology (Heywood, 2012). This belief, that all nations should be self-governing, spread from the French Revolution of 1789, so that countries previously thought of as 'realms' or 'kingdoms' began to be thought of as 'nation states', and their inhabitants as 'citizens' rather than 'subjects'. As an idea, nationalism straddles the political spectrum; at various times and places, nationalism has been associated with democratic and authoritarian governments, and with left-wing and right-wing political movements. For example, ideas about nationalism have been employed to promote the importance of social cohesion, order and stability by right-wing parties in Britain and France, while they have also been adopted by left-wing (Marxist) movements advocating 'national liberation' in countries like China and Vietnam. This is partly because the concept of a 'nation' is difficult to pin down, sometimes being used interchangeably with 'state', 'country' and even 'race' (Heywood, 2012).

Nationalism is an embedded feature of most modern societies as demonstrated in the pervasiveness of flags, national anthems, public ceremonies and national currencies and languages. However, important debates about nationalism remain. On the one hand, some commentators suggest that the growing importance of regional and global institutions (such as the EU and the UN) mean that nationalism is becoming irrelevant. On the other, the devolution of power to countries such as Wales and Scotland and the persistence of some separatist movements, for example the pressure for Basque independence in Spain, suggest that nationalism is alive and well.

An extreme interpretation of some of the ideas involved in nationalism form the basis of fascism, which focuses on establishing the dominance of a particular community or social group (often referred to as the 'dominant race'). Under fascism, subservience to the glory of a particular 'nation' or 'race' is demanded and, consequently, individual liberties are eliminated. Fascism is therefore extremely elitist and patriarchal – the dominance of one group over others is seen as desirable and inequality between this group and others is actively promoted. Aside from this central belief, many of the ideas involved in fascism are vague and inconsistent; it is more identifiable with particular movements and individuals, such as the fascist dictatorships of Hitler (Germany, 1933–40), Mussolini (Italy, 1922–43) and Franco (Spain, 1938–75), than with any systematic ideology.

It could be argued that some level of shared national identity is likely to be beneficial for health, on the basis that it is seen to promote social cohesion (Wilkinson and Pickett, 2010). However, as nationalist ideas have been employed by such a wide variety of political movements, it is difficult to draw any clear conclusions about nationalism's implications for health.

Feminism

There are a number of different forms of **feminism**, such as liberal, socialist or radical, and each has a different approach to politics, reflecting the fact that feminism is an evolving social movement.

Chapter 5 discusses explanations for gender inequalities in health.   **connections**

The origins of feminism date back to the French Revolution in the late eighteenth century and Mary Wollstonecraft's tract on the rights of woman. In the context of the nineteenth century and early twentieth century, women (particularly those in wealthier countries with emerging democracies) argued for the same legal, political and economic rights that men had begun to obtain. In the UK, women gained the same voting rights as men in 1928, the Equal Pay Act was passed in 1970 and the Sex Discrimination Act in 1975. By contrast, it wasn't until 1990 that the Federal Supreme Court of Switzerland declared the principle of equality between men and women was guaranteed by the federal constitution.

This equal rights approach of liberal feminists – to gain access to the public sphere on the same terms as men by overcoming discrimination – was challenged in the 1960s and 70s by socialist and radical feminists. Socialist feminists argued that women would only gain full equality with men under socialism and that the oppression of women was a vital element of the capitalist system; in this context, the legal equal rights gained during the twentieth century could only have a limited impact on the systemic power inequality between the sexes. Feminists drew attention to conduct within the domestic sphere as demonstrating how 'the personal is the political' and how the private domestic and family sphere can be oppressive. Only the removal of the private sphere altogether, by the collectivization of domestic work and childcare, would ensure equality (Randall, 2010).

Radical feminists shifted attention further, to the nature of domestic relations between men and women, and other more cultural aspects of male domination and oppression. They highlighted the 'oppressive dualism of gender' and argued that we live in a patriarchal society, in which women are systematically dominated by men in all areas of life (Randall, 2010). The goal was no longer to be 'just like men', but to challenge societal assumptions about masculinity and femininity, arguing that they were social constructs rather than fixed natural phenomena. They also drew attention to the limits that unequal and restricting traditional gender roles placed on women (and also men). This meant that women's individual experiences of oppression were collectivized and considered as a consequence of their political relationship of subordination and oppression by men and therefore something that could be changed – primarily by women's political empowerment and liberation from gender socialization. Recent protests in England against public objections to breastfeeding reflect far more than mere social conventions but are embedded in a much deeper set of power structures. These cultural conventions are tied to gendered notions about what is appropriate behaviour for women and reflect patriarchal power structures that restrict behaviour for women.

> **thinking about** Female genital mutilation or female circumcision can be seen as a reflection of patriarchal oppression or, as in a UN resolution in 2012, as a human rights issue in which women should be able to consent. What is your view?

example 8.7

Patriarchy and health

Patriarchy is the systematic domination of women by men and domination of men by other men. It might be expected that better health might follow from men's power and privilege. However, an international study by Stanistreet et al. (2007) found that the effects of patriarchy are more complex: in societies in which women are still unequal but beginning to gain equality in areas such as employment, increased economic activity by women correlated with increased mortality from injury and poisoning among men but not women. As women increasingly occupy traditionally masculine roles, thus challenging the stereotypes of hegemonic masculinities, some men engage in compensatory risky behaviours as a means of asserting what appears to be a diminishing masculine identity. Thus, men in the top 25% of most patriarchal societies are twice as likely to die from a behavioural cause such as accidents and homicides (Scott-Samuel et al., 2009).

Environmentalism

Many, if not all, of the political ideologies discussed so far have tended to perceive nature as nothing more than a resource for human beings to exploit. However, since the 1960s, when Rachel Carson published *The Silent Spring* ([1962] 2000), there has been an ever-increasing awareness of a growing ecological crisis. As the number of human beings and the demand for higher standards of living increase, an increasing number of people are predicting that a global catastrophe (e.g. through climate change) will soon challenge the way we live. As with all the other ideologies discussed, the term 'environmentalism' is often applied to a broad range of ideas and theories, from those that fundamentally question conventional assumptions about nature to far less radical responses to specific environmental issues. Generally, environmentalists claim that, by conceiving of nature as an ever-plentiful resource, humans have placed not only their own future in jeopardy, but that of the whole global ecosystem. To avoid disaster, environmentalists advocate that all policies should be judged by their sustainability, that is, the extent to which a particular policy can be maintained without damaging the fragile ecosystem.

Chapter 6 illustrates the human impact on the environment and its effects on health through the toxic, infectious and physical aspects of the places in which we live.   connections

This ideological perspective criticizes a basic assumption of the other ideas discussed in this section, namely the central position of human beings. This sets environmentalists apart from the usual left–right political spectrum. Since the 1980s, 'Green' parties have emerged in most industrialized countries, including the UK, with the aim of moving environmental concerns up the political agenda. Pressure groups such as Greenpeace and Friends of the Earth have also helped increase awareness of environmental concerns such as acid rain and nuclear waste. Currently, most major political parties in Britain claim to be concerned with the environment, but their various responses tend to suggest environmental concerns can be accommodated without the need for radical change. In contrast, an increasing number of scientists and environmentalists believe that the damage to the ecosystem caused by humans is now so great that significant climate and environmental change is inevitable. If this is the case, all humans can hope to achieve, even with radical change, is damage limitation (Lovelock, 2006). Despite increasingly pessimistic predictions by these groups, the more radical branches of environmentalism are unlikely to be taken seriously by mainstream politics because they suggest that there are limits on human, material ambitions; a suggestion that challenges the core of many influential ideologies.

An awareness of links between the environment and human health is not new; for example, many nineteenth-century achievements in improving public health were a result of changes to the environmental conditions in which people lived, such as sanitation and air pollution. Following the success of environmental activists in promoting the political nature of their cause, from the 1960s onwards, clear links between the public health and environmental movements began to develop. In 1990, Maurice King wrote a now-famous commentary in the medical journal, *The Lancet*, in which he argued that an ecological approach to public health was essential in order to avoid the likelihood of humans being caught in a 'demographic trap'. Increasingly, it became clear that public health could not afford to focus solely on human health, for without a sustainable, healthy environment in which to live, human health would inevitably decline. By the mid-1990s, the term 'ecological public health' was being used as a means of highlighting the dependence of public health on the survival of the ecosystem (Nutbeam, 1998). Since then, it has become increasingly accepted by mainstream public health activists that the two issues ought to be viewed as a shared agenda.

At the 2012 UN Conference on Sustainable Development, Sustainable Development Goals were called for to supplement the UN's Millennium Development Goals (MDGs), signed by most of the world's nations in 2000, and are being considered in current discussions around what the post-MDG agenda should look like. While reducing atmospheric CO_2 concentrations, protection against rising water levels and increased food security may seem desirable, they are not clear-cut choices. They are illustrative of all political choices that involve trade-offs: for example, industrialized, high-income countries can set emission targets but, depending how such targets are set, they may limit the activities of low- and middle-income countries that are seeking to industrialize.

case study the politics of 'fat'

Tackling obesity involves tough political choices. Food choices are often seen as personal choices, and this notion is deliberately pursued in advertising and has also become part of political rhetoric. The notion of choice now dominates the discourses around health and social care, education and lifestyles (DH, 2010). This prominence of individual choice is itself part of political discourse, premised on neoliberal concepts of individualism. Yet, the choices people make that lead them to be overweight or obese are not free ones at all. Patterns of food consumption are strongly linked to socioeconomic status, as well as displaying national trends. The link between obesity and poverty in the UK has a political dimension and is in part fuelled by the political lobbying and influence of food processing companies and fast-food chains. The term 'obesogenic' is now used to describe a toxic environment that encourages obesity. This case study explores the decisions of the UK's regulatory bodies regarding food price, availability, marketing and advertising; the influence of lobbying by the food industries; and the broader political context of globalization and how this affects food choices and obesity.

The exponential increase in media coverage and the inherently individual blaming tone adopted in relation to obesity seem to have the elements of what social scientists call a 'moral panic'. Moral panics are typical during times of rapid social change and involve projecting increased anxiety onto vulnerable or marginalized groups.

As Guthman and Dupuis (2005) note, such unprecedented media attention on obesity and health has resulted in obesity becoming more than simply a threat to individual and public health. Obesity reportedly raises airline costs through increased fuel costs, affects worker productivity through ill health and disability, and is even a security threat, as fitness levels among armed and civilian or public security personnel fall due to overweight. Thus, obesity per se is far bigger than fat. *It is a moral, social and political issue.*

Food choices are determined by multiple factors, many of them subject to legal regulations and controls. These factors include price, availability, promotion, marketing and advertising. Price and availability are key determinants of food choices, and the growth of cheap and readily available fast food and calorie-dense processed food has been linked to the rising levels of obesity (Griffith et al., 2013). Within free-market economies, price levels are set by the producers and there is no regulation by government, except during wartime. The only way in which governments can intervene is to tax products deemed to be unhealthy or unsafe – the route used in the case of tobacco and alcohol. Several countries have attempted to introduce so-called 'fat taxes'. Mexico has a tax of one peso (about 5 pence) on every litre of sugary drinks. In the US, New York assemblyman Felix Ortiz proposed a 'fat tax' on foods and entertainments such as video games that contribute to a sedentary lifestyle. Denmark put a tax on saturated fat products in 2011 and Finland introduced a confectionary tax in the same year. However, the Danish 'fat tax' was abandoned 15 months later as it was so unpopular and had limited impact on consumption, and the Finnish confectionary tax was only applied to some products and the rate was subsequently reduced. In some contexts, and without the appropriate measures in place, regulation can lead to smuggling. Moreover, taxing consumable products, such as food

and tobacco, is 'regressive'. This means that people with less money end up spending more of their (relatively lower) incomes on these products, so leaving them with less available for other important costs such as rent, food and utilities. Therefore, while price increases on unhealthy products may be accompanied by some health benefits, the impact on income can have negative health impacts, raising important ethical dilemmas (Wilson and Thomson, 2005; Smith, 2013).

Most liberal governments balk at such proposals, which they see as interfering with individual liberties. As J.S. Mill observed in 1859, in his classic treatise *On Liberty*, the harm principle holds that each individual has the right to act as he wants, so long as these actions do not harm others. If the action is self-regarding, that is, if it only directly affects the person undertaking the action, then society has no right to intervene. The extent to which unhealthy foods ought to be understood as having broader societal impacts (through costs to the NHS) is a matter for debate. However, the underlying political principle that has governed food policy in the UK (and most other high-income countries) to date is liberalism, in which freedom of economic activity and choice are prioritized.

The UK government has acted in a limited number of areas – food labelling, advertising to children and school meals. The Food Labelling Regulations, introduced in 1996, require food manufacturers to list the ingredients and processes used in their food products, as well as other details such as geographical origin (www.food.gov.uk). The UK uses a traffic light system of food labelling, showing fat, salt, sugar and calories but this scheme is voluntary and many major companies, such as Tesco, Kellogg's, Unilever and Kraft, use other schemes showing guideline daily amounts, which consumers may find harder to understand. In 2011, the government set up public health responsibility deals with the food industry to remove artificial trans fats and reduce salt and sugar but, again, these are voluntary agreements.

Marketing and advertising are also thought to affect people's food choices. Research has shown that TV advertising has a modest direct effect on children's food choices (Paliwoda and Crawford, 2003; Cairns et al., 2009). Given this knowledge, whether or not to regulate TV advertising and promotion becomes a salient political issue. This long-running debate has been framed in terms of protecting children from undue pressures to eat unhealthily versus the freedom of legal commercial enterprises to advertise and market their products. A TV ban on fast-food adverts before, during and after programmes aimed at children was implemented in 2007. Increasingly, advertisers are turning to online advertising or 'branding', where the food or drink will not be explicitly advertised but children will view characters (such as 'Tony the Tiger' for Frosties cereal) associated with the products, or play games on sponsored sites such as this one by Macdonald's (www.happymeal.com. au/en_AU/index.html#/Home).

connections	The ethical issues and principles of harm and freedom raised by a ban on advertising are discussed in Chapter 12.

Advertising in the media is the end product of food industries' marketing activities, which also encompass sponsorship of public events, political lobbying and funding of research. Nestle (2002) has documented her first-hand experience as a nutritionist confronting the food industry regarding healthy eating messages. Given the fact that almost twice as much food as is required is produced annually in the US, the priority of the food industry is to get people to buy more of their products, regardless of any health messages. Nestle (2002) illustrates how food companies use the political system, marketing strategies and nutrition experts to encourage people to buy their products, regardless of their impact on health. Paradoxically, Campos et al. (2006) argue that overweight and obesity are not significant public health problems, but that they have been represented as such due to the influence of the pharmaceutical and weight-loss industries. These industries obviously stand to gain financially if obesity increases and becomes seen as a medical issue. Here again, the influence of private industries on food policy debates is a dominant factor, it is just that different types of business have different interests in the debate. According to Guthman and Dupuis (2005), many of the world's leading authorities on obesity, who operationalize criteria and definitions of obesity, happen to be funded by the pharmaceutical and weight-loss industries, as have certain members of the International Obesity Task Force (responsible for WHO reports). Indeed, the pharmaceutical, weight-loss and food industries all have a vested interest in maintaining the narrow public health focus on obesity that is currently evident and the broader efforts to frame obesity as a costly epidemic, which is leading to moral panic.

Once again, the political priorities of free-market economies and free individual choices appear to be the dominant principle and philosophy guiding policy decisions in most countries. Even when confronted with such a significant and avoidable public health issue as obesity, governments are loath to regulate and legislate to improve nutrition and diets. In order for such regulations to be implemented, there needs to be evidence of health risks, significant positive media coverage of the proposed regulations, and indications of public support.

The attention given to the rising trends in obesity reflects the neoliberal agenda of global public health in its insistence on analysing health issues in terms of individual behaviour, exaggerating the extent to which people control their lives (Rayner et al., 2010). Being obese reflects underlying moral assumptions that fat people are irresponsible and reinforces neoliberal rationalities of self-governance and bodily control (Guthman, 2009).

The processes driving the integration of global food markets and their impact on health have been relatively ignored. During the twentieth century, food production began to be heavily corporatized and production shifted from small farmers to large, centralized agricultural complexes (Lang, 2004; Lang et al., 2006). In a neoliberal, free-market context where the primary incentive for producing food is profit, this has led to changes in the composition of food, placing more emphasis on foods that appeal to mass markets and comprise cheap ingredients, such as high fructose corn syrup. Additionally, globalization processes have directly contributed to dietary changes in all countries through the production and trade of international goods, foreign involvement in retailing and processing food, and global marketing campaigns.

Transitions in diet that took more than five decades in Japan have occurred in less than two in China (Chopra and Darnton-Hill, 2004). For example, between 1989 and 1993, the share of rich urban Chinese households consuming a low-fat diet (less than 10% of calories from fat) fell from 7% to less than 1%. There is a transition worldwide from problems of underconsumption to those of overconsumption and malconsumption, and no longer is there a situation where the rich world is fat and the developing world is thin. The World Health Organization has estimated that by 2015, 2.3 billion adults will be overweight and 700 million adults will be obese (WHO, 2013). Even sub-Saharan Africa is not immune to the obesity epidemic, despite the continued burden of undernutrition and the millions who lack food security and are without access to sufficient safe and nutritious food. Building sustainable and secure food supplies to feed the world's population remains a global political and economic priority.

Summary

- There are a number of different definitions of politics. These underpin different approaches to political science and competing political ideologies. Politics focuses on the debates, ideas and institutions that surround community organization and collective decision-making about resources

- Politics has not traditionally focused on health. There are various reasons for this, including the prominence of debates about healthcare. Political analysis has much to offer our understanding of population health and health inequalities and how they can be improved. The political analysis of health suggests that politics could be an important contributory discipline to health studies in the future

- Political ideologies offer competing definitions of politics, and have differing perspectives on population health and whether/how it should be improved. The role of political ideology on health and public health policy is beginning to be examined by researchers. Examples in this chapter suggest that ideology underpins how health is viewed and the extent to which it is considered to be a political issue

- Political ideology is also important when it comes to everyday debates about issues such as obesity

Questions for further discussion

1. Over the next few days, examine media reports about health:
   - What issues are up for discussion?
   - Do they relate to health or healthcare?
   - What ideological values underpin the issue, how it is presented and the solutions that are proposed?
   - How are health issues framed by different actors and why might this be?
   - Which political interests are being promoted?

2. 'As anyone who has lived among villagers or slum-dwellers knows only too well, the health of the people is influenced far more by politics and power groups and by the distribution of land and wealth than it is by the prevention and treatment of disease' (Werner, 1981). Discuss this proposition with particular reference to obesity.

3. Health is far too important to be decided by politicians. Why do people say this? How realistic is the suggestion?

4. The mix of voluntary codes and self-regulation together with some regulatory codes used to tackle obesity is typical of a neoliberal approach to politics and food. How would an environmentalist, or a socialist, approach differ?

Further reading

There are several introductory books on politics and political ideologies. These will enable you to follow up general points related to the discipline.

Heywood, A. (2007) *Key Concepts in Politics* (3rd edn). Basingstoke: Palgrave Macmillan.
An accessible and readable guide to political concepts and how they are used as tools for analysis.

Heywood, A. (2012) *Political Ideologies: An Introduction* (5th edn). Basingstoke: Palgrave Macmillan.
Essential textbook for any student wishing to understand contemporary ideological discourse, including 'new' ideologies such as feminism and environmentalism, and covers the impact of developments such as globalization.

Marsh, D. and Stoker, G. (eds) (2010) *Theory and Methods in Political Science* (3rd edn). Basingstoke: Palgrave Macmillan.
Discussion of different methodologies used in political science.

In addition, these accessible journal papers discuss the role of politics, and political science, in the study of health.

Bambra, C., Fox, D. and Scott-Samuel, A. (2005) 'Towards a politics of health'. *Health Promotion International* 20(2): 187–93.

Bambra, C., Fox, D. and Scott-Samuel, A. (2007) 'A politics of health glossary'. *Journal of Epidemiology and Community Health* 61(7): 571–4.

Smith, K.E. and Katikireddi, S.V. (2013) 'A glossary of theories for understanding policymaking'. *Journal of Epidemiology and Community Health* 67(2): 198–202.

Acknowledgements

This paper draws on Bambra et al. (2005, 2007). We would therefore like to acknowledge the co-authors of these publications, Debbie Fox and Alex Scott-Samuel, as well as other members of the Politics of Health Group (www.pohg.org.uk).

References

Bambra, C. (2011) *Work, Worklessness and the Political Economy of Health*. Oxford: Oxford University Press.

Bambra, C., Fox, D. and Scott-Samuel, A. (2005) 'Towards a politics of health'. *Health Promotion International* 20(2): 187–93.

Bambra, C., Fox, D. and Scott-Samuel, A. (2007) 'A politics of health glossary'. *Journal of Epidemiology and Community Health* 61(7): 571–4.

Barr, D., Fenton, L. and Edwards, D. (2004) 'Politics and health'. *QJM: An International Journal of Medicine* 97(2): 61–2.

Borrell, C., Espelt, A., Rodríguez-Sanz, M. and Navarro, V. (2007) 'Politics and health'. *Journal of Epidemiology and Community Health* 61(8): 658–9.

Cairns, G., Angus K., and Hastings G (2008) The extent, nature and effects of food promotion to children: a review of the evidence. Available at www.who.int/dietphysicalactivity/Evidence_Update_2009.pdf (accessed 2/12/2014).

Campos, P., Saguy, A., Ernsberger, P. et al. (2006) 'The epidemiology of overweight and obesity: pharmaceutical crisis or moral panic?' *International Journal of Epidemiology* 35(1): 55–60.

Carpenter, M. (1980) 'Left orthodoxy and the politics of health'. *Capital and Class* 11: 73–98.

Carson, R. ([1962] 2000) *Silent Spring*. London: Penguin Books.

Chopra, M. and Darnton-Hill, I. (2004) 'Tobacco and obesity epidemics: not so different after all?' *British Medical Journal* 328(7455): 1558–60.

Commission on Social Determinants of Health (2008) *Closing the gap in a generation: Health equity through action on the social determinants of health*. Available online at www.who.int/social_determinants/thecommission/finalreport/en/index.html (accessed 1/7/2014).

Dearlove, J. and Saunders, P. (2000) *Introduction to British Politics* (3rd edn). Cambridge: Polity.

DH (Department of Health) (2010) *Healthy Lives, Healthy People*. London: DH.

Freeman, R. (2000) *The Politics of Health in Europe'*. Manchester: University of Manchester Press.

Friedman, M. and Friedman, R. (1980) *Free to Choose*. London: Martin Secker and Warburg.

Fukuyama, F. (1989) 'The end of history?' *The National Interest* 16: 3–18.

Galvin, R. (2002) Disturbing notions of chronic illness and individual responsibility: towards a genealogy of morals. *Health: An Interdisciplinary Journal for the Social Study of Health, Illness and Medicine* 6(2): 107–37.

Giddens, A. (1998) *The Third Way: The Renewal of Social Democracy*. Cambridge: Polity.

Giddens, A. (2002) *Where Now for New Labour?* Cambridge: Polity.

Gramsci, A. (1971) *Prison Notebooks*. New York: International Publishers.

Griffith, R., O'Connell, M. and Smith, K. (2013) *Food Expenditure and Nutritional Quality over the Great Recession*. London: Institute for Fiscal Studies.

Guthman, J. (2009) Neoliberalism and the constitution of contemporary bodies, in E. Rothblum and S. Solovay (eds) *The Fat Studies Reader*. New York: New York Press, pp. 187–97.

Guthman, J. and Dupuis, M. (2005) 'Embodying neoliberalism: economy, culture, and the politics of fat'. *Environment and Planning D: Society and Space* 24: 427–48.

Heywood, A. (2007) *Key Concepts in Politics* (3rd edn). Basingstoke: Palgrave Macmillan.

Heywood, A. (2012) *Political Ideologies: An Introduction* (5th edn). Basingstoke: Palgrave Macmillan.

Horton, R. and Lo, S. (2014) 'Protecting health: the global challenge for capitalism'. *Lancet* 383(9917): 577–8.

Katz, A. (2004) 'The Sachs Report: investing in health for economic development or increasing the size of the crumbs from the rich man's table, Part 1'. *International Journal of Health Services* 34(3): 751–73.

King, M. (1990) 'Health is a sustainable state'. *Lancet* 336(8716): 664–7.

Lang, T. (2004) *Food Industrialisation and Food Power: Implications for Food Governance*. Available online at http://pubs.iied.org/pdfs/9338IIED.pdf (accessed 1/7/2014).

Lang, T., Rayner, G. and Kaelin, E. (2006) *The Food Industry, Diet, Physical Activity and Health: A Review of Reported Commitments and Practice of 25 of the World's Largest Food Companies*. London: Centre for Food Policy, City University.

Laswell, H.D. (1936) *Politics: Who Gets What, When, and How*. New York: Peter Smith.

Ledwith, M. (2001) 'Community work as critical pedagogy: re-envisioning Freire and Gramsci'. *Community Development Journal* 36: 171–82.

Leftwich, A. (1984) *What is Politics? The Activity and its Study*. Oxford: Bkackwell.

Lovelock, J. (2006) *The Revenge of Gaia: Why the Earth is Fighting Back – and How We Can Still Save Humanity*. London: Allen Lane.

Marmot, M., Allen, J., Goldblatt, P. et al. (2010) *Fair Society, Healthy Lives: Strategic Review of Health Inequalities in England Post-2010*. London: The Marmot Review.

Marshall, T.H. (1963) *Sociology at the Crossroads and other essays*. London: Hutchinson.

Mill, J.S. (1869) *On Liberty*. London: Longmans, Green, Reader and Dyer.

Millett, K. (1969) *Sexual Politics*. London: Virago.

Navarro, V. (ed.) (2004) The *Political and Social Contexts of Health*. New York: Baywood.

Navarro, V. and Shi, L. (2001) 'The political context of social inequalities and health'. *The Politics of Policy* 31(1): 1–21.

Nestle, M. (2002) *Food Politics: How the Food Industry Influences Nutrition and Health*. Berkeley, CA: University of California Press.

Nutbeam, D. (1998) 'Health promotion glossary'. *Health Promotion International* 13(4): 349–64.

Paliwoda, S. and Crawford, I. (2003) *An Analysis of the Hastings Review: The Effects of Food Promotion on Children*. Available at www.adassoc.org.uk/hastings_review_analysis_dec03.pdf (accessed 1/7/2014).

Randall, V. (2010) Feminism, in D. Marsh and G. Stoker (eds) *Theory and Methods in Political Science* (3rd edn). Basingstoke: Palgrave Macmillan, pp. 114–35.

Rayner, G., Gracia, M., Young, E. et al. (2010) 'Why are we fat? Discussions on the socioeconomic dimensions and responses to obesity'. *Globalization and Health* 6:7. Available at www.globalizationandhealth.com/content/pdf/1744-8603-6-7.pdf (accessed 1/7/2014).

Secretary of State for Social Services (1988) *Public Health in England. The Report of the Committee of Inquiry into the Future Development of the Public Health Function*, Cm 289. London: HMSO.

Scott-Samuel, A. (1979) 'The politics of health'. *Community Medicine* 1: 123–6.

Scott-Samuel, A., Stanistreet, D. and Crawshaw, P. (2009) 'Hegemonic masculinity, structural violence and health inequalities'. *Critical Public Health* 19(3/4): 287–92.

Scott-Samuel, A., Bambra, C., Collins, C. et al. (2014) 'The impact of Thatcherism on health and wellbeing in Britain'. *International Journal of Health Services* 44(1): 53–71.

Smith, K.E. (2013) 'Understanding the influence of evidence in public health policy: What can we learn from the "tobacco wars"?' *Social Policy and Administration* 47(4): 382–98.

Smith, K.E., Fooks, G., Collin, J. et al. (2010) '"Working the system"? British American Tobacco's influence on the European Union Treaty and its implications for policy: an analysis of internal tobacco industry documents'. *PLoS Medicine* 7(1): e1000202.

Stanistreet, D., Swami, V., Pope, D. et al. (2007) 'Women's empowerment and violent death among women and men in Europe: an ecological study'. *The Journal of Men's Health and Gender* 4: 257–65.

Stoker, G. (2010) Introduction, in D. Marsh and G. Stoker (eds) *Theories and Methods in Political Science* (3rd edn). Basingstoke: Palgrave Macmillan, pp. 15–23.

UCL Institute of Health Equity (2012) *The Impact of the Economic Downturn and Policy Changes on Health Inequalities in London*. Available at www.instituteofhealthequity.org/projects/demographics-finance-and-policy-london-

2011-15-effects-on-housing-employment-and-income-and-strategies-to-reduce-health-inequalities (accessed 1/7/2014).

UN (United Nations) (1948) *Universal Declaration of Human Rights*. New York: UN.

Veeken, H. (1995) 'Cuba: plenty of care, few condoms, no corruption'. *British Medical Journal* 311(7010): 935–7.

Werner, D. (1981) 'The village health worker: lackey or liberator?' *World Health Forum* 2(1): 46–68.

WHO (World Health Organization) (2013c) *Obesity and Overweight*. Available at www.who.int/mediacentre/factsheets/fs311/en/index.html (accessed 07/11/2013).

Wilkinson, R. (2005) *The Impact of Inequality: How to Make Sick Societies Healthier*. New York: The New Press.

Wilkinson, R. and Pickett, K. (2010) *The Spirit Level: Why Equality is Better for Everyone*. London: Penguin.

Wilson, N. and Thomson, G. (2005) 'Tobacco taxation and public health: ethical problems, policy responses'. *Social Science and Medicine* 61(3): 649–59.

Winslow, C. (1920) 'The untilled fields of public health'. *New Scientist* 51(1306): 923–33.

chapter

Social policy and health

9

Overview   294

Introduction   294

Part 1 The contribution of social policy to health studies   295
The organization of welfare   296
The changing role of the state in welfare   298
Britain becomes a welfare state, 1945–50   299
Challenging welfare, 1979–97   301
Healthcare and New Labour, 1997–2010   302
Coalition government health reforms since 2010   306
Current health issues on the social policy agenda   306

Part 2 Theoretical and research approaches   312
The development of the discipline   312
From consensus to critique   313
International and comparative social policy   314
Research methods in social policy: in understanding health   318
Policy analysis   320
The policy process   321

Case study A policy analysis of obesity in the UK   325
Summary   327
Questions for further discussion   328
Further reading and resources   328
References   329

Learning outcomes

This chapter will enable readers to:
- Understand the organization and development of social policies
- Examine the process of social policy-making
- Understand the role of social policies in influencing health
- Assess the contribution of social policy to health studies

Overview

The discipline of social policy examines how and why certain issues relating to the welfare of people come to be seen as the legitimate focus of state intervention. Social policy also critically examines the consequences, intended and unintended, of state intervention, regulation and legislation. Part 1 considers the contribution of social policy to health studies. It looks at the historical development of social policies, including health policies, identifying key issues such as the extent of state involvement in the provision of welfare and the ways in which changing political ideologies have affected views on this. Part 2 considers the methods and analytical tools of the social policy discipline. It traces the development of social policy and examines some of the key theoretical and methodological approaches, with a particular focus on the relevance of these for health studies. It looks at the policy process, how certain issues become part of the policy agenda and how policies are negotiated, formulated and implemented. Lastly, the case study on obesity examines how this topical health issue has become a legitimate focus for policy development.

Introduction

Social policy includes the study of how **welfare** is organized in any society, in particular of the role of the state in relation to the welfare of its citizens. The term 'social policy' is used in two senses. It sometimes refers to a particular kind of decision, such as that relating to education or health. It may also refer to the academic discipline that studies such policies. In order to avoid confusion, in this chapter the term 'social policy' refers to the academic discipline; otherwise, the plural form, 'social policies' will be used.

The term 'social policies' is conventionally used to describe **policy** in relation to welfare benefits, unemployment, education, housing, health and social care services. All these areas are related and also influenced by other government policies, particularly economic policy and others such as transport and environmental policies. For example, a study of state intervention in health might explore transport policy and congestion charging, given concerns about poor air quality and rising rates of asthma.

Much academic focus is on the provision and reform of healthcare systems. The development of state welfare and the establishment of the NHS in the UK in 1948 is a major area of study. This has raised certain key questions, which are still relevant today:

- What is the role of the state? When and how far should it be involved in people's lives?

- How should welfare be organized and funded?

- How are contemporary social problems identified?

- Who benefits from social policies?

- Whose values do social policies reflect?

- What are the broader functions of social policies?

- How efficient and effective are policies in providing welfare?

Social policy is informed by economics in relation to the allocation of resources for welfare and by politics through decision-making that determines the provision of welfare. Decisions about whether the NHS should fund treatment that has a low chance of success, whether services should be based on users' views, and whether people should be forced through legislation and regulation to choose a healthier lifestyle are value judgements. The rising costs of health and social care services and the increasing needs and demands of an ageing population provide a challenge to policy-makers.

Chapter 11 explores health economics as a discipline that focuses on the allocation of resources for health. Chapter 8 explores how political ideology influences healthcare delivery.

connections

Part 1 The contribution of social policy to health studies

example 9.1

The application of social policy to contemporary health issues

- Immunization, for example the promotion and use of vaccines for diseases such as measles, mumps and rubella (MMR) or meningitis B
- Disability, for example work capability assessments to get people with disabilities into employment and assess their eligibility for benefits
- Obesity, for example tackling child obesity
- Pricing of alcohol, for example setting a minimum cost per unit

- Smoking, for example the introduction of plain packaging for cigarettes
- Drug misuse, for example reclassification of cannabis as a Class B drug within the criminal justice system
- A&E treatment, for example introduction of waiting time targets, walk-in centres and use of phone lines such as NHS 111
- Patient care, for example quality of medical and nursing care in hospitals
- Private provision of healthcare services, for example the sale of the state-owned UK supplier of blood products to a US company

Social policy is concerned not just with what the state provides, but also the broader issues of entitlement and responsibility in society. The provision of healthcare is based on considerations about who is entitled to receive state support and at what level. A core concept is that of **need**.

> **thinking about** How would you define need? Are different people or population groups more in need than others? How do you decide?

The concept of human need is basic to understanding human health and welfare, yet it is a problematic concept. Attempts to define human need have raised questions about whether need is, or should be, an objective, universal concept, or whether it is, or should be, determined by variable historical, geographical and cultural factors (Doyal and Gough, 1991).

How any society sets about meeting human needs raises further problematic concepts, such as those of **social justice** and **equity**. These refer to criteria of fairness – who 'ought' to get what when resources are being allocated. Criteria of fairness may take into account the level of need or be based on some notion of merit.

This raises the question of whether welfare should be regarded as a right. Marshall (1950) identifies social rights as essential to **citizenship** and the full membership of any society. Social rights include economic security, a share in good living standards and cultural heritage. Access to welfare was, for Marshall, a matter of citizen rights. However, the degree of entitlements and how citizens' rights to welfare can be enforced remain the subject of political and ideological argument. Examples are the current debates about who receives free health and social care and whether asylum-seekers or non-EU migrants and their families should have access to state benefits.

Where a welfare system embraces the idea of rights, to what extent is meeting human needs the responsibility of families, communities or the state? Margaret Thatcher, prime minister in the 1980s, referred to the UK as a 'nanny state', by which she meant that the welfare state had taken over functions that were more properly carried out by families, and had encouraged people to neglect their responsibilities. The concept of 'welfare dependency' is used by some politicians and policy-makers to describe those who are perceived to be content to rely on state benefits instead of seeking to provide for themselves.

Welfare systems are capable of enhancing or diminishing individual autonomy. A basic principle of community care policies is that individual needs should be recognized and met in ways that enhance the individuality and autonomy of service users, in contrast to institutionalized forms of care. For example, the introduction of direct payments for disabled people under the Community Care (Direct Payments) Act 1996 (Great Britain, 1996) enabled them to spend as they wished on their care once their needs had been assessed.

The organization of welfare

> **thinking about** What do you understand by the term 'welfare'? Whose responsibility is the welfare of others?

There are different views about responsibility for the provision of social welfare, ranging from those who believe the state should provide for those in need to those who believe individuals should prove their eligibility for support.

Chapter 8 considers the ideological differences that give rise to these differences in policy.   **connections**

The term 'welfare state' is something of a misnomer since there are many different providers of individual welfare. Welfare can be understood as a system that comprises five main spheres of activity. This **mixed economy of welfare** providers refers to:

- the state

- informal welfare

- the private sector

- the voluntary sector

- occupational welfare.

Figure 9.1 shows how all five spheres contribute to welfare in the case of Alice James. Alice is 80 years old and lives alone. She has recently returned home after being discharged from hospital following treatment for a fractured hip. Her ability to remain at home is likely to depend on services being provided on a more long-term basis in order for her daughter to return to work. However, unless Alice has access to her own financial resources and is able to purchase these for herself, she will be dependent on the state (the local adult social care services department) for help. Her daughter's financial security in old age is likely to be affected if she decides to give up work to care for Alice, as contributions to her occupational pension scheme will stop. Without the informal care provided by her daughter, Alice may not be able to remain at home and may have to sell her home to help pay towards residential care supplied by the private sector. The extent and importance of informal care, which is domestic and private, is often underestimated (Ungerson, 2003).

There are many obvious ways in which people benefit from welfare, for example through the receipt of benefits, education and NHS services. It is common to think that people living on the lowest incomes benefit the most from welfare, yet some argue welfare spending benefits better off people most (Duffy, 2012).

The state has a fluctuating relationship with all other sectors in the organization and management of people's welfare. Take, for example, its regulatory role. In the private sector it has taken on responsibility for regulating tobacco advertising, in the voluntary sector it places controls on the way in which charities raise funds, while in the occupational sector it imposes rules on health and safety at work. State intervention in the informal sector is a highly contentious

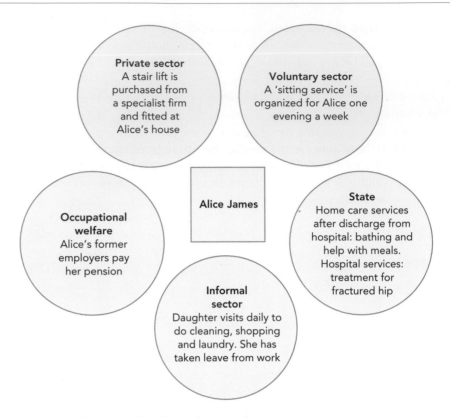

Figure 9.1 **Spheres of welfare: the mixed economy**

area. In cases of neglect or violence, intervention is widely accepted and, indeed, expected. At other times, however, the state's role is questioned, for example in the extent and nature of financial support it offers carers (Glendinning, 2006).

thinking about Should the state provide financial recompense to carers?

Financial recompense would recognize the support provided by carers who are family members or friends, but it might cloud the caring relationship and make it harder for carers to take on this role. The giving of time, money and expertise are key elements in the provision of welfare. While there is a concern that informal care provides core services that should be provided by the state, informal care is also promoted on the moral grounds that something other than the pursuit of financial gain should be a dominant force in society. In other words, carers might be motivated more by duty, altruism or love than by money.

The changing role of the state in welfare

Historically, the role of the state in planning, funding, regulating and providing welfare services has varied. Values and organizational traditions have influenced the particular form of state welfare. This section outlines the changing roles of different welfare sectors and the socioeconomic and political context of welfare.

In the UK, state involvement in welfare goes back centuries. In 1601, during the reign of Elizabeth I, a Poor Law Act was passed that was intended to control and organize payments from parish funds to destitute people. In 1834, the Poor Law Amendment Act established the Victorian workhouses that became notorious for their treatment of the poor. Under the principle of 'less eligibility', conditions in the workhouses were intended to be harsh and punitive in order to deter people from asking for help. The 'workhouse test' ensured that those seeking help had no other means of looking after themselves or their families and that the state was their last resort.

In the late nineteenth century, the workhouse system was under a great deal of strain, unable to cope with the level of need but also more widely regarded as an unacceptable approach to providing welfare (Crowther, 1983). Problems such as poverty, unemployment, infant mortality, ill health and poor housing conditions led to pressure for state action. The realization that epidemic diseases, such as cholera, spread through inadequate water and sewage services and poor housing conditions to affect everyone was an important factor in promoting and legitimating state intervention.

Welfare services in the nineteenth century demonstrate how different values applied in practice. For example, the Charity Organization Society, which worked with families in poverty, maintained an individualistic approach. It was concerned with identifying the 'deserving poor', distinguishing between the 'helpable' and the 'unhelpable'. From a different perspective, campaigners such as Charles Booth and Joseph Rowntree argued that poverty was the outcome of the economic and industrial system rather than individual idleness or immorality and therefore social reforms were needed.

In the early twentieth century, the Liberal government of Prime Minister Lloyd George introduced a series of measures, including the first retirement pension in 1908 and a limited health insurance scheme in 1911. After the First World War, welfare schemes based on the principle of social insurance were developed. Individual contributions paid from wages into an insurance scheme entitled workers to claim benefits when they were unemployed, sick or retired (Fraser, 2009).

Britain becomes a welfare state, 1945–50

The postwar period (1945–50) saw the development of Britain's welfare system. The British model differs from that of most of Europe in its approach to social policy and is a distinctive example of a comprehensive and universal welfare system. It reflects the principles of the postwar period and the pragmatic influence of regeneration.

The basic principles underpinning the development of the welfare state in the 1940s were **universalism**, comprehensiveness and **collectivism**. In practice, these principles meant that every citizen should be included within the system of benefits and services and the range of services should cater for all their needs 'from cradle to grave'.

connections   Chapter 8 discusses whether political ideology influences the changing provision of welfare.

Collectivism, demonstrated through the taxation of those in work to pay for services, represented a major shift from the Victorian position on individual responsibility for welfare. Welfare services were established on the basis of rights rather than charity. The provision of free education and healthcare could be seen as a means of reducing social and economic inequality by compensating for low wages and raising the standard of living of poorer people. Because the resources for the new system came from income tax, there was a redistribution of resources from the better off to the poorer, thus reducing overall economic inequality.

example 9.2

The Beveridge Report

William Beveridge was appointed by the wartime coalition government to review the range of insurance schemes that had developed since the turn of the century. The report he produced in 1942 (Beveridge, 1942) was a plan for a comprehensive reform of social policies, in which healthcare would be universally available and funded from taxation. He identified what he considered to be the major social problems of the day, which he termed the 'five giants stalking the land': want, ignorance, squalor, disease and idleness.

Beveridge's report formed the basis of the postwar Labour government's welfare state. Key policies included the Education Act 1944, the Family Allowances Act 1945, the National Health Service Act 1946, the National Insurance Act 1946 and the National Assistance Act 1948. These Acts established sickness and unemployment benefits, retirement pensions for men at 65 and women at 60, maternity benefits and widows' benefits. In addition, the Town and Country Planning Act 1947 offered government grants to local authorities that enabled a programme of council house building, and full employment was made possible by the buoyant economy after the war. The five giants were tackled, although not destroyed.

The state became the dominant player in the formal UK welfare system, with the private and voluntary sectors occupying a more peripheral position. Influenced by the ideas of Marshall (1950), there was a widespread consensus across the political parties that a welfare state was desirable in the development of a civilized society.

The NHS, established in 1948, was a classic example of the principles of universalism, comprehensiveness and collectivism. It was based on the following:

● Healthcare should be provided according to people's needs and free at the point of delivery to ensure that people seek help when they need it

- Healthcare should be universal and equally available to all sectors of the population and in all areas of the country

- Healthcare should be comprehensive to cover the whole range of people's health needs in one centrally planned service

- Healthcare should be collectively financed from general taxation.

In addition, other principles, such as social justice, were evident in the view that the NHS should be concerned with reducing inequalities in health.

> **?** In what ways have the principles of universalism, comprehensiveness and collectivism in the NHS been challenged?

The principle of universal provision has proved difficult to achieve and regional variations in mortality and morbidity rates remain a problem. An expanding system of welfare has had little impact on social and health inequalities. Government and research reports testify to ongoing health inequalities (Townsend and Davidson, 1992; Marmot et al., 2010).

The assumption that improved health would lead to a reduction in demand for healthcare was shown to be wrong, given medical advances and raised public expectations. There is concern that some areas and populations gain more from the NHS than others. For example, there is debate over 'postcode prescribing', whereby individuals or groups in some areas receive NHS treatment for conditions such as infertility, whereas others have to seek private treatment for the same conditions. NICE provides advice and guidance on what should and should not be provided by the NHS.

The principle of comprehensiveness has not been put fully into practice in the NHS. There have always been contested areas, such as dentistry, optical services and chiropody, which are neither fully incorporated into the NHS nor fully privatized. The 1990 reforms to the NHS presented a new approach to the allocation of resources. The introduction of an **internal market** of purchasers and providers of services aimed to facilitate the flow of funds for treatment. NHS districts were encouraged to trade with each other on a contractual basis, through which the funds followed the patients. There was less emphasis on calculating the amount allocated to the regions and more on encouraging competition between providers so that money would be provided for services rendered.

Challenging welfare, 1979–97

The election of a Conservative government in 1979 provided a challenge to the principles of universalism, comprehensiveness and collectivism that underpinned the creation of the welfare state in the UK. Prime Minister Margaret Thatcher argued that welfare spending was too high, and that the near-state monopoly in welfare provision had stifled entrepreneurial activity and created inefficient and unresponsive bureaucracies. Welfare was characterized as having sapped the moral fibre of the nation and created a culture of dependency. The Conservative programme sought to 'roll back the state' and stimulate the private market. The Conservatives viewed the NHS as a large and inefficient bureaucracy, where poor management systems had created funding problems and professionals had too much power and autonomy.

connections	Chapter 8 discusses conservatism and the New Right as political ideologies and Chapter 10 discusses how the NHS has changed from an administered service to a managed one.

Key NHS reforms included the introduction of competitive tendering for ancillary services such as laundry and catering to stimulate private provision. The NHS and Community Care Act 1990 led to a reorganization of the NHS and separation of the providers and purchasers of healthcare, where providers included hospitals and purchasers were health authorities or GPs. Reforms in community care aimed to end institutional care for older and disabled people and those with mental health problems or learning disabilities as a means of cutting costs and restoring civil rights and dignity to marginalized groups and individuals. Public health, with a focus on prevention and wellness, was addressed with the publication of two policy documents – *Promoting Better Health* (DH, 1987) and *The Health of the Nation* (DH, 1992).

In the 1990s, Conservative policies promoted a consumerist approach by focusing on service user rights and expectations with the introduction of the Patient's Charter, service standards, performance indicators, league tables and target setting to reduce the length of hospital stays and empty beds, and to provide quicker treatment. In 1992, the government introduced the private finance initiative (PFI) to encourage the private sector to make capital investment in the NHS, in return for a contract of, usually, 30 years, to design, build and operate services. Overall, health policy from 1979 to 1997 can be characterized as a search for greater efficiency, choice and quality in healthcare, driven by a managerialist approach to controlling financial costs and resources.

Healthcare and New Labour, 1997–2010

The 1997 election of New Labour under Prime Minister Tony Blair saw a change in approach and emphasis towards welfare. New Labour stated its intention to modernize welfare provision, with the creation of services that were efficient, transparent, accountable, tailored to individual needs and made use of information technology (Miller, 2004). Two White Papers (DH, 1997, 1999) signified a re-emergence of some original aims of the NHS such as universal provision and a reduction in health inequalities (see Table 9.1).

Table 9.1 **Key changes in health policy, 1997–2010**

- *The New NHS: Modern, Dependable* (DH, 1997) and *Saving Lives: Our Healthier Nation* (DH, 1999) introduced primary care groups and trusts to work with local authorities to develop more integrated services; health improvement programmes to establish local strategies for implementing national targets for health and healthcare; and NICE, an independent organization providing guidance on effective prevention and treatment interventions

- Health action zones were established to reduce health inequalities and promote better access to services in areas of poor health and high levels of deprivation. Further innovations included NHS Direct for healthcare advice and information by phone (and later the internet) and NHS walk-in centres for quick access without appointment for the assessment and treatment of minor injuries, or for advice and information

- National service frameworks, developed with the assistance of health professionals, service users and carers, managers and agencies or organizations, set out the principles and standards of provision for a range of conditions (coronary heart disease, diabetes, renal) and groups (mental health, older people)

- The NHS Plan (DH, 2000) restated the principle of free care at the point of delivery and established nursing care as free to all in residential and nursing homes. It restated a commitment to reduce the major causes of mortality and morbidity, and set targets to reduce health inequalities. The plan set further targets for new hospital schemes, extra beds and frontline staff (nurses, consultants, GPs) by 2010. Primary care trusts (PCTs) were given responsibility to commission care services and those that performed well were allowed more financial freedom. Calls were made for greater patient or user involvement on trusts, committees and boards to develop services. Private sector management teams were offered opportunities to take over failing hospitals

- The NHS Reform and Health Care Professions Act (DH, 2002) brought in structural and organizational changes through reform of the distribution of functions between strategic health authorities and PCTs; reform of structures for patient and public involvement in the NHS; and reform of the regulation of healthcare professions

- The Health and Social Care (Community Health and Standards) Act (DH, 2003) allowed NHS trusts and non-NHS bodies to apply for independent foundation trust status. In response to concerns regarding the inaccessibility of dental services, PCTs were able to commission NHS dental treatment by paying dentists for the number of patients seen. Foundation status made trusts accountable to a board of employers, staff and local residents and gave trusts more financial and organizational freedom. Foundation hospital trusts operate in England as independent not-for-profit hospitals

- The NHS Redress Act (Great Britain, 2006) proposed a redress package in clinical negligence cases that offered compensation, explanation, apology and a report on action taken to prevent similar cases in future

- The Health Act (DH, 2006) prohibited smoking in certain premises and locations, and amended the minimum age of persons to whom tobacco could be sold. It also covered the prevention and control of healthcare infections and how NHS organizations ensure patients are cared for in a clean environment with low risk of infection from MRSA or *Clostridium difficile*

- The Darzi Review (DH, 2008a) recommended developing an information base to monitor health services using a broad range of outcomes to cover elements of treatment, such as dignity, respect and autonomy, and patient involvement

- The NHS Constitution (DH, 2009) reaffirmed the right to NHS services free of charge and with equal access for all. It introduced free choice of any provider offering NHS quality and price standards and imposed a legal duty on all NHS organizations to take account of the constitution in their work

- The Marmot Review (Marmot et al., 2010) proposed introducing new indicators to highlight inequalities within as well as between areas

> **?** In what ways could it be said that New Labour was reintroducing the original principles of the NHS?

New Labour's Third Way approach from 1997 was a mixture of state welfare and market provision, with examples in Table 9.1 demonstrating elements of continuity and change from previous Conservative policies. New Labour showed commitment to continuing the PFI when it announced a new wave of hospital building at a cost of £1.5 billion in 2007. There remained a strong emphasis on ensuring value for money or 'best value', with the Health-care Commission being responsible for reviewing and rating performance. The roles of PCTs and foundation hospital trusts meant decisions on health services were made locally with service user involvement. Consumerism was evident in the legislation tackling redress in cases of clinical negligence, while state intervention was deemed permissible to regulate the professions and individual behaviour, for example the smoking ban.

The objectives of the New Labour health reforms were to:

- make improvements in efficiency, quality, responsiveness of services and equity of access

- increase treatment rates

- reduce unnecessary demand.

These objectives would be achieved by:

- encouraging competition between NHS and independent hospitals

- introducing wider choice of providers to patients

- allowing hospitals greater managerial and financial freedom

- developing innovative alternatives to hospitalization.

However, Brereton and Gubb (2010, p. xii) argued that 'the market, by and large, has failed thus far to deliver such benefits on any meaningful or systematic scale'.

A 2011 review of New Labour's health reform programme (Mays and Dixon, 2011) concluded:

- There was limited growth of new providers and potential for competition in, for example, elective hospital services

- Despite increases in spending and staffing levels following the NHS Plan in 2000, which aimed to employ 50,000 more doctors and 100,000 more nurses and midwives, there was a decline in productivity

- There were improvements in waiting lists and waiting times for hospital services

- There was an increase in overall public satisfaction with the NHS

- There were reductions in rates of smoking and hospital-acquired infections

- There was only limited progress in reducing health inequalities

- Equitable access to services showed little improvement

- Harm due to alcohol misuse and overeating did not reduce.

During New Labour's third term (2005–10), the rate of increase in healthcare expenditure slowed alongside the pace of organizational change, leading to a period of relative stability and consolidation. There was a refocusing on improving care and patient outcomes, for example with a new cancer strategy. Rather than initiating and implementing a range of new policies, the government instigated inquiries into NHS reforms (the Darzi Review) and health inequalities (the Marmot Review), which produced recommendations for further reforms (see Table 9.1). The Darzi Review (DH, 2008a) offered 'an alternative to a top-down, target-driven approach to performance management' (Vizard and Obolenskaya, 2013, p. 29). The Marmot Review (Marmot et al., 2010) called for investment in the early years when inequalities in health are determined.

When considering UK healthcare policies under New Labour, it is important to remember these policy changes were mostly implemented in England. The devolution of power from central government to the Scottish Parliament and assemblies in Northern Ireland and Wales has resulted in key policy differences:

- Prescription charges were abolished in Wales in 2007

- Since 2002, care at home has been free for those aged over 65 living in Scotland

- The ban on smoking in public places was first introduced in Scotland (March 2006), then Wales and Northern Ireland (April 2007) before England (July 2007)

- There has been less emphasis on choice and competition in Northern Ireland.

Chapter 10 illustrates the turbulent changes in the NHS in Table 10.2.   **connections**

Coalition government health reforms since 2010

The White Paper *Equity and Excellence: Liberating the NHS* was published in July 2010 (DH, 2010). After much public and parliamentary debate, the Health and Social Care Act (Great Britain, 2012) was enacted from April 2013. Key elements are the replacement of PCTs with clinical commissioning groups (CCGs) and moving all NHS trusts to foundation trust status. CCGs give groups of GP practices and other professional healthcare workers the budgets to purchase health and social care on behalf of their local communities. The legislation aims to:

- safeguard the future of the NHS by putting health professionals such as GPs at the centre as commissioners of health provision

- free up providers to innovate

- empower patients by giving them a greater voice

- offer a new focus to public health, through the newly created body Public Health England, to improve the nation's health and address inequalities.

The policy context is the 'rising demand and treatment costs', the 'need for improvement' compared to other European countries, and the 'state of the public finances' (DH, 2012).

?   What might be some of the critiques of these reforms?

A key area of debate is the direction of change, with the expansion of marketization and competition moving away from centrally planned national systems of health and care provision.

Concerns have been expressed about the fragmentation of the NHS and the loss of its duty to provide a *national* health service, replaced by a duty of CCGs to make or arrange provisions for their local population. For example, Shadow Health Secretary Andy Burnham views the Health and Social Care Act as 'a path towards fragmentation, competition and privatisation' and argues that 'there's another path, marked integration and collaboration' (cited in Hough, 2013).

Current health issues on the social policy agenda

Funding of health and social care

The question of how healthcare should be funded, and how comprehensive services should be, continues to be a problem for policy-makers. Public expectations of health services continue to rise as medicine develops new techniques and treatments to which the public demands fair and equitable access.

example 9.3

Fair and equitable access to treatment: in vitro fertilization (IVF) provision in the UK

Since the WHO recognizes infertility as a disease of the reproductive system, some argue there needs to be a greater acceptance of IVF as a legitimate clinical need (Ghevaert, 2012). The All Party Parliamentary Group on Infertility (Johnson, 2011) reported that there was continuing inequality of access to IVF treatment by area ('postcode lottery'), by group (e.g. obese women, lesbians), by age and by childlessness. The report noted that the NICE guideline recommending the offer of three free cycles on the NHS was not followed by all PCTs. Some PCTs have added their own stringent restrictions on who is eligible for treatment to the guideline, for example in the number of cycles of treatment offered.

In Wales, the minister for health and social care declared that all eligible couples would be entitled to two NHS cycles of treatment from 2010. In May 2013, the Scottish government announced that women in their forties would be able to get one free cycle of treatment for the first time by raising the age limit from 40 to 42. In Northern Ireland, current NHS provision offers one fresh cycle and one frozen embryo transfer to those eligible for treatment (www.infertilitynetworkuk.com).

Chapter 11 examines the rational basis for resource allocation within the NHS.   **connections**

Example 9.2 illustrates the problem faced by the different areas and countries of the UK that might accept, in principle, the NICE guideline for three cycles of IVF treatment free on the NHS, but in reality find that the finance and resources are not available. **Rationing** is not simply a consequence of health service reforms, but is also one of professional judgement. GPs decide which patients to refer to specialist services, based on their own ideas, beliefs and interpretation of need. Research on access to renal dialysis and other kidney treatments, for example, has shown that older people are systematically discriminated against by decisions not to refer them for specialist treatment (New and Mays, 1997).

Increasing numbers of older people

The increase in the number of older people being supported by a diminishing working population is seen as putting a strain on available welfare resources. The high social value given to independence places older people in a position of relative powerlessness and low social status, whereby they become characterized as a burden. Despite this stereotyping, ageing is not a uniformly experienced phenomenon due to varying factors such as health, access to physical and emotional support, class, gender and race (Giddens, 2006). While retirement is likely to lead to a loss of income, living standards and status, there is a view of older people as gaining greater political influence ('the grey vote') as they experience more independence in this 'third age', free from the responsibilities of employment and parenthood. Thus, policies are required to promote the health and independence of people when they are in the third age, while being responsive to their needs when their health declines.

The provision of healthcare for older people demonstrates the difficulty of determining what is a health issue. The relationship between social factors and health is shown particularly clearly in old age. Medical advances and an improvement in the standard of living have led to increased longevity in general, but social inequality tends to become more pronounced in old age.

A goal of *Saving Lives: Our Healthier Nation* (DH, 1999) was to increase the length of people's lives and the number of years that people spend free from illness. Longevity continues to be a policy goal but is seen as increasingly problematic. There are about 3 million people in the UK aged over 80, and this is projected to double by 2030. The average NHS expenditure on retired households in 2007–08 was twice that of non-retired households, and in 2010–11 two-thirds of benefits from the Department for Work and Pensions went to those over working age pensioners (Cracknall, 2010). Higher levels of need and demand for healthcare in old age have been presented as an economic problem.

> **thinking about** If there are criteria for the allocation of healthcare, should age be a criterion? Williams (1997) argued that age should be a criterion for rationing decisions and older people should not assume a right to healthcare equal to that of younger people. Do you agree?

When policies for community care were developed in the late 1980s, older people were regarded as a priority for attention. There was widespread agreement that an alternative to institutionalized regimes in geriatric hospital wards and residential care homes was needed (Means and Smith, 1998). Enabling older people to live in their own homes through reorganized services had, and still has, widespread appeal.

Integration of care

Community care is organized through a system of professional practice known as 'care management'. The care manager (from the purchasing local authority) establishes what an individual's needs are and then develops a 'package of care' that suits them, which is then purchased from a range of providers. Care management should ensure that the older person's needs are met in an integrated way, the individual having some say in how services are delivered, and the mixed economy of care offering a degree of choice. The reality has been more problematic. The 1990 NHS and Community Care Act maintained the organizational and financial separation between health and social care services, which has militated against integrated service provision. There are important differences in older people's entitlement to services, with healthcare being free and social care being means-tested. An example of this is that one older person may be bathed for free by a district nurse, whereas another may have to pay social services for a care assistant to bathe them. This has had implications for older people's access to services where some have been moved from one service to the other as each attempts to cut costs.

In Scotland, free personal and nursing care for those aged over 65 living in their own homes was introduced in 2002. Not all members of the Scottish Parliament agreed this new policy, arguing that it subsidizes the better off (Christie, 2002). People in care homes receive varying levels of payments depending on need that substantially reduce their costs. In effect, this created a two-tier system of care for older people within the UK. It resulted in older people in Scotland being better off than those in the rest of the UK, where entitlement to personal care continues to be means-tested.

Costs of care

Personalization was introduced by New Labour as the 'cornerstone of public services' to enable those receiving adult social care to be 'empowered to shape their own lives and the services they receive' (DH, 2008b). The introduction of personal budgets offers choice and control for service users to tailor services to their needs. It is seen as transforming the social care system by allowing service users, as budget holders, to take on the role and responsibilities of the care manager (Dickinson and Glasby, 2010). This illustrates a consumerist model where individuals compete in the market to secure the 'best deal', which undermines collective principles of public service provision and is likely to favour the more articulate and educated (Lymbery, 2012). However, a key principle underpinning the disability movement is evident in acknowledging service users as experts in their own lives and being given greater control.

In February 2013, in the context of increasing numbers of older people having to sell their homes in the face of unlimited costs of care, the health secretary announced plans for a cap of £75,000 on the amount they will have to pay for social care in England from 2017. The cap and other proposals are based on the principles and recommendations of the Dilnot Commission's (2011) report into the future of social care. The key principle is a shared responsibility model, dividing the costs of adult social care between the individual and the state. Recommendations included:

- raising the means-tested threshold at which people are liable for their full care costs

- devising national eligibility criteria across England for consistency and fairness

- ensuring parity by getting individuals to contribute a standard fixed amount to their living costs in residential care (Dilnot, 2011).

These proposals can be seen as an attempt to tackle the problems and unfairness created in the current system by means-testing thresholds, postcode lottery differences, rationing and quality of services.

Quality of care

A public inquiry report on failings at the Mid Staffordshire Hospital NHS Foundation Trust (Francis, 2013) prompted a public outcry.

connections	Chapter 12 discusses the ethical and legal issues involved in the inquiry into Stafford Hospital and the extent to which there can be an expectation of care by patients and carers and of professional standards by healthcare workers.

example 9.4

Stafford Hospital

An investigation by the Healthcare Commission looked into high mortality rates among patients admitted as emergencies to Stafford Hospital from 2005 to 2008. Evidence of inadequate care and other failings led to a further independent inquiry and then the announcement of a full public inquiry by the new coalition government in June 2010. Both inquiries were chaired by Robert Francis QC, who heard evidence of patient abuse, lack of basic care, an atmosphere of fear, low morale and defensiveness among professionals, and management thinking dominated by financial pressures that preferred statistics and reports to data on patient experiences. Francis (2013, p. 3) refers to a story 'of appalling suffering of many patients' failed by a system that was focused on reaching national targets, financial balance and foundation trust status 'at the cost of delivering acceptable standards of care'.

In February 2013, Prime Minister David Cameron initiated the Keogh Review into the quality of care and treatment provided in hospital trusts in England with higher than average mortality rates over the previous two years (Keogh, 2013). The Keogh Review acknowledges that over 90% of deaths in hospital occur when patients are admitted as emergencies rather than in planned procedures. It also recognizes the complexity of interpreting data and understanding the causes of high mortality in the 14 trusts under scrutiny. It led to some immediate actions to protect patients, such as the closure of some operating theatres, changes to staffing levels, and dealing with backlogs of complaints from patients. The problem is then dealing with public anxiety in replacing services lost or downgraded, particularly those based around A&E.

Access to healthcare

Health reforms and policies introducing greater competition and choice have led to concerns about equity of access to healthcare in a market that could be exploited by those with money or better educated, and discriminate against more costly, high-risk patients. As Mays and Dixon (2011, p. 126) observe, patients want 'guaranteed access to high-quality local services' and not to have to shop around. Further, they note the difference between healthcare and other markets. In markets, some providers get into financial difficulties or fail. What happens when a hospital 'fails' can lead to political fallout between politicians, policy-makers and the public where there is a threat of hospital closure or downgrading of service provision. For example, the Save Lewisham Hospital campaign in south London was started in 2012, supported by patients, community groups, GPs and health professionals, to fight proposals to reduce services at the hospital, including closure of the A&E department (www.save-lewishamhospital.com). The proposal came as part of cost-saving measures presented by a neighbouring trust that was in financial difficulties. In July 2013, the High Court overturned the decision by the secretary of state for health to downgrade and close services.

> Chapter 12 discusses whether individuals' right to healthcare can be upheld in law and discusses the judicial review of Lewisham Hospital.
>
> **connections**

Consumerism and empowerment

There is ongoing debate whether policy should take a consumerist or empowerment approach to the provision of welfare. Consumerism may be characterized by customer, choice, complaint and compensation and can be seen in policies such as direct payments and personalization, referred to above. An empowerment approach is apparent in policies encouraging service user involvement and control over services. Empowerment can be collectivist through the promotion of support systems, networks and self-help groups.

Need and risk

A different way of framing and developing policy would be to use the concept of welfare risk rather than welfare need. This would require policy-makers to define those at risk or regarded as vulnerable, such as children and older people, and then devising protection policies. The concept can be extended into areas of health risk such as smoking, high cholesterol, obesity and heart disease.

This historical outline has shown how ideas and values concerning the role and relative responsibilities of the state, individuals, families and the private and voluntary sectors have been developed to deal with social problems. Policy-making and implementation are part of a political process influenced by pragmatism and expediency as well as ideology. Part 2 turns to the policy process and presents perspectives and frameworks for analysis to help the reader develop a critical view of proposed and actual social policies.

Part 2 Theoretical and research approaches

example 9.5

Examples of research in health policy

- Comparative health systems and the ways these are shaped by political, cultural and historical influences
- Evaluation of healthcare policy and related initiatives to help policy-makers improve the analysis underlying their choices
- Policy analysis
- Study of societies in transition and the impact on health policy
- The challenges posed for health systems by austerity, health technologies, longevity and chronic conditions

The development of the discipline

The discipline of social policy is inextricably linked with the processes of policy-making and practices in welfare provision. Its roots can be traced to the early twentieth century, when there was an upsurge of interest in the education and training of emerging occupational groups in the developing public sector welfare services. Because there were no texts written at the time, academic courses relied on casework records, including those of the Charity Organization Society, as sources of data. Other sources included government statistics, census data and official reports. Empirical research data, such as those produced by Booth (1902) and Rowntree (1901) were important to the development of the academic study of welfare. However, the intention was that the data they produced should not simply be available for study but also be a means of stimulating government action to address social problems.

This conceptual linkage in social policy between academic work and action by the state was influential in the development of welfare state policies in the Fabian Society and the Labour Party in the early twentieth century. In the UK, the concept of a 'welfare state' had an increasingly broad appeal and in the postwar years, all political parties had plans to develop welfare services along broadly similar lines. This period of intense political activity was reflected in academic circles, as the discipline of social administration flourished in British universities. The broad consensus over the role of the state in developing welfare services was evident in the style and content of the discipline, which was concerned with the design and development of effective services, informed by professional ideas relating to the best ways of meeting human need.

Welfare systems of this time were classified by Titmuss (1974) as 'residual' or 'institutional':

1. *Residual systems* offer welfare as a last resort, or safety net, to those in danger of becoming destitute. Individual responsibility for welfare is encouraged, and welfare services are targeted at those in greatest need.

Recipients may be means-tested. In residual systems, welfare is often experienced as stigmatizing to recipients.

2. *Institutional systems*, in contrast, favour universal benefits, and services collectively financed through taxation. These are less likely to be experienced as stigmatizing because they benefit a wide cross-section of society and are intended to reduce socioeconomic inequalities. Universal benefits include retirement pensions and disability benefits, while universal services include education or health provided free at the point of delivery.

> **?** Institutional welfare characterized Britain in the postwar years. How has it been challenged?

From consensus to critique

Welfare as social control

During the 1960s, there was also a growing realization that the welfare state was not necessarily benevolent and included some highly questionable practices. The concept of 'institutionalization' – the loss of personal identity that occurs when people are subjected to institutional regimes – was developed (Goffman, 1961). Evidence of abuse of patients in psychiatric hospitals, residents of institutions for people with learning disabilities and older people was also publicized. Undignified treatment of frail older people in hospitals included removing their dentures and spectacles and leaving them to 'vegetate' (Robb, 1967). The growing awareness of the harm done to people through welfare institutions raised important questions about their human rights and contributed towards the drive to deinstitutionalize welfare services in the 1970s and 80s and the provision of care and support in people's own homes. These revelations raised more fundamental questions concerning the role of the welfare state as an instrument of social control, engaged in oppressive acts against vulnerable people. It was at this time that the discipline became known as 'social policy' rather than 'social administration', indicating a shift in perspective from a study of how to deliver welfare to a critical analysis of welfare policies and the role of the state.

Universalism and service users

A number of important critiques of welfare come from services users that question whether needs can be met within a universalist model of welfare. The uniformity of services and lack of understanding of the differences between service users were often targets of criticism (Duffy, 2012). These highlighted the incorrect assumptions that were often made about the needs and expectations of women, black and minority ethnic groups, and disabled and older people. For example, within mental health, the varying needs and demands of patients from different ethnic groups are often neglected as services are organized along rigid lines.

There is also evidence that the health problems of older people are frequently given low priority or simply assumed to be the normal consequence of ageing. Twigg (2006) points to the low priority given to continence services in the NHS, despite the effect that problems with continence can have on physical and mental wellbeing. The need for greater awareness of the differences between service users was highlighted in a report published in 2013 from a confidential inquiry into the premature deaths of people with learning disabilities (CIPOLD, 2013). This identified that among people with learning disabilities, illness was often not diagnosed and this contributed to a greater likelihood of premature death. The inquiry also found that preventive action was often inadequate and people with learning disabilities were often overlooked by health promotion campaigns.

International and comparative social policy

Social policy has increasingly developed an international focus. Comparative social policy has highlighted similarities and differences between the welfare systems of different countries. Esping-Andersen (1990) developed a model of 'ideal types' of welfare regime (see Table 9.2), in which two dimensions of comparison are of particular importance:

- the extent to which the state enables individuals to enjoy an acceptable standard of living independent of the labour market ('decommodification')

- the extent to which the state promotes equality and social integration through welfare.

A simple comparison of spending on welfare does not answer these questions. In the US in 2004, for example, healthcare absorbed 15.3% of GDP compared with 10.9% for Germany and 8.3% for the UK; yet state welfare is residual and minimal in the US but relatively well developed in the UK. However, by looking at sources of funding, one sees different values at play. In the UK, 86% of health spending was funded by public sources in 2004, while in the US the figure was 45%, reflecting a greater reliance on private healthcare (OECD, 2006).

Esping-Andersen's (1990) model classifies welfare regimes according to the approach taken to policy-making within different countries as well as the overall scope of welfare and citizens' entitlement to welfare. He first identified three ideal types: *social democratic,* characteristic of Scandinavian countries, *conservative/corporatist,* characteristic of Germany and France, and *liberal welfare*, characteristic of the US.

Classifications such as Esping-Andersen's are useful in helping us to identify similarities and differences between countries. The model was open to criticism, however, because it excluded countries such as Greece and Italy,

Table 9.2 **Comparative welfare regimes**

Regime type	Characteristics	Example
Liberal	State welfare provided at a minimal level, targeted at the poorest. The voluntary and informal sectors are expected to play a major role, and the private markets are relatively unregulated. Also known as 'residual' or 'laissez-faire' welfare states	US
Conservative/ corporatist	Government involvement in the organization of welfare through private and state insurance schemes and the voluntary sector. Tends to be conservative in its approach to family values	Germany, France
Social democratic	Emphasis on the government's role in providing comprehensive welfare services funded by taxation, so a high level of employment is necessary. Social equality is an important aim	Sweden, Denmark

which have low levels of formal welfare. It was also pointed out that the model focuses on income maintenance, the labour market and formal welfare provision, which neglects the contribution of the informal sector and the family in producing welfare (Barnes, 2012). Since the family is the most significant provider of welfare in all welfare states, this is an important omission. The collapse of the Soviet bloc in the late twentieth century and the re-emergence of independent nation states in Eastern Europe has seen a transition in welfare provision, from the Soviet state-managed secure economy with guaranteed employment and service provision to more liberal, democratic, market-oriented but insecure systems that do not guarantee employment or rights to services (Deacon, 2000).

? What other factors would need to be taken into account if comparisons were to include developing countries?

Gough (2004) expands Esping-Andersen's classifications to include developing countries. In distinguishing between welfare regimes, he notes different patterns of colonization and decolonization:

1. The *insecurity* welfare regimes of sub-Saharan Africa are characterized by late decolonization and independence. In these countries, the main livelihood comes from agriculture, families and clans take care of welfare needs, and key roles are played by political or military elites and external agencies such as the UN or the World Bank.

2. The *productivist* welfare regimes of East Asia, such as Taiwan and Malaysia, have different patterns of colonization. These are dynamic emerging capitalist economies where the aim is high economic growth, with social policy regarded as social investment, and the state acts as a regulator rather than a provider of welfare.

3. The *conservative-informal* welfare regimes of South America experienced early decolonization and independence. Their economies were principally driven by exports that led to wealth and the development of a capitalist class and urban workers. While those in the formal employment sector benefited from the emergence of social insurance and protection schemes, those in the informal economy remained unprotected and unregulated.

The United Nations Development Programme (UNDP) provides useful data for comparisons between countries and produces an annual Human Development Report. Its Human Development Index is calculated from data on the per capita GDP, life expectancy and adult literacy in any country. It is used to indicate whether a country is developed, developing or underdeveloped. Giving a world overview, the *Human Development Report 2013* (UNDP, 2013) noted how rapidly some countries are developing and how their economic output is set to surpass that of the currently richest countries in the world. However, it also notes how economic progress does not automatically translate into human welfare. It calls for sustained investment in education, nutrition, health and employment.

> **?**   Why is comparative social policy useful when undertaking health studies?

Comparative social policy contributes to our understanding of both how and why welfare is organized in a particular way. In Ireland, for example, there is a long tradition of church involvement in healthcare. In Sweden, women's participation in paid employment has been higher than in many other European countries, which affects how the informal sphere operates. Comparative approaches demonstrate how concepts such as needs, rights, equity, autonomy and responsibility are expressed through policies in different ways and in different contexts.

The globalization of economic, political, social and cultural life has transformed policy-making and the discipline of social policy. Deacon (2007) identifies how globalization has influenced the social policies made by individual countries at all standards of socioeconomic development. In addition, policies are increasingly made at a supranational level. For example, in the 1990s, the World Trade Organization actively pursued reform of trade in services, including health services. The 1995 General Agreement on Trade in Services (GATS) is intended to promote international competition in health services. The healthcare services of individual countries are thus expected to be open to foreign providers. The GATS enables individuals to travel to other countries to obtain healthcare, enables healthcare workers to travel to work in different countries, and enables companies based in one country to set up services in others. There are clear differences between countries, dependent in part on general socioeconomic status. For example, the International Monetary Fund or the World Bank might make international competition a condition of any aid provided to a socioeconomically disadvantaged country. Countries with highly developed social democratic welfare systems might be less open to international competition.

The era of globalization necessitated a major shift in thinking in social policy and has reawakened interest in the questions that shaped the early development of the discipline, including those concerned with the role of the state in providing for its citizens. At a deeper level, a focus on globalization compels us to consider questions of fairness, equity and justice and how social policies in one part of the world might have a negative effect on welfare in other parts of the world. The UN's *Human Development Report 2013*, referred to above, identified important areas for sustaining development: enhancing equity, including gender equity, enabling citizen participation, including by young people, confronting environmental pressures, and managing demographic change. The report also noted how increasingly interconnected and complex policy decisions are and how the impact of a decision in one part of the world will resonate in others (UNDP, 2013). This means that the pressing issues of our time require international collaboration and coordinated action.

example 9.6

Migrant health and care workers

An example of the increasing interconnectedness of policy-making can be seen in the health and social care systems of high-income countries, which have come to depend to a large extent on the supply of health workers from low-income countries. Pond and McPake (2006) analysed trends in this type of migration and note how it is influenced by policy developments. Thus, in the UK, when public expenditure on healthcare rose in the late 1990s, there was an increase in the number of workers migrating to work in the NHS. The opening up of employment opportunities for professional workers might be seen as a positive enhancement of their rights. However, the drain of skilled workers from low-income countries further undermines their already overstretched and underresourced healthcare systems. In 2008, the World Health Assembly, a decision-making body of the WHO, developed a voluntary code in an attempt to control this practice. As was pointed out, the right of freedom of movement of labour should not be used to undermine people's right of access to healthcare.

A related development is the migration of care workers (mainly women), who now constitute a high percentage of the staff of care homes in high-income countries. Indeed, this phenomenon clearly illustrates the importance of looking beyond national boundaries to understand the social policies of individual countries. Once again, we can see how policies in one part of the world have affected conditions in other parts. In countries such as the US, Canada and the UK, a number of trends have increased the demand for care workers and nurses. These include demographic trends, the drive towards quicker hospital discharges, more 'personalized' care provided in people's own homes, as well as the growth of private care homes.

It has been observed that these migrant workers are often highly vulnerable to exploitation, with low pay, poor working conditions and insecurity being common experiences (Lund, 2006; Redfoot and Houser, 2008). For example, in 2011, a scandal erupted in Norway when it was discovered that migrant care staff at nursing homes run by a multinational corporation were working up to 100 hours a week without overtime pay, sometimes up to 20 hours a day, and with some being housed in a bomb shelter in the basement of one of the nursing homes. These workers did not have valid contracts and their rights to holiday pay and pensions were also violated (Lloyd et al., 2014). Of course, the poor conditions of employment experienced by the staff also have an impact on the quality of the care received by the older people living in the care homes. This case points to an overwhelming interest in reducing the *costs* of care to the detriment of the *quality* of care and the quality of life of staff and residents.

Through globalization, the long-standing disadvantageous position of women as care workers has thus become a racialized and international matter. The migration of women care workers highlights the connection between the global and the personal. The individual care relationship in a British care home between a worker from the Philippines and an older resident encapsulates many present-day global trends and policies.

Research methods in social policy: in understanding health

A range of methodologies, empirical and non-empirical, qualitative and quantitative, can be identified in social policy. For example, the works of social researchers, such as Townsend's (1979) surveys of poverty, contributed significantly to theory development. Townsend's research led to the development of the concept of 'relative deprivation', which describes the standard of living of any individual or group compared to the vast majority of the population. Townsend argued that policies to tackle poverty needed to take into account social and cultural factors as well as individual human needs. In an increasingly globalized world, the challenge is to develop such policies, recognizing that policies in one county might contribute towards the relief of poverty in another or might exacerbate it.

Surveys form a central part of the data that inform social policy on topics as diverse as food expenditure, carers, health behaviours, sexual attitudes and lifestyles and gambling prevalence. The UK Data Service provides access to some of these data at http://ukdataservice.ac.uk/get-data/themes/health.aspx.

---

example 9.7

Using textual analysis to understand policy

'Policy is both text and action, words and deeds' (Ball, 1994). Scott (2000, p. 18) observes that 'policy texts are characterized as official texts which operate to influence public perception of a policy agenda'. He notes how words are used and positioned to sound authoritative and present a case for policy change as though there is no challenge or room for debate. The type of words used

when communicating policy can also be analysed for the 'hidden' messages or ideas and associations that are conveyed. A close reading of policy texts is a useful way to begin policy analysis.

A starting point is a 'content analysis' through a systematic reading of a policy document. A quantitative approach involves counting the number of times key words or ideas are used. A qualitative approach or 'narrative analysis' considers the meanings, contexts, subjects and descriptions of the policy, such as who the policy is talking about and what is intended for them.

For example, *The Mandate: A Mandate from the Government to the NHS Commissioning Board: April 2013 to March 2015* (DH, 2013) set out the objectives the newly formed NHS Commissioning Board (renamed NHS England in 2013) is obliged to pursue. Of itself, the use of the term 'mandate' is of interest, because it reflects an authority or commitment – the mandate here is a commitment to preserve the principles of the NHS.

One of the objectives within this mandate is 'Enhancing the quality of life of people with long-term conditions'. The document sets out the approach government expects service providers to adopt in their services to support people with long-term conditions. The first statement refers to the need to 'empower' people living with long-term conditions. Elsewhere, the language adopted emphasizes self-care. While the language may suggest independence as positive, it also suggests a personal responsibility. The role of services is described as being there to enable people to manage their own conditions. The document links convenience, needs and choice, and suggests achieving this through more use of technology, such as electronic communication with GPs and other health professionals. Personalized care and maximum choice and control reflect a consumerist approach to social policy in which services provided through, or by, the state should be characterized by good consumer experience, such as smooth seamless transitions from one healthcare setting to another and good integration of services. The values implicit in such terms could be seen as in conflict, for example maximum choice for patients could lead to increased costs and greater reliance on services.

Research that enables the voice of the service user to emerge presents a particular problem to policy-makers and service providers as the demand to be more sensitive to service users' own constructions of their needs sits uncomfortably with demands to provide more efficient and cost-effective services. Data from qualitative research, such as that published by the Joseph Rowntree Foundation and others, have encouraged service users' voices to be included in social policy theorizing. Williams et al. (1999) argue that there is a need to understand the relationship between the personal history and experiences of people who use welfare services and the material and social world. The idea of welfare users as passive recipients or victims of the system has been profoundly challenged by a range of organizations, such as disabled people's and women's groups. Glasby and Beresford (2006) argue that the 'practice wisdom' of health and social care practitioners and the lived experiences of service users are as valid a means of developing knowledge as formal research.

? Percival and Hanson (2006) reported unease among service users about the use of technologies to support the self-management of long-term conditions. In their research, participants experienced telecare as an infringement of their privacy and a form of surveillance. Why would a policy continue to be developed when service users have expressed dissatisfaction with it?

Telehealth and telecare are seen as ways of reducing the number of visits people need to make to their GP practice or hospital. This policy is typical of a broader social policy agenda in which the values of independence and personal responsibility are emphasized and collective responsibility through tax-funded provision is reduced. It emphasizes efficiency and cost reduction in services.

Research methods in social policy: policy analysis

Social policy analysis concerns not only welfare systems but also individual policy development. As discussed above, the critical analysis of policy is a core activity of research and theory-building. Policies may be analysed on the basis of whether they achieve their objectives. Glendinning et al. (2008) evaluated the pilot project of individual budgets, a policy of the Labour government of the time. As they argued, the policy on individual budgets represented a potentially profound shift in the organization and culture of services. Their report pointed out that while there were many positive aspects to individual budgets, different service user groups experienced them differently, and organizational difficulties also impeded their implementation.

However, policy analysis goes deeper than simple evaluations of policies against their stated aims and objectives. Policy analysis can be divided into analysis *for* policy and analysis *of* policy (Hill, 2009):

- Analysis *for* policy contributes to solving social problems through a focus on evaluating the impact of policy, gathering data and information to assist policy-makers, and advocacy to present policy options or choices.

- Analysis *of* policy is an academic activity concerned with advancing understanding and knowledge through studies of policy content, outputs and processes such as decision-making.

Although this distinction is useful, there is a relationship between the two types as each influences the other: the development of knowledge has implications for policy-making, and policy-making is the subject of academic analysis.

Hudson and Lowe (2009) suggested a framework for policy analysis that considers policy at a macro-, meso- and micro-level. These levels should be understood as interconnected, and although the focus of analysis will be on one or other level, the connections to other levels are also important:

- *A macro-level analysis* considers concepts such as globalization, the political economy, and changes in the world of work, technology and governance. The discussion above of care worker migration is an example of a policy that has been the subject of macro-level analysis, with globally agreed policies on the movement of labour as the primary concern.

- *A meso-level analysis* looks at the structures of power, policy networks, institutions and policy transfer; for example, the differential power exerted by the state and various policy stakeholders such as political elites, organizations, pressure groups and service users in introducing, shaping or undermining social policies. Policy transfer is about the exchange or sharing of policy ideas. Once again, the spread of ideas underpinning social policy happens at national and global levels, but the ways in which these ideas are put into practice will be influenced by distinctive local cultures.

- *A micro-level analysis* focuses on decision-making and decision-makers, implementation and delivery, and evaluation and evidence. Decision-making is limited by the choices available in the chaotic real world of policies developing incrementally and building on what has gone before, rather than being a rational choice that starts with a blank sheet of paper. Individuals and charismatic leaders have an impact, such as Minster of Health Aneurin Bevan in establishing the NHS, and the frontline workers or 'street-level bureaucrats' (Lipsky, 1980) who implement and deliver social policies. The latter's role may be crucial in promoting, interpreting, hindering or delaying a policy.

Research methods in social policy: the policy process

Social policies can be understood as dynamic processes influenced by a range of groups and individuals with a stake in the process. Understanding the policy process enables us to understand the power relationships between the people involved and, beneath the surface, the relationship between policies and social divisions and inequalities.

A traditional approach to the policy process as a system is shown by the model developed by Hogwood and Gunn (1984), which lists the stages in a policy cycle:

1. deciding to decide

2. deciding how to decide

3. issue definition

4. forecasting

5. setting objectives and priorities

6. options analysis

7. policy implementation, monitoring and control

8. evaluation and review

9. policy maintenance, succession and termination.

This is a useful model but policy development is rarely neat and tidy, moving in orderly linear fashion from one completed stage to the next. Kickbusch (2010, p. 263) argues that policy agendas are 'actions triggered by windows of opportunity which can be opened by policy entrepreneurs'. She maintains that activists for health promotion should become engaged in the policy process and opportunities to do so should be seized wherever possible. The most difficult aspect of engagement is the political because this involves the skills of bargaining, compromise and negotiation. Kickbusch's approach is a good example of pragmatic policy analysis, with its emphasis on analysis *for* policy.

Figure 9.2 shows different elements of the policy process and how they affect each other. The relationship between policy-making and output, for example, may be examined to assess the efficiency of implementation systems. On the other hand, understanding the way in which issues get on the policy agenda in the first place can shed light on outcomes. There are several elements to the process.

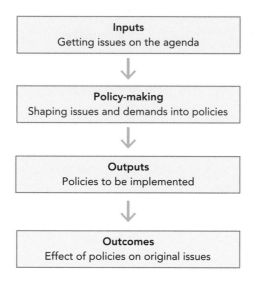

Figure 9.2 **The policy process**

Inputs

The way in which issues emerge as problems requiring government action reflects particular social and cultural values. Human needs and suffering do not always attract attention, and even where there is an awareness of a problem, this does not always translate into political action. Social phenomena may be perceived as problems by some but not others. Lone parenthood, for example, is consistently characterized as a social problem, but this characterization is open to dispute.

Policy inputs may come from within governments or international bodies as well as external interest groups. Getting an issue onto the agenda requires effective organization and access to sources of power and influence. The ability of any group to lobby effectively is crucially important. Some groups are more privileged than others in having access to formal or informal networks of power. Powerful transnational corporations, for example, have enjoyed greater influence over health policy than health service users. On the other hand, it was the actions of pressure groups that galvanized governmental and intergovernmental action on HIV/AIDS and led to the education of health and care professionals, the shifting cultural perceptions of the disease, and the coordinated demand for access to life-saving antiretroviral drugs in sub-Saharan African countries.

Policy-making

The process of formulating issues or demands into policy proposals comes next in the policy process. Policy-makers have to consider how any issue fits in with their overall agenda, what the political implications of adopting an issue as policy might be, and how likely it is that proposals will gain wider support and pass through the legislative process. Consultation enables policy-makers to test and listen to opinion. In the UK, this might be through a Green Paper, which tests opinion on policy ideas. A White Paper sets out government policy more specifically than a Green Paper but is still part of a process of consultation. For example, the government's White Paper *Equity and Excellence: Liberating the NHS* (DH, 2010) was regarded as part of a consultation on the way the intended policies would work in practice. Since the policy heralded a major change in the organization of the NHS, it was necessary to consider potential pitfalls in implementation. Following this, a bill is introduced to Parliament – the Health and Social Care Bill 2011, in this example – which is debated in both Houses of Parliament, and finally legislation follows (Great Britain, 2012).

example 9.8

Policy-making: the example of a smoking ban in workplaces and public places

In July 2007, a ban on smoking in virtually all workplaces in England came into effect following the passage of the Health Act in 2006. The ban in England followed smoking bans introduced in Scotland (March 2006) and in Wales and Northern Ireland (April 2007).

The call for a ban was based on scientific evidence that exposure to other people's smoke is dangerous to health. Reports such as the government's Scientific Committee on Tobacco and Health and studies such as Jamrozik (2005) had raised public awareness of the risks of passive smoking. The pressure group Action on Smoking and Health (ASH) commissioned a MORI poll in 2004 that

showed overwhelming public support for new legislation to end smoking in the workplace. A government report on public health (Wanless, 2004) considered the evidence of smoking bans implemented in other countries such as Ireland. In November 2004, the government responded with the White Paper *Choosing Health: Making Healthier Choices Easier* (DH, 2004), which included proposals to end smoking in the majority of workplaces and public places except for private clubs and pubs not serving food.

Ultimately, the smoking ban went further than the government intended. Concern in the Cabinet that many Labour MPs would not support the exemptions of clubs and pubs led to the decision to allow a free vote, where MPs make up their own minds rather than follow the party line. This resulted in a total ban in all enclosed areas. The legislation introduced fines for individuals caught smoking in a banned area and for those in charge of premises failing to stop people smoking in a restricted area (ASH, 2011).

While welcomed by anti-smoking groups like ASH, trade unions concerned for the health and safety of their members, and the government, others regarded it as an infringement of civil liberties. This included organizations such as the Tobacco Manufacturers' Association and Forest (Freedom Organisation for the Right to Enjoy Smoking Tobacco).

In 2011, the Department of Health commissioned Linda Bauld (2011) to conduct a review of the evidence on the impact of smoke-free legislation in England. This concluded that smoke-free laws are effective in reducing exposure to second-hand smoke and the effect was most marked among bar workers and children.

More recently, attempts have been made to introduce plain packaging of cigarettes to deter people from smoking. In the process of developing the legislation, the government changed course and decided to wait until more evidence was obtained about the effectiveness of plain packaging. This was regarded by some as an example of the power of pro-smoking lobby groups to steer policy in a particular direction. Evidence from Australia, where plain packaging has been in operation for over a year, suggests that this is an important strategy, particularly in deterring young people from starting to smoke (*BMJ*, 2013).

Outputs

If a bill goes through all the stages mentioned above, it becomes an Act of Parliament that requires implementation through central or local government or other agencies. At this stage, there is scope for further modification. Local conditions and priorities differ, and this will influence the implementation process. For example, the relationship between the overall strategic aims of the Department of Health and health authorities is not straightforward. The government may give guidance on putting policies into operation, but how this is interpreted at the local level varies. The relationship between central and local government is an important focus for analysis in social policy. So, too, are the resources put into the enforcement of policies. As policy implementation is increasingly in the hands of nongovernmental and commercial organizations, enforcement and regulation become all the more necessary. For example, in the wake of the collapse of Southern Cross Healthcare in 2011, the government is considering ways to strengthen governance of care home finances. Southern Cross, a major private, for-profit provider, ran over 750 care homes country-wide, with over 30,000 residents and employing around 41,000 staff. It ran into financial difficulties and went into liquidation in December 2011 after more than two years of uncertainty about its long-term viability. As reported by the BBC at the time, this created major anxieties for residents and their families about where the older people could go (BBC, 2011).

Outcomes

What difference does a policy make to people's lives? Given the scope for modification at all stages of the process, it is not surprising that policy outcomes can be quite different from what was envisaged by stakeholders at the beginning. This often means that the process of campaigning and lobbying begins again as further reforms and changes are demanded. Policies also often have unforeseen consequences that may stimulate pressure for further policy action.

At this stage, the experiences of patients and service users also need to be taken into account. Policies to improve efficiency in the NHS have, for example, led to problems over the discharge from hospital of frail and chronically sick people, who may be regarded as 'bed-blockers'. How do individual patients experience problems over hospital discharge? How does it feel to be a 'bed-blocker'? In what way can such feelings and experiences be articulated and heard by policy-makers and service providers?

The policy process is therefore not neat and linear but continuous and complex, influenced by the context in which it occurs. This involves social policy analysts in identifying the links between policy processes and broader economic, political and social systems, as well as taking into account service users' experiences.

case study a policy analysis of obesity in the UK

This case study takes up themes identified in the chapter, including the application of frameworks for policy analysis, and answers key questions:

- How is obesity as a health issue defined?
- Who should address obesity and how?
- Whose views and values are reflected in policy decisions?

Defining the issue

Obesity is defined as a health issue in relation to rising trends and its impact on health status. For example, in 2011–12, as a result of obesity there were 11 times more hospital admissions than there were in 2001–02.

It is also such a high priority because it is seen as preventable. Figures for 2011 supplied by the Health and Social Care Information Centre show that there was a marked increase in obesity rates (obesity being calculated as having a BMI of over 30) from 13% of men and 16% of women in 1993 to 24% of men and 26% of women in 2011 (www.hscic.gov. uk/catalogue/PUB13219). In 2011, 9.5% of children attending reception class at school were obese.

Media stories can help initiate or maintain a policy drive. The TV series *Jamie's School Dinners* (Channel 4, 2005) revealed poor quality and low investment in school meals, which generated a widespread audience reaction in support of the celebrity chef Jamie Oliver's campaign to improve school dinners. The emphasis on healthy school dinners as a strategy for promoting child health is still strong.

Addressing the problem of obesity

When considering who is responsible for addressing the problem of obesity, a number of important questions arise concerning the extent to which individuals should be held responsible for their own body weight. The current government's (NHS Choices, n.d.) perception of underlying causes is as follows:

- There is easy access to cheap, high-energy food that is often aggressively marketed to people.
- People's lifestyles and jobs are much less active than in the past and many leisure activities such as watching television, playing video games and browsing the internet are usually done sitting down.

- People drive or use public transport and walk a lot less than they used to.

We can see from this that individual as well as social and cultural factors are implicated in increased levels of obesity. While individuals are regarded as responsible for their weight, together with their activity levels and lifestyles, there is also recognition of the availability of cheap, high-energy food as a contributing factor.

Views and values reflected in policy decisions

The term 'aggressive marketing' draws a distinction between different approaches to the selling of food that contributes to obesity and suggests that it is the form of marketing, rather than the easy access to food, that is the underlying problem. This perspective is reflected in the Department of Health's policy on tackling obesity, which established a Public Health Responsibility Deal (https://responsibilitydeal.dh.gov.uk). This policy is intended to encourage businesses to make it easier for individuals to make healthier choices – focused on alcohol, food, health at work and physical activity. The strategies include the provision of more information for consumers, including food labelling and calorie information on menus. Local councils are included in the policy – also being involved in spreading information that will enable people to make healthier choices. Thus, a range of organizations, including public, commercial and community, are perceived as having responsibility to act on obesity.

A question arises, however, about the *effectiveness* of this policy. A report by the Academy of Medical Royal Colleges (2013) argued for much stronger measures. While it regarded the Responsibility Deal and campaigns on food labelling as having positive aspects, it argued that, overall, the government's 'programme to tackle obesity had been largely piecemeal and disappointingly ineffective' (p. 7). The report refers to the UK's 'obesogenic' environment and calls for more urgent action. This would include more mandatory measures, including a ban on TV advertising of foods high in saturated fats, sugar and salt before 9 pm, as well as more resources put into the promotion of active living and the creation of green spaces for children to play. Perhaps the most contentious recommendation is for a 20% levy on the price of sugary soft drinks to be piloted for one year.

While the government has a strong impetus to stop the rise in health expenditure associated with obesity, the overarching policy context at national and global levels requires that regulation over commercial activity should be as light as possible. Hence, the Responsibility Deal attempts to persuade, but not require, commercial companies to behave in particular ways. Indeed, it would be extremely difficult for an individual government to take on a powerful multinational food corporation and force it to change.

connections	Chapter 8 discusses the relationship between the state and industry in working for the public's health in the context of neoliberal ideology and the importance of the free market.

There is also a question about whether individuals should be made to behave in particular ways. For example, there have been suggestions over the years that parents should be blamed for childhood obesity and that their failure to keep their children healthy should be judged in the same way as currently would be the case if they neglected their children. This perspective places the responsibility for healthy eating entirely on the individual and exonerates food producers, retailers, government, schools and others from sharing that responsibility. A different take on this is that parents do not act in isolation and that their choices about the food they give to their children are influenced more by TV advertising than health promotion messages. However, the emphasis on parental responsibility is entirely consistent with the more individualistic approach to social policy discussed earlier in this chapter.

Chapter 12 discusses the ethical issues involved in the banning of food advertising to children.

connections

This case study has illustrated how obesity becomes defined as a health issue requiring a policy response and how that response is based on a mixture of evidence and political values. What emerges is not consistent or consensual, but comprises a policy strategy informed by popular beliefs and values as well as scientific evidence, economic imperatives and political agendas. The policy agenda is never static, but constantly shifting and evolving.

Summary

- The discipline of social policy provides a method for understanding the relationship between global and local influences on welfare

- Social policy enables us to understand how ideas about people's health and wellbeing are put into practice through welfare systems

- Social policy also enables us to recognize that interventions are not always beneficial and that policies may not, in practice, enhance health and wellbeing

- Critical approaches in social policy probe deeper to analyse the complex nature of welfare systems

- An analysis of the policy process provides further illumination of the relationship between policies and the economic, political and social contexts in which they are developed

- Social policy includes fundamental philosophical questions about the way in which a society secures the health and wellbeing of its most vulnerable members, such as older people

- Social policy continues to experience a tension between the need to analyse and critique welfare policies and the need to provide information that can be used to develop policies. Social policy is, simultaneously, about values, principles and pragmatism

- The importance of social policy to health studies is that it enables us to see how ideas about people's health and wellbeing are shaped into policies and practices, and how this is a dynamic process that is continually being analysed and changed

Questions for further discussion

1. Over the next two or three days, study reports or articles on health issues in one of the broadsheet newspapers. Think about the following:
   - Who is raising the issue and whom do they represent?
   - Is the issue on the policy agenda locally, nationally or internationally?
   - Where is pressure being directed?
   - What values are being expressed through this issue?

2. 'On the principle of the equal moral worth of all people, healthcare should not be rationed.' Discuss this proposition, with particular reference to old age.

Further reading and resources

There are several useful introductory texts on social policy. These will enable you to follow up general points related to the discipline.

Blakemore, K. and Warwick-Booth, L. (2013) *Social Policy: An Introduction* (4th edn). Buckingham: Open University Press.
Readable text looking at the general themes of welfare and at particular areas. Chapter 7, on health policy and health professions, will enable you to explore this issue in greater depth.

Blank, R.H. and Burau, V. (2013) *Comparative Health Policy* (4th edn). Basingstoke: Palgrave Macmillan.
Wide-ranging introduction to the provision, funding and governance of healthcare across a variety of health systems.

Buse, K., Mays, N. and Walt, G. (2012) *Making Health Policy* (2nd edn). Buckingham: Open University Press.
Hill, M. (2009) *The Public Policy Process* (5th edn). Harlow: Pearson Education.
These two textbooks provide an overview of the making of health policy and health policy analysis.

Crinson, I. (2009) *Health Policy: A Critical Perspective*. London: Sage.
Critical assessment of developments in health and healthcare policy within the UK and Europe. Each chapter integrates conceptual themes drawn from the fields of sociology and political science to offer a unique combination of theory, historical detail and wider social commentary.

Dean, H. (2012) *Social Policy: Short Introduction* (2nd edn). London: Polity.
Snappy and enthusiastic style, aimed at newcomers to the field.

Fraser, D. (2009) *The Evolution of the British Welfare State* (4th edn). Basingstoke: Palgrave Macmillan.
Classic text on social policy and social ideas in Britain since the Industrial Revolution.

www.gov.uk
The Department of Health website explores current and recent activities by central government in health. Some publications can be downloaded at no cost at www.gov.uk/government/organisations/department-of-health.

www.kingsfund.org.uk
The King's Fund is a good source of information.

http://www.kingsfund.org.uk/library
The King's Fund's Information and Knowledge Services provide a free source of information on health and social care policy and management.

http://hdr.undp.org
Provides access to the United Nations Development Programme's annual Human Development Reports.

References

Academy of Medical Royal Colleges (2013) *Measuring Up: The Medical Profession's Prescription for the Nation's Obesity Crisis*. Available at www.aomrc.org.uk/doc_view/9673-measuring-up (accessed 15/8/2014).

ASH (Action on Smoking and Health) (2011) *Smokefree Legislation*, Fact sheet, November. Available at http://ash.org.uk/files/documents/ASH_119.pdf.

Ball, S. (1994) *Education Reform: A Critical and Post-Structuralist Approach*. Buckingham: Open University Press.

Barnes, M. (2012) *Care in Everyday Life: An Ethic of Care in Practice*. Bristol: Policy.

Bauld, L. (2011) *The Impact of Smokfree Legislation in England: Evidence Review*. Bath: University of Bath. Available at www.gov.uk/government/uploads/system/uploads/attachment_data/file/216319/dh_124959.pdf.

BBC News (2011) 'Southern Cross set to shut down and stop running homes', 11 July. Available at www.bbc.co.uk/news/business-14102750.

Beveridge, W. (1942) *Social Insurance and Allied Services* (The Beveridge Report). London: HMSO.

BMJ (2013) 'UK government's delay on plain tobacco packaging: how much evidence is enough'. *British Medical Journal* 347: f4786.

Booth, C. (1902) *Life and Labour of the People of London*. London: Macmillan.

Brereton, L. and Gubb, J. (2010) *Refusing Treatment: The NHS and Market-based Reform*. London: Civitas.

Channel 4 (2005) *Jamie's School Dinners*, TV series broadcast from 23 February

Christie, B. (2002) 'United Kingdom divided as Scotland introduces free personal care for elderly people'. *British Medical Journal* 324(7353): 1542.

CIPOLD (2013) *Confidential Inquiry into Premature Deaths of People with Learning Disabilities*. Available at www.bris.ac.uk/media-library/sites/cipold/migrated/documents/fullfinalreport.pdf (accessed 3/10/2014).

Cracknall, R. (2010) *Key Issues for the New Parliament 2010: The Ageing Population*. Parliamentary briefing paper, pp. 44–5. Available at www.parliament.uk/business/publications/research/key-issues-for-the-new-parliament/ (accessed 8/8/2013).

Crowther, M. (1983) *The Workhouse System 1834–1929: The History of an English Social Institution*. London: Methuen.

Deacon, B. (2000) 'Eastern European welfare states: the impact of the politics of globalization'. *Journal of European Social Policy* 10(2): 146–61.

Deacon, B. (2007) *Global Social Policy and Governance*. London: Sage.

DH (Department of Health) (1987) *Promoting Better Health*. London: HMSO.

DH (1992) *Health of the Nation*. London: HMSO.

DH (1997) *The New NHS: Modern, Dependable*. London: TSO.

DH (1999) *Saving Lives: Our Healthier Nation*. London: TSO.

DH (2000) *The NHS Plan*. London: HMSO.

DH (2002) *NHS Reform and Health Care Professionals Act*. London: HMSO.

DH (2003) *Health and Social Care (Community Health and Standards) Act*. London: HMSO.

DH (2004) *Choosing Health: Making Healthy Choices Easier*. London: TSO.

DH (2006) Government response to report on tackling childhood obesity. Press release 2006/0077. London: DH.

DH (2008a) *High Quality Care for All: NHS Next Stage Review Final Report*. Report by Lord Darzi. London: TSO.

DH (2008b) *An Introduction to Personalisation*. Available at http://webarchive. nationalarchives.gov.uk.

DH (2009) *The NHS Constitution: The NHS Belongs to us All*. London: DH.

DH (2010) *Equity and Excellence: Liberating the NHS*. London: DH

DH (2012) *Overview of the Health and Social Care Act fact sheet*, 15 June. Available at www.gov.uk/government/publications/health-and-social-care-act-2012-fact-sheets (accessed 7/8/2013).

DH (2013) *The Mandate: A Mandate from the Government to the NHS Commissioning Board: April 2013 to March 2015*. London: DH.

Dickinson, H. and Glasby, J. (2010) *The Personalisation Agenda: Implications for the Third Sector*, Working Paper 30. Birmingham: Third Sector Research Centre.

Dilnot, A. (2011) *Fairer Care Funding: Report of the Commission on Funding of Care and Support*.

Doyal, L. and Gough, I. (1991) *A Theory of Human Needs*. Basingstoke: Macmillan – now Palgrave Macmillan.

Duffy, S. (2012) 'Who really benefits from welfare?' Available at www. centreforwelfarereform.org/library/by-az/who-really-benefits-from-welfare. html (accessed 25/7/2013).

Esping-Andersen, G. (1990) *The Three Worlds of Welfare Capitalism*. Cambridge: Polity.

Francis, R. (2013) *Final Report of the Mid Staffordshire NHS Foundation Trust Public Inquiry*. Available at www.midstaffspublicinquiry.com/report (accessed 8/8/2013).

Fraser, D. (2009) *The Evolution of the British Welfare State* (4th edn). Basingstoke: Palgrave Macmillan.

Ghevaert, L. (2012) 'The IVF postcode lottery must stop'. Available at www. bionews.org.uk/page_155601.asp (accessed 1/7/2013).

Giddens, A. (2006) *Sociology* (5th edn). Cambridge: Polity.

Glasby, J. and Beresford, P. (2006) 'Who knows best? Evidence-based practice and the service user contribution'. *Critical Social Policy* 26(1): 268–84.

Glendinning, C. (2006) Paying family caregivers: evaluating different models, in C. Glendinning and P. Kemp (eds) *Cash and Care: Policy Challenges in the Welfare State*. Bristol: Policy, pp. 127–40.

Glendinning, C., Challis, D., Fernandez, J. et al. (2008) *The National Evaluation of the Individual Budgets Pilot Programme*. York: Social Policy Research Unit.

Goffman, E. (1961) *Asylums: Essays on the Social Situation of Mental Patients and other Inmates*. Harmondsworth: Penguin.

Gough, I. (2004) Welfare regimes in development contexts: a global and regional analysis, in I. Gough and G. Wood with A. Barrientos et al. (eds) *Insecurity and Welfare Regimes in Asia, Africa and Latin America: Social Policy in Development Contexts*. Cambridge: Cambridge University Press, pp. 15–49.

Great Britain (1996) *Community Care (Direct Payments) Act 1996*. London: HMSO, Ch. 30.

Great Britain (2006) *NHS Redress Act 2006*. London: HMSO.

Great Britain (2012) *Health and Social Care Act*. London: TSO.

Hill, M. (2009) *The Public Policy Process* (5th edn). Harrow: Pearson Education.

Hogwood, B. and Gunn, L. (1984) *Policy Analysis for the Real World*. Oxford: Oxford University Press.

Hough, K. (2013) 'NHS on a path towards "fragmentation, competition and privatisation"'. www.commissioning.gp.

Hudson, J. and Lowe, S. (2009) *Understanding the Policy Process* (2nd edn). Bristol: Policy.

Jamrozik, K. (2005) 'Estimates of deaths attributable to passive smoking among UK adults: database analysis'. *British Medical Journal* 330(7495): 812–17.

Johnson, G. (2011) 'Holding back the British IVF revolution? A report into NHS IVF provision in the UK today' by All Party Parliamentary Group on Infertility. Available at www.bionews.org.uk/page_96927.asp (accessed 1/10/2013).

Keogh, B. (2013) *Review into the Quality of Care and Treatment by 14 Hospital Trusts in England: Overview Report*. Available at www.nhs.uk/NHSEngland/bruce-keogh-review/Documents/outcomes/keogh-review-final-report.pdf (accessed 1/10/2014).

Kickbusch, I. (2010) 'Health in all policies: where to from here?' *Health Promotion International* 25(3): 261–4.

Lipsky, M. (1980) *Street-level Bureaucracy: Dilemmas of the Individual in Public Service*. New York: Russell Sage Foundation.

Lloyd, L., Banerjee, A., Fadnes, F. et al. (2014) 'It's a scandal!: comparing the causes and consequences of nursing home media scandals in five countries'. *International Journal of Sociology and Social Policy* 34: 2–18.

Lund, F. (2006) Working people and access to social protection, in S. Razavi and S. Hassim (eds) *Gender and Social Policy in a Global Context: Uncovering the Gendered Structure of 'the Social'*. Basingstoke: UNRISD/ Palgrave Macmillan, pp. 217–33.

Lymbery, M. (2012) 'Social work and personalisation: fracturing the bureau-professional compact?' *British Journal of Social Work* 1: 1–17.

Marmot, M., Allen, J., Goldblatt, P. et al. (2010) *Fair Society, Healthy Lives: Strategic Review of Health Inequalities in England Post-2010*. London: The Marmot Review.

Marshall, T.H. (1950) *Citizenship and Social Class and other Essays*. Cambridge: Cambridge University Press.

Mays, N. and Dixon, A. (2011) Assessing and explaining the impact of New Labour's market reforms, in A. Dixon, N. Mays and L. Jones (eds) *Understanding New Labour's Market Reforms of the English NHS*. London: King's Fund, pp. 124–42.

Means, R. and Smith, R. (1998) *From Poor Law to Community Care: The Development of Welfare Services for Elderly People 1939–1971*. Bristol: Policy.

Miller, C. (2004) *Producing Welfare: A Modern Agenda*. Basingstoke: Palgrave Macmillan.

New, B. and Mays, N. (1997) Age, renal replacement therapy and rationing, in *Health Care UK 1996/7: The King's Fund Annual Review of Health Policy*. London: King's Fund, pp. 205–23.

NHS Choices (n.d.) Latest obesity stats for England are alarming. Available at www.nhs.uk/news/2013 (accessed 1/8/2014).

OECD (2006) 'Rising health costs put pressure on public finances, finds OECD'. Available at www.oecd.org/general/risinghealthcostsputpressureonpublic financesfindsoecd.htm (accessed 1/8/2014).

Percival, J. and Hanson, J. (2006) 'Big brother or brave new world? Telecare and its implications for older people's independence and social inclusion'. *Critical Social Policy* 26(4): 888–909.

Pond, B. and McPake, B. (2006) 'The health migration crisis: the role of four Organisation for Economic Cooperation and Development countries'. *Lancet* 367: 1448–55.

Redfoot, D.L. and Houser, A.N. (2008) 'The international migration of nurses in long-term care'. *Journal of Aging and Social Policy* 20(2): 259–75.

Robb, B. (1967) *Sans Everything: A Case to Answer*. London: Nelson.

Rowntree, B.S. (1901) *Poverty: A Study of Town Life*. London: Macmillan.

Scott, D. (2000) *Reading Educational Research and Policy*. London: Routledge Falmer.

Titmuss, R.M. (1974) *Social Policy: An Introduction*. London: Allen & Unwin.

Townsend, P. (1979) *Poverty in the United Kingdom*. Harmondsworth: Penguin.

Townsend, P. and Davidson, N. (eds) (1992) *Inequalities in Health: The Black Report* (2nd edn). Harmondsworth: Penguin.

Twigg, J. (2006) *The Body in Health and Social Care*. Basingstoke: Palgrave Macmillan.

UNDP (United Nations Development Programme) (2013) *Human Development Report 2013*. New York: Oxford University Press.

Ungerson, C. (2003) Informal welfare, in P. Alcock, A. Erskine and M. May (eds) (2003) *The Student's Companion to Social Policy* (2nd edn). Oxford: Blackwell, pp. 200–6.

Vizard, P. and Obolenskaya, P. (2013) *Labour's Record on Health (1997–2010)*. Working Paper 2. Available at http://sticerd.lse.ac.uk/dps/case/spcc/wp02.pdf (accessed 02/08/13).

Wanless, D. (2004) *Securing Good Health for the Whole Population: Final Report*. London: HMSO.

WHO (World Health Organization) (2002) *Global Strategy on Diet, Physical Activity and Health*. Geneva: WHO.

Williams, A. (1997) 'Rationing health care by age: the case for'. *British Medical Journal* 314: 820–2.

Williams, F., Popay, J. and Oakley, A. (1999) *Welfare Research: A Critical Review*. London: UCL Press.

VICKI TAYLOR, HILARY SCOTT and MARTIN WALTER

Organization and management of health and healthcare

Overview   335

Introduction   335

Part 1 The contribution of management to health studies   337
Understanding organizations   337
Working across organizations   351
Managing healthcare services   352
Working in groups and teams   352
Leadership   354
Managing change   357

Part 2 Theoretical and research approaches   357
Scientific management   358
Bureaucracy and organizations   359
The human relations approach to understanding people and organizations   360
Behavioural theory   361
Situation theory   361
Contingency theory   362
Motivation theories   362
Systems theory and the sociotechnical system approach   366
Chaos (or complexity) theory   368

Case study Formulating an obesity strategy   369
Summary   371
Questions for further discussion   371
Further reading   372
References   373

Learning outcomes

This chapter will enable readers to:

- Gain a sound understanding of modern management theories and relate them to examples of practical situations and issues, particularly in relation to healthcare
- Better understand the nature and operation of health services and how they can be managed
- Understand the influences on large, complex organizations and the skills and abilities needed by practitioners

Overview

Management – the professional administration of business concerns, public undertakings and organizations in general – is a topical subject, particularly in relation to health and healthcare services. This chapter will explore why this topic should form part of the health studies curriculum for students, regardless of their professional background or personal inclination to be involved in management. The chapter outlines some of the major theoretical concepts relating to organization and management studies, and applies these to the NHS in the UK. The NHS is a unique organization with a huge and diverse remit and workforce, and its scale of operations means that many different organizational and management styles have been tried and tested. Part 1 focuses on theories relating to organizations and how they operate within a broad political and policy context. Part 2 discusses different management theories and models and their relevance to the NHS, and discusses contemporary issues such as what best motivates workers, and how leaders can enthuse their staff. The chapter concludes with a case study on the development of a local obesity strategy.

Introduction

We all relate to organizations of various kinds – the local authority, the GP practice, local retailers, online stores, schools and colleges – and we are all affected by the way they are managed, the way they interact with us and deliver (or not) the goods and services we seek. The more we are aware of the way these organizations operate and how they are structured and managed, the more successful we are likely to be in our dealings with them.

Organizations vary enormously in their size and complexity. The UK's NHS is one of the largest and arguably most complex organizations in the industrialized world, with responsibility for prevention, curing and caring, and employing a huge and diverse workforce. Furthermore, the provision of healthcare in the UK accounts for almost a fifth (18% or £129.7 billion) of Treasury expenditure, and reflects the high priority afforded it by the voting public (UK Public Spending, n.d.). As such, it demands serious attention in the shape of good management. Moreover, health and healthcare services compete for resources with other major government responsibilities, such as education, welfare, defence and local authority funding. Applying theories that examine organizations, their structure and culture, management of the workforce and leadership to the NHS is therefore a good test of the theories' adequacy and usefulness.

Management is the act – or art – of managing resources, whether they are human, technological or financial. It is about conducting business, from initiating and developing ideas for new or improved products to leading, supervising and delivering the result. It is concerned with the arrangements for carrying out organizational processes and executing work (Mullins, 2013) and depends on the skill, competence, knowledge, dedication, vision and integrity of those who manage. Managers' skills are closely connected to the success, or otherwise, of the organization's work.

Almost a century ago, Fayol described the central tasks of management (Pugh and Hickson, 1996) as:

- planning
- organizing the structure
- organizing human resources (people)
- coordinating or harmonizing the various functions
- controlling the operation and outcome of the organization.

Most healthcare systems have, at various times, problems with one, more, or all of these tasks. The pace of change in the NHS has accelerated over the past 30 years, with frequent changes to organizational structures and systems, efforts to develop the workforce, including creating new sorts of practitioner that differ from the traditional nurse and doctor roles, treating people safely and effectively, and variable success in achieving financial balance and managing complex budgets and processes. Before 1948, healthcare services were usually paid for either by individuals or charities. This gave way to a nationalized system in 1948, the NHS, which is free at the point of delivery. From 1948 until the 1980s, the NHS provided the most cost-effective and influential economic model for state-funded healthcare services. There were periodic efforts during the 1950s and 60s to adjust the new system so that it provided care in the most economical way, but the 1970s brought the first focused effort on effective and rational management of healthcare in the wake of the oil crisis, recession and the squeeze on all services funded from taxation.

Two essential management attributes mark out successful organizations: effective management and appropriate organizational structure. Effective management enables the organization to adjust and respond to the pressures placed on it. It could be argued that the largest public sector health service organization in the world was slow to wake up to these essentials. Regional strategic planning was not formally introduced into the NHS until about 1970 and the concept of management, as differentiated from administration, came largely as a result of the 1983 Griffiths Report (DHSS, 1983). It was only after this report was adopted by the government in 1984 that, for example, fully developed personnel departments became the norm, and this was in an organization of well over 1 million workers. The past 50 years have seen the development of a market-based approach to healthcare – healthcare that improves people's lives at a price the economy can bear – by changing the way healthcare is organized and managed.

connections   Chapter 9 explores the development of the NHS and systems of welfare.

Part 1 The contribution of management to health studies

example 10.1

The application of organization and management to contemporary health issues

- Understanding the specific nature of leadership in healthcare – over the years a number of different approaches to leadership have been taken, from the notion that leaders are born through to the development of leaders, transformational leadership and the more recent distributed approach to leadership
- Change management and the factors that enable or hinder change in large organizations such as those in the NHS and social care system. Understanding how to bring about change effectively is essential to providing effective care. Analysing readiness for change and understanding why people resist change are key areas of study in the management of change
- Understanding the environments in which organizations exist and operate and how they can develop their organizational structure and culture in order to deal with these challenges
- Understanding how organizations plan, manage and control the activities that take place is critical. Understanding what motivates staff is also important, as are the recruitment and retention strategies, and induction and socialization processes that all staff experience
- The nature of good governance and performance accountability is an integral component of effective staff management, as is innovative coaching and mentoring in leadership development
- Understanding what factors contribute to making a team more effective and the dynamics of teams
- Setting and making the most effective use of a budget is critical to ensuring cost-effectiveness and best value

Understanding organizations

What is an organization? On the surface, this seems to be a straightforward question but the term 'organization' often means different things to different people. Various answers have been advanced, but it comes down to there being a set of rules, or social arrangements, for achieving agreed goals. In the NHS, such goals include the prevention of illness, caring for and/or healing the sick and advancing our knowledge of health and illness. Some key features are common to all organizations (Taylor, 2013):

- Organizations consist of people
- Organizations exist for a purpose
- Organizations are designed to achieve objectives
- Organizations exist in relationship to others
- Organizations have ways of working shaped by shared attitudes.

All organizations consist of people

Organizations are necessary because individuals are unable to accomplish the same outcomes as effectively, if at all, as an organized group (Mullins, 2013). Some organizations require extensive premises from which to deliver services, such as hospitals or local authority 'one stop shops', while others are focused around community-based activities and have more modest accommodation requirements. The organization refers to the way the individuals who comprise the staff are organized to work together. These people often have shared values and views about the purpose of the organization.

The NHS currently employs more than 1.7 million people, around half of whom are clinically qualified, 'including 39,780 GPs, 370,327 nurses, 18,687 ambulance staff and 105,711 hospital and community health service medical and dental staff. Only the Chinese People's Liberation Army, the Wal-Mart supermarket chain and Indian Railways directly employ more people' (NHS Choices, n.d.). Given the size and complexity of the NHS, it may at first seem difficult to understand how the different professions can work together effectively, and this is one of the reasons why it is important to study organizations.

Organizations exist for a purpose, or number of purposes

This is often expressed as a hierarchy of purposes with a set of organizational goals and specific objectives. At the top of the hierarchy, there is an account about why the organization exists, often referred to as its 'vision' or 'mission statement', then some broad statements about what the organization is trying to do. At a lower level, there are specific objectives that set out how these activities are going to be undertaken. Usually, specific measures, often referred to as 'performance data' or 'key performance indicators', are used to monitor and evaluate the extent to which these objectives are achieved. The NHS 'exists to improve the health outcomes and care for all people in England' (NHS England, 2013a). The vision that 'everyone has greater control of their health and their wellbeing, supported to live longer, healthier lives by high quality health and care services that are compassionate, inclusive and constantly-improving' (NHS England, 2013b) articulates this and provides a framework (the NHS Outcomes Framework) against which objectives for all staff and performance, of individuals and the organization as a whole, can be measured. Key performance indicators for NHS England are captured in the NHS Outcomes Framework (NHS Commissioning Board, 2012), which is organized across five domains:

- Domain 1: Preventing people from dying prematurely

- Domain 2: Enhancing quality of life for people with long-term conditions

- Domain 3: Helping people to recover from episodes of ill health or following injury

- Domain 4: Ensuring that people have a positive experience of care

- Domain 5: Treating and caring for people in a safe environment and protecting them from avoidable harm.

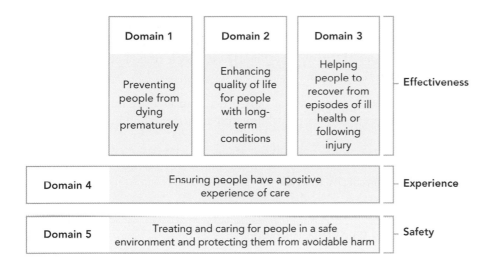

Figure 10.1 **The NHS Outcomes Framework**
Source: NHS England, 2014

thinking about Consider an organization you are familiar with. What is its purpose? Does it have a clear vision or mission statement? Do individuals have clear objectives that relate to the organization's overall purpose or part of the organization they work in? How is performance measured or monitored?

Organizations don't just happen, they are designed

Organizations have some control over how they organize themselves to achieve their objectives, usually referred to as 'organizational structure'. Mintzberg (1979, p. 2) defined organizational structure as 'the sum total of the ways in which it divides its labour into distinct tasks and then achieves coordination among them'. This refers to a set of roles and recognized relationships between them, usually interdependent, where each role depends on others to achieve the organizational purpose. Organizational structure provides the framework to enable an organization to divide and carry out its work. In complex structures with large numbers of staff, organization is important. Everyone within the organization needs to understand their role and how they fit into its overall structure. Organizations can be structured in many different ways, for example divided up on the basis of functional groups such as finance, communications and so on. This is particularly useful when people in functional departments need to communicate regularly with one another. Other arrangements include grouping people together on the basis of the product or service area. Staff within health and social care settings are often organized on the basis of the client group, for example services for older people or children and young people. This type of organizational structure is referred to as a 'product or service structure'.

> **thinking about** How would you find out how an organization such as a university or your workplace is structured?

An organization's structure not only gives it an identity but also a framework for the allocation of responsibility and authority, showing:

- the span of control and command
- the shape of hierarchy (tall, flat)
- the degree of centralization
- the degree and type of specialization
- the degree of job definition.

Example 10.2 explains these terms.

example 10.2

Organizational structures

- *Span of control:* refers to the number of people reporting directly to a manager. This is influenced by the nature of the work, the degree of specialization and functional groupings or where individuals are working on similar tasks
- *Shape of hierarchy:* a classic bureaucracy (like many NHS organizations) can be represented as a hierarchy with a number of layers of staff at different levels of seniority. Organizations with many levels are called 'tall', those with few, 'flat'. Two-thirds of organizations have between five and eight levels of management (Pugh, 1988)

- *Degree of centralization:* refers to the degree of centralized decision-making, which inevitably takes longer as decisions have to be referred up the chain of command. Decentralized decision-making is quicker and usually provides greater flexibility. This form of decision-making is also more responsive to differing situations
- *Degree and type of specialization:* refers to the extent to which jobs are specialized and/or require specialist knowledge
- *Degree of job definition:* in bureaucratic organizations, there is a greater tendency for tighter definition and delineation of roles, responsibilities and accountabilities

> **thinking about** Consider an organization you are familiar with. How many people report to each manager (their span of control)? How many layers or levels of management are there? Is the hierarchy tall or flat? How much autonomy does each worker have? Is authority centralized or decentralized?

Does the organization employ functional experts for some tasks, for example a finance department? How clear is the definition of jobs? Do some of them overlap? How many people do employees report to? What are the implications of this?

Since its inception, the NHS has been organized in some form of hierarchy, with local organizations (for the most part) providing services within a largely centralized policy framework. Figure 10.2 shows the structure of the NHS following the radical reorganization of the Health and Social Care Act 2012. Currently, the NHS in England comprises some 211 organizations known as clinical commissioning groups (CCGs), which commission community-based and hospital services from, largely, 261 NHS provider organizations – 161 acute trusts (including 101 foundation trusts), 56 mental health trusts (including 41 foundation trusts), 34 community providers (18 NHS trusts and 16 social enterprises), 10 ambulance trusts and 8,000 GP practices.

The organizational structure of the NHS has increased in size and complexity in response to changes in demand. As previously indicated, the structure of an organization underpins how it operates, alongside organizational 'rules' that do or do not enable participation. Weber (1964) argued that the most effective form of organizational structure, described as a 'bureaucracy', was one where the roles and relationships of employees were clearly defined. A bureaucratic organizational structure is characterized by a belief that rules and legal order provide legitimacy for the authority of managers and is designed, just like a machine, to achieve organizational goals and objectives. It follows that larger organizations need clear rules and regulations to hold them together and, among other things, prevent loss of budgetary control.

thinking about Consider a large organization you are familiar with. How is the work divided up?

While there are large organizations bound by relatively few rules, public services in the UK have tended to develop a greater degree of bureaucracy. These types of organization have hierarchies, rules, regulations and job descriptions that demarcate responsibility and ensure order and rigidity. The more complex an organization is, the more complex the processes for dividing up the work or tasks that need to be undertaken to achieve the organizational purpose, and to coordinate and integrate these activities. The methods used to achieve this also ensure that there are clear ways of undertaking the various tasks and protect the individual working within the organization. Lawrence and Lorsch (1967) referred to these methods and processes as 'differentiation' and 'integration'. They defined differentiation as the 'state of segmentation of the organizational system into subsystems' and integration as the 'process of achieving unity of effort among various subsystems in the accomplishment of the organization's task' (Lawrence and Lorsch, 1967, pp. 3–4).

The health & care system from April 2013

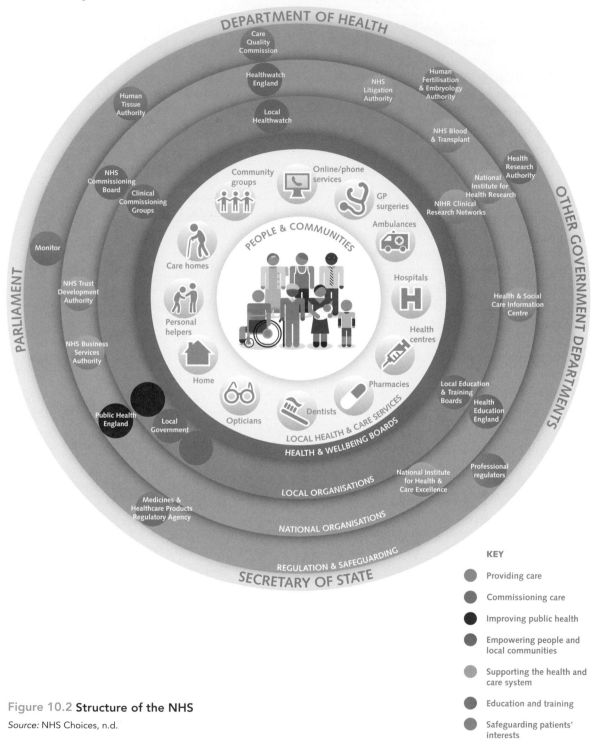

Figure 10.2 Structure of the NHS

Source: NHS Choices, n.d.

Organizations are affected and shaped by factors in the wider external environment. For example, changes in the economy, social trends and the political climate can have an important impact on organizations. An understanding of the external environment is particularly critical because it provides a source of many threats and new opportunities as well as drivers for change.

Organizational effectiveness is dependent on successful management of the opportunities and threats presented by these external influences for change, together with the internal response to these challenges. Public sector organizations, and the NHS in particular, seem to have gone through endless change in the past decade. The NHS is constantly subject to change as the policy context and available resources change. Organizations do not operate in a vacuum (Buchanan and Huczynski, 2010; Mullins, 2013) but continually interact with the external environment. This is particularly so for the NHS, which is subject to intense political scrutiny and has been affected by differing ideologies and policies concerning the best way to provide healthcare and healthcare services.

Chapters 8 and 9 discuss the influences and shaping of the NHS and welfare systems.   **connections**

The external environment is usually regarded as everything that lies outside an organization's boundaries. This external environment can be divided into two: the 'near' and the 'far' external environment:

- The *near* external environment can be influenced, but not controlled, by the organization. The near environment includes groups and organizations that the organization interacts with, such as local politicians, suppliers and local interest groups.

- The *far* external environment refers to factors that cannot easily be controlled or influenced directly from within the organization. They include a wide range of political, environmental, sociocultural, technological, legal and economic factors, such as the overall economic performance of the country, the labour supply, and the costs of other government commitments such as defence and education. There may be political pressure to match government spending on healthcare with those of comparable EU countries, such as France and Germany.

All organizations need to be aware of, and respond to, the impact of these external factors.

The PESTLE (political, economic, sociocultural, technological, legal and environmental) analysis can be used to assess the potential impact of external influences that might influence, or be influenced by, an organization (Table 10.1).

Table 10.1 **PESTLE analysis of environmental pressures**

PESTLE factor	Far environment	Health environment
Political	Government policy Taxation policy Acts of Parliament	Policy on smoking cessation and obesity
Economic	Money supply Interest rates Employment Financial wellbeing	NHS budget Local health services priorities Prices of drugs
Sociocultural	Demographics Social mobility Culture	Prevailing patterns of ill-health: the health burden Health-related behaviour
Technological	Research and development New discoveries	New drugs and their availability New treatments and procedures
Legal	Laws	Employment law, for example Working Time Regulations
Environmental	Environmental protection laws, for example disposal of asbestos	Healthy/unhealthy environment affecting health of the population

connections   Chapter 5 examines the socioeconomic patterns of health and ill health, Chapter 11 looks at issues of rationing and public spending and Chapter 12 looks at the legal context for health service delivery.

?   How does increasing globalization affect the internal and external environments of organizations?

Instability in the environment may give rise to various degrees of turbulence for organizations. An important part of good management is being vigilant regarding forthcoming changes and taking anticipatory action. Ansoff and McDonnell (1990) proposed five levels on which to consider environmental turbulence, from level 1, when the organization can easily respond to an environmental event (as in 1948, when the NHS was set up), to level 5 when major changes are introduced so quickly that the organization is overwhelmed. Table 10.2 shows how the environment for health and social care has increased in turbulence since the beginnings of the NHS in 1948 to the present day.

connections   Chapter 9 describes the development of the welfare state and some of the political drivers influencing change.

?   Practitioners in the NHS may point to numerous reorganizations in the past decade, including the establishment of foundation hospitals, proposals for 'poly clinics', changing roles towards more generic workers, as well as many changes in structure. What accounts for this level of turbulence?

Table 10.2 Environmental turbulence and the NHS

Date	History	Level of turbulence	Events
1948	Start of the NHS	*Level 1: Predictable* – a repetitive environment characterized by stability of markets; where the challenges repeat themselves; change is slower than the organization's ability to respond; the future is expected to be the same as the past	Pre-existing health facilities were nationalized, but not rationalized. Funding levels remained unaltered and followed historic patterns. Healthcare provision essentially low tech. Health services now free at the point of use, including prescriptions. Demand for health services rose steeply. Unanticipated costs rose but general inflation low, at around 2.5%. The NHS run by administrators and doctors
1960s	Several attempts made to rationalize the NHS. Only minor changes made	*Level 2: Forecastable by extrapolation* – complexity increases but managers can still extrapolate from the past and forecast the future with confidence	Rise in technical development. Big increases in NHS clinical support staff. Heart–lung machine, kidney dialysis now widespread and experiments with transplantation; first kidney transplant. Variety and costs of available drugs increase. NHS funding increased, but spending deficits made up by the Treasury's system of secondary estimates. Inflation mostly low
1970s	First major reorganization of the NHS to change the national structure. A top-down bureaucratic imposition to achieve uniformity of structure and grading (1974)	*Level 3: Predictable threats and opportunities* – complexity increases further when the organization's ability to respond becomes more problematic; however, the future can still be predicted with some degree of confidence	Continued rise in technical development and application and in numbers of clinical support staff. NHS planning system introduced. First attempt to rationalize funding to local areas. Steep rise in inflation. IMF loan conditions ended the secondary estimates scheme and imposed cash limits. Rise of NHS manger and managerial function of senior clinical staff and clinical support staff. Reforms opposed by many clinicians
1980s	Second reorganization of the NHS (1982), rescinding some of the 1974 reforms. The 1983 NHS Management Inquiry (Griffiths Report) introduced general managers who were in charge of clinical staff. Further reforms introduced in 1989 to differentiate providers from purchasers or commissioners of healthcare	*Level 4: Partially predictable opportunities* – turbulence increases with the addition of global and sociopolitical changes. The future is only partly predictable	Reforms introduced in the context of other reforms of Conservative Thatcher government, attempting to make public services function similar to those of the private sector. Many non-NHS managers introduced to the NHS for the first time. Many funding cutbacks and bed numbers reduction. Introduction of the private finance initiative. Further cost escalation. Inflation high
1990s	Full implementation of 1989 reforms and many other changes introduced by central government. GP fundholding. Further reforms under the New Labour government	*Level 4–5:* turbulence increased with unexpected events occurring more quickly than the organization can respond	Strict imposition of cash limits led some local health authorities to selectively cut services. Postcode provision arose and became a political issue. Regional health authorities abolished, functions shared between regional offices and expanded health authorities. Several high-profile 'scandals' (paediatric cardiac surgery, mistaken cancer test results) with consequences for healthcare safety agenda. NHS trusts and GP fundholding introduced. Fundholding subsequently abolished. Local primary care groups established. Clinical governance and modernization agenda established
2000s	Further changes to NHS structure imposed by government. Significant additional funds applied to the NHS, which serve mostly to fill long-standing deficits. Trend to establish 'independent' organizations to oversee NHS practice, in the form of regulators (Healthcare Commission and Commission for Social Care Inspection) and 'guiders' – National Institute of Health and Clinical Excellence, National Patient Safety Agency	*Level 5: Unpredictable surprises* – turbulence increases further with unexpected events and situations occurring more quickly than the organization can respond	NHS Plan published, promoting patient and public involvement in decisions about healthcare, reintroduction of market-like principles to NHS through payment by results and practice-based commissioning. Primary care groups become primary care trusts. Abolition of Community Health Council, establishment of the Commission for Patient and Public Involvement in Health; then its abolition in favour of locally based organizations. Health authorities combine into strategic health authorities, then reduce in number from 28 to 10. Greater client focus illustrated though Choose

>

Date	History	Level of turbulence	Events
2000s cont'd			and Book, sharing doctor's letters with patients and decreased time to treat initiatives. Direct payment for social care services takes hold. First NHS foundation trusts established in 2004, given increased freedom and control over financial and operational matters. Market economy and decentralization of services promoted. The Health Act 2006 brought in smoke-free legislation. Increased patient choice introduced in 2008 for outpatient services. New NHS Constitution launched in 2009, with overall aim of bringing high-quality care to all and free to all
2010s	Present-day NHS undergoing major changes in its core structure, including who makes decisions about NHS services, service commissioning, and the way money is spent. Extension of the market approach to healthcare is evident	*Level 5: Unpredictable surprises* – turbulence increases further with unexpected events and situations occurring more quickly than the organization can respond	To date, the 2010s have seen great medical breakthroughs and healthcare innovations. The NHS was celebrated at the London 2012 Olympic Games, and marked its 65th anniversary on 5 July 2013. The Francis Report and the Keogh Review increase public concern about the quality of the provision of care. *Putting Patients First: The NHS England Business Plan for 2013/14–2015/16* explains how NHS England's commitment to transparency and increasing patients' voices is fundamental to improving patient care. Describes an 11-point scorecard that NHS England will introduce for measuring performance of key priorities, focused on receiving direct feedback from patients, their families and NHS staff. Supports the cultural change needed to put people at the centre of the NHS, a key theme in the Francis Report, by making sure patients' voices are heard and used to deliver better services. The Health and Social Care Act 2012 was passed. It was argued that it was passed to safeguard the future of the NHS by placing clinicians at the centre of commissioning, by freeing up providers to innovate, and to empower patients and give a new focus to public health. Led to abolition of PCTs and strategic health authorities and establishment of clinical commissioning groups, Public Health England and the transition of public health into local government

The NHS became the social equivalent of mass production; largely state directed and managed, built on a paternalistic relationship between state donor and individual recipient. Patient expectations were a low or nonexistent priority. The National Health Service Act 1946, which led to the establishment of the NHS in 1948, had, however, encapsulated doctors' clinical freedom in their right to prescribe and refer, that is, to spend the NHS budget, in the interest of their patients, as they saw necessary. The size and complexity of the NHS has led to an extensive bureaucratic structure, which includes relevant Acts of Parliament, the decisions of boards, standing financial instructions, health and safety regulations, codes of practice and human resources policies. The NHS is constantly subject to change as the policy context changes, as do the resources and materials received. Top-down initiatives designed to promote changes in clinical activity – such as national service frameworks or the public health outcomes framework – introduce monitoring systems that may be viewed as signs of a lack of trust, thus eroding commitment to the NHS itself and often resulting in resistance to change.

Organizations also exist in relationship with others

Organizational boundaries may be clear or blurred – the provision of care by the NHS and social care services and the boundaries between health and social care are not always clear-cut, as evidenced by the frequent debate about whether the provision of a 'bathing service' is a social care or healthcare service. The NHS, together with social care, is the largest organizational enterprise in the UK and consists of many different types of smaller component organizations, each having to work together. They, in turn, are made up of smaller organizational departments and units, which must also work together if people are to have coherent services. It is at the interface of these organizational boundaries that problems and inefficiencies often occur. For example, an older person finds that they are not able to cope at home following treatment in hospital and may need residential care in the longer term. The consultant makes a referral to social care services when the patient has completed their treatment. The adult social services department of the local authority gives the referral a low priority because the case is complex, there are more urgent cases, and the patient is 'safe in hospital'. The consultant believes that institutionalization and the possibility of a hospital-acquired infection mean that the patient is not at all safe and makes their views plain. The local authority believes the NHS is trying to shift responsibility, and cost, to social services, and that seamless care is being compromised. Part of this clash is due to the organizational 'culture' in which professionals such as doctors and social workers work. However, the distinction between health and social care is becoming increasingly blurred.

Organizational ways of working are shaped by the shared attitudes, behaviours and values of those who work in them

In the NHS, the values of working together for patients – compassion, respect and dignity, commitment to quality of care, improving lives and the belief that 'everyone counts' – are enshrined in the NHS Constitution (DH, 2013). These values form the basis of **organizational culture**. Organizational culture includes everything from the visible structures and processes to more deeply held values that underpin observed behaviour – captured succinctly by Deal and Kennedy (2000) as the 'way things are done around here'.

Trice and Beyer (1992) suggest that culture is manifested in and through the symbols of organizations. 'High-profile symbols' such as logos, mission statements and annual reports are more obvious. 'Low-profile symbols', like practices, communications, physical attributes, such as the way offices are organized, and common languages, are less visible (Table 10.3).

> **?** Consider Table 10.3 and consider how symbols contribute to, communicate and shape the overall representation of an organization you are familiar with.

Table 10.3 Categories of low-profile symbols in organizations

Categories	Examples
Practices: defined as the rites, rituals and ceremonies	Tea/coffee-making practices, annual office party/office outings, doctor's ward hospital round, director's visit to a regional office, long-service and annual award ceremonies
Communications: the stories, myths and symbols	Stories that are repeated by members of the organization/department/work group and influence colleagues' behaviour
Physical forms: office layout, dress code	Physical arrangement and layout of offices, furniture, art works, accepted dress code and so on
Common language	Jargon used within an organization, which provides some of its identity and affects how and in what way people respond to their work

Source: Adapted from Trice and Beyer, 1992

Handy (1993, 1995) proposed that culture was a product of the shared rules of behaviour in organizations and identified four distinct types of culture: power (or club), task, person and role cultures based on four Greek gods (see Table 10.4).

Table 10.4 Analysis of organizational culture

Type of culture	Characteristics	Health services
Person culture: Dionysus	Professionals who thrive on autonomy and personal decision-making. Their organizations exist to serve their needs and are flexible. A person culture puts individuals and their interests first and sees the organization as a means to an end. Represented as a constellation of loosely clustered stars. A consulting partnership and many virtual organizations are typical of this type of culture	GPs and other doctors and practitioners who have developed a degree of clinical autonomy
Role culture: Apollo	An organization based on rules and rule-following with defined and limited degrees of enterprise and discretion. Staff and job functions are clearly defined. Formalized communication, systems and procedures and clearly delegated authorities within a defined structure. Certainty, stability and regulation are important organizational values. Illustrated as a building supported by columns and beams, representing specific roles in keeping up the building	NHS attempts to define roles, for example Knowledge and Skills Framework, Agenda for Change

Type of culture	Characteristics	Health services
Club or power culture: Zeus	An organization based on a single autocratic person who makes all the rules (which may be varied at any time) and who is intolerant of disloyalty. The organization is likened to a club, enabling the decisions of those at the centre to be undertaken. Communication is between people as individuals rather than more formal communication. A charismatic figure who characterizes the culture is important. A high level of person/organization match is key, with a family feel to the organization	Most frequently found in some hospital consultants running clinical 'firms' or departments
Task culture: Athena	A team whose members acquire recognition through expertise and skill rather than grade. Tends to focus exclusively on the task in hand and favour collective decision-making. Likened to a net in which groups are put together and assembled in different ways depending on what needs to be done. The intersection of the nets represents the place where power and influence lie. Competent people who enjoy new challenges and are stimulated by joining different teams for different purposes often prefer a task culture	Research departments, A&E departments and other specialist units where there are few status differences among staff. However, being essentially fluid, they are often managed by Zeus people

Source: Based on Handy, 1995

Handy declares that no organization consists of a single culture, but within a smaller unit, there will be a more or less consensual culture, for example regarding the degree of individual autonomy. When a change in values is required, resistance to that change is very likely. More recently, Schein (2010) identifies three levels of culture, illustrated in Table 10.5.

Table 10.5 **Levels of organizational culture**

Level of organizational culture	Characteristics
Artefacts	Tangible, easily seen and manifested by products, language, technology, clothing, myths and stories, published values, rituals and ceremonies and the physical environment. Surface level of organizational culture
Espoused beliefs and values	Include goals, norms, beliefs, shared assumptions and values. Usually developed from the beliefs and values of leaders and founders of the organization
Basic underlying assumptions	Unconscious, taken-for-granted assumptions that are shared with others. Any challenge to these assumptions will result in anxiety and defensiveness, which may explain why attempts at change fail. Base level of organizational culture

Source: Adapted from Schein, 2010

Organizational culture can have a negative as well as positive impact on the provision of care, as demonstrated by the culture at Mid Staffordshire NHS Foundation Trust. The report of the public inquiry chaired by Robert Francis QC into the role of the commissioning, supervisory and regulatory bodies in the monitoring of Mid Staffordshire NHS Foundation Trust was published in 2013. The key findings were:

> a culture focused on doing the system's business – not that of the patients [and an] institutional culture which ascribed more weight to positive information about the service than to information capable of implying cause for concern … the extent of the failure of the system shown in this report suggests that a fundamental culture change is needed. (Francis, 2013, p. 5)

In a large-scale survey of the NHS, Dixon Woods et al. (2013) conclude that a key priority is attention to systems, cultures and behaviours and identify the following strategies for senior leaders to create a positive culture:

1. Continually reinforce an inspiring vision of the work of their organizations

2. Promote staff health and wellbeing

3. Listen to staff and encourage them to be involved in decision-making, problem-solving and innovation at all levels

4. Provide staff with helpful feedback on how they are doing and celebrate good performance

5. Take effective, supportive action to address system problems and other challenges when improvement is needed

6. Develop and model excellent teamwork

7. Make sure that staff feel safe, supported, respected and valued at work.

connections   Chapter 9 discusses the implications of the Francis Report in relation to changing views on welfare. Chapter 12 discusses the ethical implications in relation to expectations of care by patients and professional colleagues.

The NHS includes many different work cultures at different organizational levels that regularly test the decision-making structures of the NHS. There have been other more recent tests:

- outsourcing or contracting out services

- developing partnerships with other organizations that have an interest in, or influence over, people's health

- the move to engage patients and the public in decisions about their own healthcare and health services in general.

Many trusts have taken decisions to outsource cleaning, catering, portering, laundry and security services. It could be argued that the use of agency nurses and other professionals also constitutes a form of outsourcing.

Outsourced workers are not NHS employees and are managed by the company employing them. Their loyalty is to their employer rather than to the organization in which they are deployed, and team working among them is dependent on the calibre of leadership available in the outsourced, as well as the 'host', company. This can present a further challenge to the main organization that has to 'manage' these workers through non-employed managers and by written contracts covering their precise duties. It also presents a challenge to developing an organizational culture, as there can be many subcultures with different values, norms and practices within one organization.

Working across organizations

Delivering services through **partnerships** between health, social care and other organizations has developed from an operational necessity (coordinating the work of health and social care professionals around the care of individual clients and patients) to a strategic goal for the organizations involved. Early experience of this way of working took the form of joint planning activities among health and local authorities providing services to the same communities. The professional, political and practical benefits of closer working led to pooled budgets, joint service management arrangements, and the more formal exercise of partner bodies' responsibilities and new organizational forms, for example health and wellbeing boards, local strategic partnerships and local drug and alcohol action teams, which include health services, local authorities, education and police services and voluntary organizations. Voluntary sector organizations, including charities, are now actively engaged in providing mainstream and specialist services, and are being commissioned by clinical commissioning groups (CCGs) using public funds. Independent for-profit organizations commissioned in the same way increase plurality in service provision. Forming effective partnerships between these agencies is not easy. Differences in approach, belief, priorities and governance obstruct the necessary commitment at all levels that partners need in order to make their partnership work for the people they serve.

? What cultural challenges to the NHS are posed by initiatives for patient and public involvement?

Perhaps the most recent cultural change in healthcare and health service provision has emerged from the policy to engage patients and the public in decisions about healthcare and health services. The policy has twin goals: to make people take more responsibility for their own wellbeing by helping them engage actively in decisions about their own healthcare; and to make health services more relevant to people who need them by involving patients and the public in designing and monitoring these services. Following the Francis Report (2013) and the Keogh Review (2013), there has been an even greater focus on putting patients first.

Managing healthcare services

For many years, health and social services were 'administered' rather than managed, with centrally devised policies carried out by publicly accountable administrators. The search for a more rational and effective way to deliver health services saw service planning emerge as a serious discipline. The first reorganization of the NHS in 1976 was based on the principle of consensus management and a new population-based system of funding for health services. In 1984, following the Griffiths Report in 1983, general managers were appointed to various levels in the health services with the expectation that they would 'manage' the semi-autonomous professional disciplines and services that constitute the NHS. Consensus management – the principle that all management decisions should be implemented only after an agreement between all stakeholders – was at an end. The years that followed saw several structural changes, not least that which created the now familiar 'super-discipline' of 'commissioning', as distinct from providing, services. But the development underpinning all these structural changes has been focused on leadership and the creation of conditions in which individuals and teams can do their best work. The most difficult challenge large organizations like the health service face is how to use their scale and strength effectively, while remaining sufficiently flexible to adapt to new circumstances. As Moss Kanter (1989) put it in her guide to successful change management: How do you teach the giant to dance?

Working in groups and teams

The organization of health services has tended to devolve into smaller and more compact groupings, for example clinical care groups, divisions and disease-specific teams, for example cancer networks and infection control teams. Teamwork is a significant factor in healthcare delivery and **team-building** an essential aspect of organizational development. Two important things flow from this; first, smaller units are often more flexible and, second, this approach requires many more 'leaders', or workers with leadership skills, at every level of the health services.

The words 'group' and 'team' are often used interchangeably. A group can be described as any collection of people defined by a common purpose: located together, classified together or sharing beliefs. In an organizational context, however, a team may be defined as a group of workers selected by an organization for a defined purpose. Teams exist in many different forms, as can be seen in Table 10.6.

Table 10.6 **A classification of teams**

Types of team	Examples
Groups reporting to the same supervisor	Departmental teams, management teams
Groups of people with common aims	Research teams
Temporary groups for specific tasks	Project teams for introducing new services
Groups of people with interdependencies that cross organizational boundaries	Community nursing teams
Groups with no formal links but members cannot accomplish tasks as individuals	Teams of experts problem-solving or 'firefighting', project teams

Difficulties may arise when team members are drawn from quite disparate disciplines. An example is health promotion teams, which might include schoolteachers, local authority staff, psychologists, nutritionists, health promotion workers, trade union representatives, shopkeepers and parents.

? What is needed to turn such a group into a team?

Team membership is different from being an employee in a large organization. Large organizations ascribe roles or job functions to each position in the hierarchy and the role is performed irrespective of who the role occupant happens to be. It is easy to feel like a cog in a wheel and the role can become mechanistic and impersonal. This can result in a weakened sense of personal responsibility for work performance and a subsequent loss of personal satisfaction from employment.

Teams are more flexible and provide support to all team members to achieve agreed goals and outcomes. Achieving these goals or outcomes requires collaboration and coordination of activities among the team's members. This, in turn, requires team members to have regular and frequent interactions with each other. This interaction builds a team identity, which is distinct from members' individual identities. Part of the team leader's task is to lessen the rigidity with which each team member regards their role, without being accused of exploitation. Tuckman (1965) observed that teams go through observable stages of development: forming, storming, norming and performing. Tuckman and Jensen (1977) added a fifth stage they called 'adjourning', to reflect the process that teams go through when they complete their tasks:

- *Forming:* interactions are polite and guarded

- *Storming:* interactions may test differences between group members. Conflicts may emerge as members may be committed to their own ways of doing things

- *Norming:* groups may get organized, confronting and resolving issues, focusing on the task instead of the group and establishing systems and procedures

- *Performing:* groups become more supportive and communicative, rely on each other more readily and combine in joint problem-solving rather than mutual blaming when problems are encountered. The norming and performing stages of groups may be dependent on leaders and their facilitation skills

- *Adjourning:* having a formalized ending and reviewing 'how we're doing' is essential for ongoing team development. For teams that come together for a single project, adjourning (sometimes referred to as 'mourning') allows a sense of closure and accomplishment.

Although it is assumed that any team will progress through all five stages, this is not always so. Changes in team composition or strong professional or political agendas may inhibit team development and thus effectiveness. The *Journal of Interprofessional Care* regularly publishes papers on interprofessional teams, where professionals are clear about their own individual roles, but perceive that their roles are not recognized or understood by other members of the team, for example Sidani and Fox (2014).

Leadership

?   Are all managers leaders?

Leading and managing are different (Taylor, 2013). Managing involves activities such as planning, organizing and controlling work. Leading is more focused on facilitating change and creating vision. While 'leaders do not have to be managers, many managers are often required to display leadership capability' (Taylor, 2013, p. 5). While management may be regarded as having responsibility for organizational structure, strategy and systems – the hard Ss as Watson (1983) identified them – leaders tend to work with people and are responsible for staff, skills, style (culture) and shared goals – the so-called soft Ss.

?   If the leader's prime function is to create followers, what power do they have?

The ability to punish or reward, also known as 'resource power', will not necessarily produce willing followers. 'Referent power', where would-be followers admire the leader's characteristics and wish to copy them, is more effective (French and Raven, 1968). In the professional world of health services, referent power is greatly enhanced by expertise or 'expert power'.

thinking about Consider people you know whom you perceive to be leaders. What personal qualities do they possess? Are they able to command respect from a wide range of different people? Why do you trust them? Why do you, or would you, follow them?

The requirement for a leader to be a charismatic superman or superwoman was one of the mythologies debunked in a survey of 2,000 NHS managers (Alimo-Metcalfe and Alban-Metcalfe, 2000). The most important leadership characteristic to emerge from this study was concern for others, followed by the ability to communicate and inspire. Emotional intelligence has also been cited as key to being an outstanding (as opposed to average) leader (Taylor, 2013). Traditionally, leaders were viewed as being 'born' with the required skills, or able to adapt their leadership style to suit the situation. Research (Hosking, 1997; Wenger and Snyder, 2000) views leadership as a dynamic social process where there is either a leader and followers (transformational leadership), or where people play different roles at different times (distributed leadership). Increasingly, transformational approaches to leadership have been criticized for too great a reliance on the notion of a heroic leader, who seeks to create the vision and gains followership, in favour of the idea that leaders exist at every level.

? What do you think will be the key challenges for leadership in healthcare?

Hartley and Benington (2010) identified some key challenges for 'leaders' or 'leadership' within the healthcare context. These include:

- changes in population demographics and disease profiles
- change in patterns of illness and financial constraints
- increased and new expectations from patients, carers and communities
- new technologies and techniques in healthcare requiring new ways of working.

As health and social care delivery has grown more complex, and expectations have increased, the requirements of leaders have had to, and will need to continue to, change. The director, general manager or chief executive must lead clinical, professional and support staff and cannot rely on shared professional experience and qualifications for credibility and authority. The requirements to listen, take advice, explain, convince and, wherever possible, secure agreement are common to all situations. Inevitably, some decisions will trigger opposition among one or more of the interested staff groups, and securing support, or acquiescence, will demand a flexible and appropriate approach. Neither a purely task nor people orientation alone is adequate to resolve the leadership complexities presented in the modern NHS. Contemporaneous expectations of leadership in the NHS have shifted in the wake of reports such as the Francis Report and the Keogh Review. Storey and Holti (2013) suggest three categories that they argue should form the basis for leadership in the NHS. Table 10.7 summarizes these and comments briefly on what will be required from leaders.

Table 10.7 **Categories that should form the basis for leadership in the NHS**

Categories	Comments
Provide and justify a clear sense of purpose and contribution	Requires a balanced attention to a clear focus on the needs of service users, efficiency, compassion. Patient safety and patient experience at the heart of service provision and decision-making
Motivate teams and individuals to work effectively	Requires clarity in setting challenging and clear goals, building team commitment and a positive emotional climate, and encouraging high staff involvement and engagement. Provision and operation of organizations with 'meaningful design' and underpinning human resource systems. Performance focus is on management and improvement, and listening and responding to staff
Focus on improving system performance	Encouraging a service improvement culture, addressing system problems and encouraging innovation. Foster a climate that encourages inquiry, modelling learning and new behaviours and ways of working, including humility and the self-doubt appropriate to genuine inquiry

Source: Adapted from Storey and Holti, 2013

These categories form the basis for the development of the healthcare leadership model (HLM) recently launched by the NHS Leadership Academy (2013). The HLM has nine dimensions, as shown in Figure 10.3. At the core of the HLM is distributed leadership, where leadership is viewed as being the responsibility of everyone at all levels in (and parts of) the organization. The type of

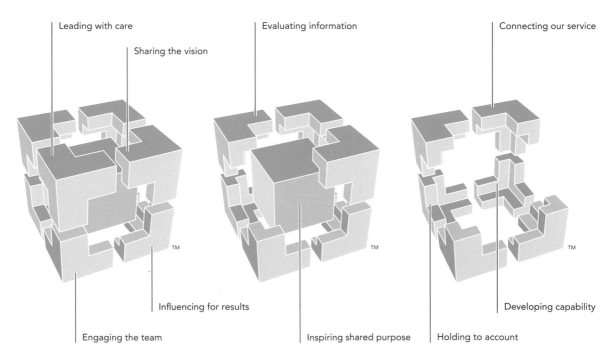

Figure 10.3 **The healthcare leadership model**
Source: NHS Leadership Academy, 2013

job someone has, the needs of the people they work with, and their role within the organization will affect which dimensions are the most important for them to use and develop, and, as such, the framework builds on the challenges faced by leaders at every level within health and healthcare organizations.

Managing change

Effecting change within any organization has been likened to managing a contest between opposing and resisting forces – the so-called force field approach (Lewin, 1951). Gleicher et al. (1987) proposed an approach known as the 'change equation': $A + B + C > D$, where

- 'A' stands for dissatisfaction with the present situation. If employees are comfortable in an inefficient situation, education is required to demonstrate its disadvantages

- 'B' represents a shared vision of a better future or way of working. This can raise morale and increase motivation and thus commitment for change

- 'C' is an acceptable first step or the least threatening way of initiating change

- 'D' is the cost to the individual or group of making the change.

Good communication is a vital underpinning of this equation. Leadership that attends to all four components of this equation is most likely to bring about the desired change. Where successful, the system will suffer minimal disruption and is likely to self-heal any damage that occurs. This commonsense formula is often forgotten in many organizations where change is announced from the top and implemented with minimal, if any, consultation. Even when the situation is urgent, for example the changes in practice concerning the retention of human organs and tissue demanded by the government and public, attention to the change equation can facilitate positive development.

Part 2 Theoretical and research approaches

example 10.3

Examples of health management research

- Embedding change in routine practice. The 'plan do study act' cycles introduced by the Modernisation Agency, then the Institute of Health Improvement, are based on cycles of improvement and lean theory (Fillingham, 2008). The use of lean thinking in the NHS in order to improve current processes and identify areas for improvement is an ongoing area of interest for the Institute of Health Improvement (superseded by NHS Improving Quality) as the driving force for improvement across the NHS in England

- What is needed to engage healthcare professionals in leadership; see, for example, the medical leadership project (www.nets.nihr.ac.uk/projects/hsdr/081808236)

- The impact of incentives in healthcare systems on the behaviour of providers and consumers of care, for example the incentives given by costing systems within organizations that produce healthcare, the impact of payment systems on market development, and the effect of choice and competition on healthcare outcomes; see, for example, the work of Imperial College Business School (wwwf.imperial.ac.uk/business-school/research/health-management)
- Enhancing performance, for example the role of boards (Chambers et al., 2013)

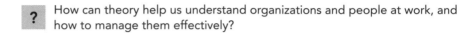 **?**   How can theory help us understand organizations and people at work, and how to manage them effectively?

Theories about the way people and organizations behave have developed over more than 100 years and reflect changing social attitudes and ideas about manufacture and service. They offer descriptions and analyses of the way employees and organizations behave in different sets of circumstances, which can help people understand what they observe around them when they are at work. There is no one 'right' theory of organization or behaviour: some were products of their age, all have proponents and critics. Attention to theory can, however, help students, practitioners and managers understand, and therefore influence, the people and organizations around them.

For example, it is obvious that not all organizations are alike and it often seems that the similarities between them are outweighed by their considerable differences. General practices and hospitals both employ clinical and support staff and deliver healthcare but are profoundly dissimilar in scale and culture. Such disparities generate distinctive variations in structure and rules, ways of working, and even value systems, which affect efficiency and people's experiences of their work. There is no one 'right' way to manage organizations: much depends on a combination of factors including the organization's history, size and function.

This part identifies the types of management and organization theory that have developed in recent times, and indicates where each might be of value to people concerned with healthcare organizations.

Scientific management

The progenitors of modern management theory were Taylor (1856–1915) in the US and Fayol (1841–1925) in France. Taylor, whose operational sphere was a steel works, prescribed precise methods and practices for his manual workers and rewarded them with pay commensurate with their compliance and output. He discounted the ability of his workers and managers to identify and use the most efficient methods for any particular task. Today, Taylor's 'scientific management' has its counterpart in many clinical procedures such as the avoidance of contamination in barrier nursing. These prescribed procedures are now carried out without any additional monetary reward but as part of accepted professional practice. Moreover, improvement in such practices can come about from research findings, often conducted by health professionals themselves. While the rather remote and directive nature of Taylor's approach is no longer deemed appropriate, its essential methodology is still reflected in professional practice informed by scientific evidence.

Fayol, also an engineer, wrote about the formal structure of organizations, with the emphasis on planning, technical requirements and the principles of management with its concomitant assumptions of logical and rational behaviour. His five elements of management – to forecast and plan, organize, command, coordinate and control – clearly stem from an era when autocracy was the predominant and accepted approach to management. Fayol, like his contemporary Weber, developed a model of the organization as a well-designed and well-run machine, which would always respond to the levers of control, provided they were correctly applied, in other words, 'good management'.

> **?** Would the levers of scientific management help today's managers?

The initial but transient enthusiasm for Taylor's ideas occurred at the time when America was attempting to re-establish her industrial base and output following the Civil War. Pure Taylorism foundered because of its rigidity and a flawed assumption of workers' rationality. However, his ideas have endured for over 100 years in efficiency surveys, work study and method study, which survive in various forms either in their own right (e.g. clinical pathway reviews) or in combination with other review methods (e.g. business process re-engineering).

Bureaucracy and organizations

The notion of an organization based on rules is popularly attributed to Weber (1864–1920), who used the term **bureaucracy** to label the phenomenon, and regarded the term as synonymous with efficiency (rather than the mildly abusive connotation of today). Although Weber (1964) did not define the term, he described the following characteristics of a bureaucracy: a hierarchy of authority, a system of rules and thus impersonality (each individual had to follow the rules rather than personal preference), and many specialized roles. One can readily recognize some of these characteristics in the larger parts of the health services, and indeed size appears to be positively correlated with bureaucratic characteristics, namely the role culture (Handy, 1995).

There have been many criticisms of bureaucracy as an organizational form, not least its potential to stifle initiative (which Weber regarded as a positive function) and restrict personal growth and development. In a bureaucracy, people are rewarded for following rules rather than attaining goals, and so the rules and associated processes can become ends in themselves. The nature of health and social care, however, demands a clear framework in which practitioners work (licensing, regulation, accreditation), and requires those same professionals to exercise clinical discretion. An accommodation is required between, for example, a list of drugs and procedures that may be prescribed under NHS arrangements, and the need to provide patients with the best care available. Rules generally allow organizations to exercise control at long range, whereas at close range there is usually someone who has been vested with sufficient discretion to give or amend a ruling.

? To what extent is the NHS a bureaucratic organization?

The human relations approach to understanding people and organizations

The mid-1920s saw the next major development in management theory – the human relations approach, frequently associated with Mayo, who was a researcher at the Graduate Business School at Harvard University. The significant work discussed below was undertaken by his colleagues Roethlisberger and Dixon (1943).

Unlike scientific management, which regarded workers as robotic servants, the human relations school discovered that workers responded to their working conditions, to leadership, group dynamics, managerial behaviour and, above all, to recognition. Where Taylorism had dehumanized workers, the human relations approach sought to humanize work organizations, sometimes to the detriment of economic efficiency. The 'discovery' of this seemingly obvious phenomenon occurred during the famous Hawthorne experiments conducted from the mid-1920s in the Western Electric Company in America.

example 10.4

The Hawthorne experiments

The Hawthorne experiments consisted of several phases. In the first phase, six women were segregated in a 'test' room and told to work normally on their assembly of relay switch gear. Over a period of two years, the physical conditions, lighting, ventilation and temperature control were changed, as were their pay arrangements, incentives, benefits, work breaks and so on. However adverse their conditions became, their productivity rose with each change of the conditions – even when all privileges were temporarily removed.

These workers were made aware that they were taking part in an experiment. Although the methodology employed was flawed, the explanation for this unanticipated finding was that the *recognition* afforded to the workers was the source of their motivation. This phenomenon became known as the 'Hawthorne effect'.

Although of enormous significance, these experiments were poorly conducted, badly flawed and subject to much criticism. The major lesson they offer, however, is the importance of managerial behaviour and the informal organizations that arise among workers trying to do good work – something Weberian bureaucracy ignores and, indeed, seeks to suppress. Mullins (2013) believes that these experiments, with all their faults, were the first approach to organization and management with an appreciation of industrial sociology.

Whereas Taylor sought to design systems of work without regard to the needs of people, the human relations approach took an opposite direction, placing the needs of people above the requirements of the organization. Both are now regarded as inadequate management models. Attaining a workable balance between these two requirements appears to be a major and necessary skill of the manager and much later research on shift working demonstrated and highlighted this fact.

Behavioural theory

Research in the 1940s in the University of Michigan and in the 1950s in Ohio State University investigated management and leadership styles. Managers were categorized as 'job centred' or 'employee centred', which were broadly aligned to the Taylorist and human relations approaches respectively. Many thought that these orientations were personality traits and reflected the way leaders regarded their subordinates and the assumptions they made about subordinates' attitude to work.

This was developed into a popular theory by McGregor (1987), which described theory X and theory Y leaders. Theory X leaders believed that their subordinates disliked work and responsibility and would avoid it if they could. These leaders would therefore become highly directional towards their staff, emphasizing task accomplishment above all else. Theory Y leaders held the opposite view and took an approach that gave greater weight to engaging with employees and their needs and preferences at work. It was clear that neither extreme was necessarily helpful and that leader behaviour, if it were to be effective, had to be flexible and appropriate for different situations. Indeed, the Ohio studies were able to demonstrate that these two characteristics were independent variables and that the most effective leaders, rather than having a fixed leadership style, selected the most appropriate style and behaviour for each situation.

Situation theory

Situation theory grew from the recognition that no one management or leadership style could serve all situations and that flexibility was required. Tannenbaum and Schmidt (1973) described a matrix that identified several factors that might influence the leadership approach in a given situation:

- factors in the manager, for example their experience, confidence, expertise

- factors in their subordinates, for example maturity and training, willingness and ability to take decisions

- factors in the situation, for example degree of urgency, nature of the task to be undertaken.

In highly complex organizations such as the NHS, the decision of direction (that is, 'what is to be done') is taken at the top of the hierarchy and imposed on the organization beneath. How that direction is to be achieved is frequently left to local leaders, and it is here that situation theory can be applied.

Contingency theory

Contingency theory provides a further development of situation theory. Extensive research by Fiedler (1967) led him to postulate that the amount of *influence* a leader possesses should determine leadership approach. Where this influence was relatively moderate, for example where a leader's technical expertise was similar to or less developed than that of subordinates, the preferred approach needed to be employee centred. Where a leader's influence was either weak or strong, a task orientation could be adopted. Fiedler's theory has been contested as far too simplistic an approach and contradicted by evidence from other sources. Nevertheless, it is interesting to note that in the complex world of health and social care, leaders may have only moderate influence in what are highly technical situations. The title, salary and budget that may go with a leadership position do not necessarily bring legitimate and ultimate authority. The goals of health and social care organizations are more often achieved collaboratively, contingent on situational factors.

> **thinking about** Does a lack of specialist expertise limit a person's ability to manage?

Motivation theories

League tables and reports of regulators' and individuals' experiences tell us that health and social care institutions do not all perform to the same standard. Many types of factors may be at work (see the PESTLE analysis above), and the issues are complex, but staff motivation, and therefore individual performance, is a significant factor in organizational performance. Motivation is a complex concept, but put simply it refers to 'the will to work', particularly when unsupervised. Quality, persistence, endurance, energy, patience and many other attributes are involved.

The motivation to work, and its link with job satisfaction, is clearly a large and important aspect of management theory. Motivation theories may be divided into two groups: content and process theories.

Content theories

Content theories postulate that all humans are driven by a similar set of needs. Good organization and management ensure that these needs are satisfied at work and can increase the motivation of workers. But to what extent is this really true? The most familiar content theorist is Maslow (1943), who suggested that there is a hierarchy of people's needs: they will first be motivated to satisfy essential physiological needs and then move on to psychological needs, via security, social and self-esteem needs. When one need is satisfied, the next higher level need becomes the motivation for action on their part.

> **thinking about** Consider the last job you enjoyed. What was the basis for your satisfaction – pay, status, autonomy, or its purpose and significance?

The salience of each need varies with the individual. Some workers value job security far more than a risky challenge. Traditionally, public sector workers have been thought to fall into this category, while others, such as entrepreneurs, are thought to do their best work in conditions of high risk. However, risk is understood differently by different people and in different situations and contexts. The dot-com entrepreneur might regard the public sector worker's daily contact with clients and patients as extremely risky, while the public sector worker might value the autonomy of the self-employed entrepreneur. Moreover, it is by no means certain that an individual will seek to satisfy all such needs in a work context. Hobbies, sports, social interests and competitions may provide the opportunity for self-actualization, which Maslow describes as the highest need of all. For self-actualization to occur at work, appropriately challenging jobs must be available during times of full employment, together with the recognition that accompanies excellent performance. Maslow's hierarchy was developed not in a management but in a clinical context and has been applied by enthusiastic management theorists (Fincham and Rhodes, 2005); however, it has not enjoyed much empirical support.

Alderfer (1972) grouped individuals' basic needs into:

- existence, for example job security, pay

- relatedness, for example social interaction

- growth, for example professional development.

These are not necessarily hierarchical needs; rather a continuum along which one might travel in either direction depending on circumstance and stage of career development. This theory might explain the importance of training and career development and the benefits they might bring in the retention and motivation of health service workers. However, Alderfer also believed that workers who could not satisfy their growth needs would settle for taking larger 'helpings' of existence and relatedness satisfaction. The worker's effort–reward 'psychological' contract with the employer would favour the worker rather than the organization, for example workers would satisfy more of their social needs at work, perhaps at the expense of efficiency. This might present a particular challenge for managers.

Herzberg (1966) thought that not all needs were motivating, because his definition of motivation included the additional effort and energy contributed by the worker, beyond the minimum normally required by the organization. He distinguished between hygiene factors that relate to the context of work and motivators that relate to work content:

- *Hygiene factors* include supervision, salary, the work environment, company policy and even relationships with colleagues

- *Motivators* include achievement, recognition for achievement, responsibility, interesting/meaningful work and an opportunity for career development and advancement.

This theory appeals to health and social care workers where, because of the high number of professionals employed, there is considerable scope for exercising professional judgement, and recognition can come from several sources, for example patients, their relatives, colleagues and managers. However, Herzberg's methodology has been criticized, as have the conclusions he has drawn from his oft-repeated research projects. Not all people are the same and ultimately his theory is limited by the same constraints that bind all the content theorists, namely the impossibility of devising a universal formula to motivate all staff.

Process theories

Process theories are based more on the precise value of the reward to the individual in exchange for particular behaviour. Adam's equity theory (1965) considers the output required for the input given: Is it worth it? What's in it for me? This is linked with social comparison: What is the effort–reward contract for other similar workers, or workers in my social comparison group? Inequitable treatment of workers can cause dissatisfaction and low morale and ultimately low output. Workers whose professional ethos will not permit a lowering of standards of their work may nevertheless lower their work rate, for example see fewer patients, to register their displeasure.

Expectancy theory (Vroom, 1964; Porter and Lawler, 1968) takes this process one step further by asking three questions:

1. If I work harder, what is the chance of my being able to achieve the standard of performance required? If there are problems with personal confidence, experience, training, or availability of equipment, which might mean that working harder will not achieve the right standard, I may decide against the extra effort.

2. If I can surmount these hurdles, what is the likelihood of my receiving my reward, intrinsic and/or extrinsic, recognition and/or treasure?

3. Will I value the reward offered?

Process theories are about cognition, how people experience and perceive their working environment and respond to it. Indeed, Handy (1993) has described it as a motivation 'calculus' – which is the person's needs, what a person is expected to accomplish and the effort needed to achieve the required work performance. These processes depend in part on the confidence each worker has in their leader's ability to deliver a working environment that allows them to do their best work.

According to Herzberg (1966), motivation comes from the satisfaction of a person's intrinsic needs, not payment. Once again, the leader is crucial in providing a supportive environment that enables self-development. Locke and Latham (2013) introduced the idea of goal-setting theory in motivating performance. In aiming to achieve goals, people look at the likelihood of achieving them. If they think their current behaviour will not allow them to achieve their goals, they will either modify their behaviour or choose different goals. Setting challenging but achievable goals that are clearly understood and have specific performance targets, and the provision of timely and regular feedback, are central. This enables employees to see clearly how their own behaviour can be changed or modified to improve performance. In considering content and process theories of motivation, effective management and leadership are key, particularly when so many health services employees are professionals and expect to be treated as such.

---

example 10.5

Job design

Where Taylor sought to impose rigidity of operation and to inhibit each worker's scope for innovation, current approaches involve the introduction of variety, autonomy and task defragmentation. A variety of tasks not only helps reduce monotony at work, but calls on a wide repertoire of skills and experience. Autonomy increases personal control, and responsibility for a complete task serves to enhance meaningfulness and satisfaction.

The trend to develop jobs in this way depends on three moderators (Hackman and Oldham, 1980):

1. The ability and skill of the worker, related to training, qualification and experience
2. The strength of the employee's growth needs (at work) – their 'comfort zone' on Maslow's hierarchy or Alderfer's continuum
3. The employee's satisfaction with the context of the work – the psychological contract, which may include issues such as pay and conditions, organizational policy and rules, ethics and intrinsic rewards such

as recognition. This third factor appears to relate as much to the process theories of motivation as to Herzberg's hygiene factors.

Horizontal job loading, where all tasks are of a roughly similar level of skill and responsibility, can increase variety, but can also increase stress if imposed at an unreasonable level for a particular individual. Higher grading and extrinsic rewards usually accompany vertical job loading, where greater responsibility for the task, such as planning, financial control and management of others, is given.

One further important finding by Katz (1978, cited by Schein, 1988) was that for those workers remaining in the same job for over 15–20 years, contextual factors such as pay and benefits, co-worker relations and compatibility with supervisors were of equal importance. Contextual factors therefore became relatively more important as job longevity increased. When this occurs, job redesign may be less motivating than better pay or working conditions. Alternatively, a step change of job function or a change of occupation may reinvigorate some employees.

Systems theory and the sociotechnical system approach

Health and social care services comprise a plethora of systems, each aimed at delivering one or more elements of care – prevention, diagnosis, treatment, rehabilitation or long-term care. Systems theory proposes that the whole is greater than the sum of its parts. This means that each component subsystem acquires a greater significance when it is part of a superordinate system. Indeed, the significance of subsystems depends on their inclusion. Von Bertalanffy (1951), a biologist who first wrote about systems theory, made the connection between biological systems, for example the homeostatic system, and organizational systems.

connections	Chapter 1 describes the basis of homeostasis as a system in balance.

Nadler and Tushman's (1984) congruency model of organizational behaviour examines the relationship between organizational components and the organization and its environment (Figure 10.4). The extent to which they are congruent with each other is an indicator of the likely efficiency of the organization and thus its survival and effectiveness. Put simply, the greater the congruence, the more efficient the organization, given its environmental constraints. Are there sufficient numbers of trained employees? Are they deployed in the most efficient manner? For example, if the government's policy is to encourage patient choice regarding home births, will there be enough appropriately trained midwives, together with appropriate back-up facilities in time to meet the introduction of the policy?

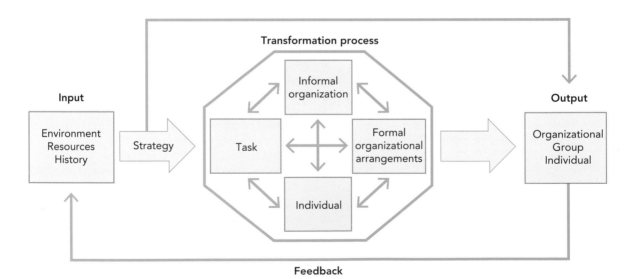

Figure 10.4 A congruency model of organizational behaviour

Source: Adapted from Nadler and Tushman, 1984

Nadler and Tushman (1984) suggest that four organizational components need to be optimized in order to achieve effective operations:

1. The formal organizational structure: relationships and responsibilities (job descriptions)

2. The tasks to be performed: caring and curing, educating and researching

3. The individual employees: sufficient, trained, qualified, experienced and competent

4. The informal structure: the way the organization works, its behavioural norms and 'culture'.

The model specifically does not include groups or technology, both of which can have an important bearing on organizational efficiency. But neither does it necessarily exclude them.

Changes made to a single element in one part of the system inevitably have repercussions for many other systems and subsystems. For example, efforts in health education, such as smoking cessation or obesity prevention, will result in longer healthier lives and less demand on curative services over the long term. However, there may be additional demands on social care services if people live longer. Changes within the healthcare organization lead to similar complex effects. For example, changes made to increase the autonomy and responsibility of frontline workers may increase anxiety within the organization with regard to budgetary control. On the other hand, withdrawal of financial control to the centre to ensure savings may well lower the morale and motivation of those same frontline workers.

A particular variant of systems theory is the sociotechnical systems approach identified by Trist and Bamforth (1951). Their context was that of coal mining following the introduction of mechanization. The social patterns of work were destroyed by the new technology, leading to a reduction in coal output. The new methods were potentially more efficient but, after investigation, further changes were required to take account of workers' social needs before output could be restored. Although coal mining and healthcare are very different enterprises, workers in both workplaces operate in teams, under stress, using technology that is still developing and continually being replaced. Technology can have a significant impact on the way we work and its introduction constitutes significant change that can extend to the psychological contract being compromised, even though job designations may remain unaltered. Technology can cause deskilling but also lead to reskilling. Not everyone will be able to accept either outcome.

There are, however, occasions when change brings unexpected consequences, or shifts in behaviour or performance arise for no apparent reason. The models described so far do not help in such circumstances: so what might do so?

Chaos (or complexity) theory

This chapter has addressed a number of theories aimed at imposing order on otherwise potentially unstable organizations. The bureaucratic approach seeks to limit discretion and impose rigidity, while the management techniques associated with motivation and leadership appear to be more flexible levers of control. But are these approaches effective in every case? If they were, then once mastered, all organizations would run like well-oiled machines, optimizing effectiveness and efficiency. Clearly, this is not the case. So, what is happening to cause such variations in performance between similar organizations and between different operational periods within the same organization?

Some NHS organizations appear to have greater competence in treating patients than others. Some improve their clinical and financial performance, while others underperform. Many experience variations over time in these and other parameters and appear to go in and out of control inexplicably. According to Tiplady (2003, p. 2):

> Chaos theory is based on the recognition that real world systems never settle down into a steady state ... All systems go through continual patterns of order and disorder, always changing, never repeating. 'Chaos' ... exhibits a kind of stability within instability.

The source of this disorder comes from the complexity within the system, the effects of which are unpredictable. For example, the emergence of HIV/AIDS in the 1980s placed considerable demands on healthcare services and ring-fenced money. New forms of treatment in the 1990s, which meant people were living with the disease (rather than dying from it), required new, more integrated forms of service delivery. Small changes in policy and managerial adjustments can often lead to significant changes over time, and this fact gives us a clue as to the manner in which change might best be achieved within organizations. Tiplady likens the initiation of change to sowing seeds in people's minds, which will bear considerable and unforeseen fruit in the future. He believes that successful change is best seen as an iterative process of small steps, rather than a heavy-handed imposition from above. Whatever the approach, however, outcomes may vary considerably from those predicted. Moreover, while the performance of the organization as a whole may be unpredictable, the same is found to apply within its component parts.

It is clear that from the earliest attempts to identify a workable management hypothesis, managers and researchers alike have seen the necessity to exercise control over workers and organizations in order to achieve planned output. While chaos theory may help us to understand why some targets are missed and others unexpectedly exceeded, there is an unremitting requirement for better management of all types of organization. The following case study on the formulation and implementation of a local obesity strategy will attempt to illustrate some of these points.

case study formulating an obesity strategy

Organization and management skills are vital for the planning and implementation of an obesity strategy. All organization and management activity takes place within a policy context. Local obesity strategies require goals and targets to be set, partnership working to be operational and effective, resources to be available, and monitoring and evaluation to demonstrate its effectiveness. The following case study uses these categories to discuss the development of an obesity strategy.

The policy context for the obesity strategy is positive and proactive. In 2004, the government set a public service agreement **target** to halt the year-on-year rise of obesity in children aged under 11 by 2010, and to reduce obesity across the population as a whole. This target was owned by three different governmental departments: the Department of Health, the Department for Education and Skills, and the Department for Culture, Media and Sport. But in 2007, the 2010 deadline was quietly abandoned and replaced by a deadline of 2020. The National Child Measurement Programme (NCMP), introduced in 2006, led to children in reception class (aged 4–5 years) and year 6 (aged 10–11 years) having their height and weight measured (HSCIC, n.d.). These data are used to inform local planning and delivery of services for children and to allow analysis of trends in growth patterns and obesity. A major report on obesity predicted that, by 2050, 60% of men, 50% of women and 25% of children in the UK will be obese (Foresight, 2007). In 2008, the government published *Healthy Weight, Healthy Lives: A Cross-Government Strategy for England* (Cross-Government Obesity Unit/DH/ DCSF, 2008). Then, in 2011, *Healthy Lives, Healthy People: A Call to Action on Obesity in England* (DH, 2011) highlighted the need for a holistic life course approach to tackling childhood obesity, with partnership working between education, local authorities and the private and voluntary sectors.

A government toolkit for developing local obesity strategies (Swanton, 2008) identifies the following general approach:

1. Understanding the problem in the area, estimating prevalence, identifying priority groups and setting local goals
2. Identifying local leadership and developing a multiagency approach to tackling obesity
3. Choosing interventions to achieve local targets
4. Monitoring and evaluation
5. Building local capabilities in promoting physical activity, good nutrition and the benefits of a healthy weight.

Under the terms of the Health and Social Care Act 2012, upper tier and unitary authorities became responsible for improving the health of their population and for local obesity strategies. Many departments in a local authority, including schools, children's services, housing, transport and planning, have a role to play in such strategies.

A childhood obesity strategy needs to provide a framework that integrates an organization's major goals, policies and actions. A strategy can be cutting edge, offering innovative approaches, but in the public sector it may become permeated by slow, cumbersome and change-resistant personnel and procedures. As we have seen in this chapter, however, all organizations operate in an environment, and a strategy merely attempts to ensure a fit between goals, resources (including staff capacity and capability) and environment.

One goal is the maintenance of an ongoing data set (the NCMP) measuring the local child population's BMI. Other relevant sources of information include data on the incidence, prevalence and duration of breastfeeding and other feeding practices from the birth of a baby to around nine months. Data are also collected on the take-up of school meals. It is recommended (WHO,

2011; NHS Choices, 2013) that children over five should engage in at least 60 minutes of moderate to vigorous physical activity every day. Local authorities will therefore monitor pupil's engagement in physical education (PE) and sport delivered by schools, although the national curriculum for PE was disapplied in 2013 and is no longer statutory.

The key requirements for a target to be agreed are that it:

- should be recognized as valid by all partners
- is based on sound evidence regarding its effectiveness
- is feasible
- can be monitored and evaluated.

Each target developed should be SMART – specific, measurable, achievable, realistic and time limited – or as SMART as possible.

A multiagency approach is critical to tackling obesity. The local area needs to decide the most appropriate arrangements for bringing together all the partners within the delivery chain in order to develop a local strategy and monitor its implementation. This includes ensuring that information, especially regarding good practice, flows up and down the delivery chain. The Children and Young People's Strategic Partnership Board has senior-level representation from key partners, reporting regularly to the council. Most multiagency programmes benefit from having a coordinator – a person who has the 'clout' to bring partners together and drive forward implementation – with all the leadership characteristics identified by Stewart (1995) – vision, values, valour, virtue, visibility, vigour and vigilance. The coordinator provides inspiration as well as the all-important people skills – the ability to communicate, listen and respond appropriately. It is also important that they are aware of team-building processes, and ensure that members have the necessary time and space to form, storm and norm before being called on to perform

(Tuckman, 1965). Instead of trying to impose uniformity and consensus on the group, the coordinator needs to allow conflicting agendas to emerge and be discussed, but also ensure that every partner has some input into the strategy and can therefore 'own' it. Being honest about the limitations of the strategy is also important, so that partners do not develop unrealistic expectations of what the strategy can deliver.

Keeping people's engagement with strategy development is crucial and maintaining the commitment of team members may be difficult. The initial group formulating a strategy is likely to be led by a public health consultant and the planning group will include health professionals. Drawing in education, leisure and other local authority colleagues may be difficult if they see the planning group as a 'doctors and nurses' group. Continuing professional development is not only essential for the delivery of the strategy but also maintains staff commitment. Neither local workforce development strategies nor service specifications within the commissioning process may have identified childhood obesity as an issue. Instead, interested frontline staff would have had to self-nominate to get involved in the childhood obesity strategy. Leadership and direction from senior management can significantly improve this.

In order to be implemented, the strategy will require funding and resources. While some of the resources (e.g. people's expertise, time and energy) are available as part of normal working patterns, other items (e.g. healthy cooking lessons in schools, exercise facilities in parks) require dedicated funding. It is important therefore that funding for the implementation of the strategy is identified and ring-fenced, even if at the outset this is for a limited period.

Through the partnership, it may be possible to map existing services but their attractiveness or suitability to meet the needs of different groups and individuals within the local community may not be known. So, in this example, it was decided to draw out the expected contribution of existing and community-based programmes and services and optimize the opportunities of the NCMP.

Monitoring and evaluation are necessary to demonstrate the effectiveness of a strategy and secure sustainable long-term funding. The BMI measurements for school children provide ongoing data that could be used to assess the effectiveness of the obesity strategy. Specific initiatives include monitoring of uptake, for example the number of children using supervised walk to school and 'cycle to school' schemes will be logged by supervisors. Different partners will also be conducting their own routine audit and monitoring activities that will shed light on the impact of the strategy to reduce obesity. However, one of the challenges of the strategy is to devise a means of collating and combining these diverse forms of monitoring and evaluation in order to provide an overall evaluation. Developing robust data-sharing protocols and mechanisms for implementing and managing

them between local NHS services (particularly midwives and health visitors) and children's services will be a priority. A second challenge is to identify what changes (if any) could be attributed to the strategy, and what changes would have happened anyway, as part of secular shifts and movements, regardless of any additional local input. These challenges pose significant dilemmas that require specialist expertise and funding to address.

The various elements of a successful strategy – a positive policy environment, setting appropriate goals and targets, strong leadership and partnership working, adequate resourcing, and ongoing monitoring and evaluation all need to be in place. Many challenges remain, not least to secure sustainable funding and establish that the strategy is effective, and to ensure sustainability in the context of constant changes to the NHS, but the basic requirements of developing an effective strategy have all been addressed.

Summary

- Theoretical and empirical work can help us understand why organizations and the people that comprise them behave as they do

- An organization's goals, strategies, structure, technology and external environment all relate to each other and this relationship is critical for its performance and effectiveness

- Managers face many challenges in managing internal dynamic processes in an organization, including the role of culture, managing change, decision-making processes, managing work in groups and teams, and power and politics

Questions for further discussion

1. You will find a doctor leading healthcare organizations in the US and many European countries. Why are there so few who do this in the UK?

2. Can members of the public have any real say in decision-making about healthcare and health services?

3. What experience, skills and competences does a manager of a healthcare service need? Are these different from those required to manage another sort of organization?

4. Could a professionally cross-trained (generic) worker such as a children's worker replace many of the current well-differentiated professions? Would this help or hinder the development of a teamwork ethos in healthcare?

Further reading

Buchanan, D. and Huczinsky, A. (2010) *Organisational Behaviour* (7th edn). New York: Prentice Hall.
Multidisciplinary text that enables students to study the behaviour of organizations and the role of management. Explores core concepts and debates in a readable and accessible manner.

Hatch, M.J. (1997) *Organization Theory: Modern, Symbolic and Postmodern Perspectives*. Oxford: Oxford University Press.
Interesting analysis of different perspectives on organizations. Discusses the ways in which organizations can be analysed including as social structures or cultures and looks at key concepts scuh as decision-making, power and change.

Iles, V. (2005) *Really Managing Health Care* (2nd edn). Maidenhead: Open University Press.
Deals with practical issues in healthcare management.

Klein, R. (2010) *The New Politics of the NHS: From Creation to Reinvention* (6th edn). Oxford: Radcliffe Publishing.
Concentrates on those issues that seem to best illuminate the analytic themes and provide the most insight into political processes.

Martin, V. (2003) *Leading Change in Health and Social Care*. Abingdon: Routledge.
Martin, V. and Henderson, E.S. (2010) *Managing in Health and Social Care* (2nd edn). Abingdon: Routledge.
Both texts look at key issues in managing and leading health and social care.

Mullins, L.J. (2013) *Management and Organisational Behaviour* (10th edn). Harlow: Pearson.
Major text dealing with all the management theories and thinking, historic and current. Does not deal specifically with the health service.

Taylor, V. (2013) *Leading for Health and Well-Being*. London: Learning Matters/Sage.
Clearly wrtten exploration of leadership and management theory related to leading for health and wellbeing.

www.leadershipacademy.nhs.uk
The Leadership Academy includes information on the healthcare leadership model, which has been developed to help staff who work in health and care to become better leaders as well as a wide-ranging programme of development targeted at all potential leaders working within the NHS. The site includes resources such as 360 degree tools and assessment frameworks, as well as information about courses and development activities for staff.

www.kingsfund.org.uk
The King's Fund is an excellent source of publications on health services change, leadership and reform. See, for example, The King's Fund (2012) *Leadership and Engagement for Improvement in the NHS: Together We Can*, at www.kingsfund.org.uk/sites/files/kf/field/field_publication_file/leadership-for-engagement-improvement-nhs-final-review2012.pdf.

http://changeday.nhs.uk/healthcareradicals
The School for Health and Care Radicals is a virtual environment sponsored by the NHS Improving Quality website. It has a series of learning modules on change management.

www.bath.ac.uk/hr/hrdocuments/change/Managing_change.pdf
Leading and Managing Change at the University of Bath: Guidance and Tool Kit is one of a number of toolkits available for change management.

References

Adams, J.S. (1965) Inequity in social exchange, in L. Berkowitz (ed.) *Advances in Experimental Social Psychology*, vol. 2. New York: Academic Press, pp. 267–99.

Alderfer, C.P. (1972) *Existence, Relatedness and Growth*. New York: Free Press.

Alimo-Metcalfe, B. and Alban-Metcalfe, R. (2000) 'Heaven can wait'. *Health Service Journal* 12: 26–9.

Ansoff, I.H. and McDonnell, E.J. (1990) *Implanting Strategic Management*. Englewood Cliffs, NJ: Prentice Hall.

Buchanan, D.A. and Huczynski, A.A. (2010) *Organisational Behaviour* (7th edn). Harlow: Pearson.

Chambers, N., Harvey, G., Mannion, R. et al. (2013) 'Towards a framework for enhancing the performance of NHS boards: a synthesis of the evidence about board governance, board effectiveness and board development'. *Health Service Delivery Research* 1(6).

Cross-Government Obesity Unit/DH/DCSF (2008) *Healthy Weight, Healthy Lives: A Cross-Government Strategy for England*. London: HMSO.

Deal, T. and Kennedy, A. (2000) *Corporate Cultures: The Rites and Rituals of Corporate Life*. New York: Perseus Books.

DH (Department of Health) (2011) *Healthy Lives, Healthy People: A Call to Action on Obesity in England*. London: DH.

DH (2013) *The NHS Constitution: The NHS Belongs to us All*. London: DH.

DHSS (1983) *NHS Management Inquiry: Report to the Secretary of State for Social Services* (The Griffiths Report). London: DHSS.

Dixon Woods, M., Bake, R., Charles, K. et al. (2013) 'Culture and behaviour in the English National Health Service: overview of lessons from a large multimethod study'. *BMJ Quality and Safety* doi: 10.1136/bmjqs-2013-001947.

Fiedler, F.E. (1967) *A Theory of Leadership Effectiveness*. New York: McGraw-Hill.

Fillingham, D. (2008) *Lean Healthcare: Improving the Patient's Experience*. Chichester: Kingsham Press.

Fincham, R. and Rhodes, P. (2005) *Principles of Organisational Behaviour* (4th edn). Oxford: Oxford University Press.

Foresight (2007) *Tackling Obesities: Future Choices – Project Report* (2nd edn). London: Government Office for Science.

Francis, R. (2013) *Final Report of the Mid Staffordshire NHS Foundation Trust Public Inquiry*. London: TSO. Available at www.midstaffspublicinquiry.com/report (accessed 20/3/2014).

French, J.R.P and Raven, B. (1968) The bases of social power, in D. Cartwright and A.F. Zander (eds) *Group Dynamics: Research and Theory* (3rd edn). London: Harper & Row, pp. 259–69.

Gleicher, D., Beckhard, R. and Harris, R. (1987) 'The change equation'. Available at www.valuebasedmanagement.net (accessed 7/6/2014).

Hackman, J.R. and Oldham, G.R. (1980) *Work Redesign*. Reading MA: Addison-Wesley.

Handy, C.B. (1993) *Understanding Organisations* (4th edn). London: Penguin.

Handy, C.B. (1995) *Gods of Management*. Oxford: Oxford University Press.

Hartley, J. and Benington, J. (2010) *Leadership for Healthcare*. Bristol: Policy.

Herzberg, F. (1966) *Work and the Nature of Man*. New York: World Publishing.

Hosking, D.M. (1997) Organizing, leadership and skillful process, in K. Grint (ed.) *Leadership: Classical, Contemporary and Critical Approaches*. Oxford: Oxford University Press, pp. 293–318.

HSCIC (Health and Social Care Information Centre) (n.d.) *National Child Measurement Programme*. Available at www.hscic.gov.uk/ncmp.

Katz, R. (1978) 'Job longevity as a situational factor in job satisfaction'. *Administrative Science Quarterly* 23: 204–23.

Keogh, B. (2013) *Review into the Quality of Care and Treatment Provided by 14 Hospital Trusts in England: Overview Report*. Available at www.nhs.uk/nhsengland/bruce-keogh-review/documents/outcomes/keogh-review-final-report.pdf (accessed 12/12/2013).

Lawrence, P.R. and Lorsch, J.W. (1967) *Organizations and Environment*. Cambridge, MA: Harvard University Press.

Lewin, K. (1951) *Field Theory in Social Science*. London: Harper & Row.

Locke, E.A. and Latham, G.P. (eds) (2013) *New Developments in Task Setting and Goal Performance*. London: Routledge.

McGregor, D. (1987) *The Human Side of Enterprise*. London: Penguin.

Maslow, A.H. (1943) 'A theory of human motivation', *Psychological Review* 50: 370–96.

Mintzberg, H. (1979) *The Structuring of Organizations: A Synthesis of the Research*. Englewood Cliffs, NJ: Prentice Hall.

Moss Kanter, R. (1989) *When Giants Learn to Dance*. New York: Simon & Schuster.

Mullins, L.J. (2013) *Management and Organisational Behaviour* (10th edn). Harlow: Pearson.

Nadler, D.A. and Tushman, M.L. (1984) A congruence model for diagnosing organisational behaviour, in D. Kolb, I. Rubin and J. McIntyre (eds) *Organisational Psychology: A Book of Readings* (4th edn). Englewood Cliffs, NJ: Prentice Hall, pp. 587–603.

NHS Choices (n.d.) The NHS in England. Available at www.nhs.uk/NHSEngland/thenhs/about/Pages/nhsstructure.aspx (accessed 25/3/2014).

NHS Choices (2013) *Physical Activity Guidelines for Young People*. Available at www.nhs.uk/Livewell/fitness/Pages/physical-activity-guidelines-for-young-people.aspx (accessed 25/3/2014).

NHS Commissioning Board (2012) *NHS Outcomes Framework and CCG Outcomes Indicators: Data Availability Table*. Available at www.england.nhs.uk/wp-content/uploads/2012/12/oi-data-table.pdf (accessed 10/8/2014).

NHS England (2013a) *Putting Patients First*. Available at www.england.nhs.uk/wp-content/uploads/2013/04/ppf-1314-1516-er.pdf (accessed 10/3/2014).

NHS England (2013b) *A Guide to our Vision and Purpose*. Available at www.england.nhs.uk/wp-content/uploads/2013/.../our-vis-and-purp.pdf (accessed 10/3/2014).

NHS England (2014) *NHS Outcomes Framework – 5 domains resources*. Available at www.england.nhs.uk/resources/resources-for-ccgs/out-frwrk/ (accessed 10/8/2014).

NHS Leadership Academy (2013) *The Healthcare Leadership Model*, version 1.0. Leeds: NHS Leadership Academy.

Porter, L.W. and Lawler, E.E. (1968) *Managerial Attitudes and Performance*. Homewood, IL: Dorsey Press.

Pugh, D.S. (1988) 'The convergence of international organisational behaviour'. Invited paper to the British Psychological Society Conference, London, and Open University School of Management Working Paper No. 2/90.

Pugh, D.S. and Hickson, D.J. (1996) *Writers on Organisations* (5th edn). London: Penguin.

Roethlisberger, F.J. and Dixon, W.J. (1943) *Management and the Worker*. Cambridge, MA: Harvard University Press.

Schein, E.H. (1988) *Organisational Psychology* (3rd edn). Englewood Cliffs, NJ: Prentice Hall.

Schein, E.H. (2010) *Organizational Culture and Leadership* (4th edn). San Francisco: Jossey Bass.

Sidani, S. and Fox, M. (2014) 'Patient-centered care: clarification of its specific elements to facilitate interprofessional care'. *Journal of Interprofessional Care* 28(2): 134–41.

Stewart, R. (1995) *Leading in the NHS: A Practical Guide* (2nd edn). Basingstoke: Macmillan – now Palgrave Macmillan.

Storey, J. and Holti, R. (2013) *Towards a New Model of Leadership for the NHS*. NHS Leadership Academy. Available at www.leadershipacademy.nhs.uk/wp-content/uploads/2013/05/Towards-a-New-Model-of-Leadership-2013.pdf (accessed 25/3/2014).

Swanton, K. (2008) *Healthy Weight, Healthy Lives: A Toolkit for Developing Local Strategies*. Produced for the National Heart Forum/Cross-Government Obesity Unit/Faculty of Public Health. Available at www.fph.org.uk/uploads/full_obesity_toolkit-1.pdf (accessed 25/3/2014).

Tannembaum, R. and Schmidt, W.H. (1973) 'How to choose a leadership pattern'. *Harvard Business Review* 51(3): 162–75, 178–80.

Taylor, V. (2013) *Leading for Health and Wellbeing*. London: Learning Matters/ Sage.

Tiplady, R. (2003) Letting go: chaos theory and the management of organisations. Available at http://tiplady.org.uk/pdfs/lettinggo.pdf (accessed 20/3/2014).

Trice, H.M. and Beyer, J.M. (1992) *The Culture of Work Organisations*. London: Prentice Hall.

Trist, E. and Bamforth, K.W. (1951) 'Some social and psychological consequences of the longwall method of coal-getting'. *Human Relations* 4(1): 37–8.

Tuckman, B.W. (1965) 'Development sequence in small groups'. *Psychological Bulletin* 63: 384–99.

Tuckman, B.W. and Jensen, M.A.C. (1977) 'Stages of small-group development revisited'. *Group and Organization Studies* 2(4): 419.

UK Public Spending (n.d.) Public expenditure. Available at www.ukpublicspending.co.uk/government_expenditure.html (accessed 22/3/2014).

Von Bertalanffy, L. (1951) 'Problems of general systems theory: a new approach to the unity of science'. *Human Biology* 23(4): 302–12.

Vroom, V.H. (1964) *Work and Motivation*. New York: Wiley.

Watson, C.M. (1983) 'Leadership, management and the seven keys'. *Business Horizons* March-April: 8–13.

Weber, M. (1964) *The Theory of Social and Economic Organisations*. London: Collier Macmillan.

Wenger, E. and Snyder, W. (2000) 'Communities of practice: the organizational frontier'. *Harvard Business Review* 78: 139–45.

WHO (2011) *Global Recommendations on Physical Activity for Health*. Available at www.who.int/dietphysicalactivity/physical-activity-recommendations-5-17years.pdf?ua=1 (accessed 25/3/2014).

Health economics

Overview	378
Introduction	378
Part 1 The contribution of economics to health studies	380
Market forces and healthcare	381
The allocation and distribution of healthcare 'off the market'	384
Part 2 Theoretical and research approaches	387
Resources and money	387
The output of healthcare	388
The economic notion of cost	388
The cost–benefit approach	389
Techniques of economic appraisal	392
Case study The use of QALYs in the treatment of obesity	397
Summary	398
Questions for further discussion	398
Further reading	398
References	399

Learning outcomes

This chapter will enable readers to:

- Appreciate why economics exists
- Understand the basic principles of economics
- Understand how these principles can be applied to health
- Be familiar with and describe the different types of economic appraisal
- Understand the contribution that health economics can make to health studies

Overview

There is a growing awareness worldwide that the resources available to maintain and improve health are finite, whereas the demands made on these resources appear to be virtually infinite. Consequently, many are looking to economics – the science of making choices in situations of scarcity – for assistance. Part 1 explains what economics is and, equally importantly, what it is not. The emphasis throughout is on how economics does not deal with problems that are uniquely 'economic' but instead addresses common issues from a different perspective. Economics is about the allocation of resources to production and the distribution of those outputs to society. The way in which this is done in unregulated markets is explained, followed by a discussion of what might make healthcare differ from other market goods. Problems in the allocation and distribution of services in non-market situations, such as with the UK NHS, are examined, with particular emphasis on the difficulties that arise when healthcare is given according to people's needs rather than their ability to pay (demand). Part 2 explains the cost–benefit approach; this being defended by a return to the basic economic principle of scarcity, the fact that choice always involves sacrifice, and the importance of being explicit about the criteria on which inescapable choices are made. Efficiency is defended as a criterion for choice on the basis that it seeks to maximize the health that can be achieved from whatever level of resources are available. There is an explanation of the three key techniques of economic appraisal: cost–benefit, cost-effectiveness and cost–utility analyses. It is emphasized that these tools ought to be employed only with a firm understanding of the principles upon which they are based. The chapter ends with an obesity-related case study of how QALYs are used in determining whether or not any intervention represents a good use of a healthcare system's scarce resources.

Introduction

Since the 1970s, healthcare expenditure worldwide has grown at an unprecedented rate. In the UK, for example, expenditure on healthcare rose from £37 per person in 1970/71 to £2,124 per person in 2010/11, with the proportion of GDP spent on healthcare increasing from 3.9% to nearly 9% (OHE, 2013).

With overall economic growth during most of that period, an increase in healthcare spending ought to be regarded as a good thing. After all, more spending on healthcare should mean more health for the population. Yet the increased spending did not appear to have been accompanied by a corresponding fall in the demands being made on the healthcare systems.

More recently, the economic downturn (now known as the Great Recession) caused by the financial crisis of 2007–08 has not only stopped the increase in healthcare expenditure, it has caused a reduction in real terms spending in many countries. Given this trend, it is not surprising that there is a growing recognition that resources for healthcare are unlikely ever to be sufficient to meet all health needs. This, in turn, means an increasing acceptance that not everything that can be done will be done and that choices are inescapable. Economics is the science of making choices.

> **?** What do you understand by 'economics'? What insights into health and healthcare provision might its study offer?

Economics has been defined as:

> the study of how men [this was 1976] and society end up choosing, with or without the use of money, to employ scarce productive resources to produce various commodities over time and distribute them for consumption, now and in the future, among various groups and people in society. It analyses the costs and benefits of improving patterns of resource allocation. (Samuelson, 1976, p. 5)

The discipline exists because the resources (inputs) available to produce goods and services (outputs) are finite, whereas humankind's desire to consume these outputs would appear to be infinite. Economics concerns how society makes a choice about how much of its scarce resources are allocated to the production of particular goods or services, and how these outputs of production are then distributed to members of society.

Economics is a discipline – a recognized body of thought – and health economics is the application of this body of thought to the topic 'health'. Thus, it deals with questions such as:

- How much of society's scarce resources should be devoted to the production of health?
- How should health outputs be distributed?

These are couched in words that make them recognizable as 'economic' questions, but what about the following?

- What is the best way of treating people with disease X?
- Should we introduce a programme to screen for disease Y?

These may appear to be clinical and policy issues respectively rather than economic ones. Indeed, decisions of this sort are regularly made without seeking the assistance of economists. Yet both can also be viewed as legitimate economic questions since they involve the use of scarce resources (inputs) and are concerned with making people healthier (outputs).

Health economics is, first and foremost, a 'way of thinking' based on a defined set of principles. It puts an economic perspective on the issues and problems concerning how to get the most from healthcare resources. The two questions above could be rephrased by asking:

- What is the most cost-effective way of treating people with disease X?

- Do the benefits of introducing a programme to screen for disease Y outweigh the costs?

> **?** What knowledge would a health economist need to answer these questions?

Health economics can be viewed as having a 'toolkit' containing a number of different appraisal techniques. All are concerned with examining policies and interventions by comparing the resources needed (*cost*) with the effects produced (*benefit*). The broad umbrella of the cost–benefit approach also includes cost-effectiveness analysis and cost–utility analysis, which are discussed later in this chapter.

If health economics is concerned with the production of health, it must be concerned with more than just interventions provided by health professionals. Public health policies such as banning smoking in public places also produce the output 'health' as do road safety and environmental measures. Macroeconomic issues, such as the effect of unemployment on health, and policy issues, such as increasing taxes to reduce the demand for unhealthy goods, are also within the remit of health economics.

Part 1 The contribution of economics to health studies

---

example 11.1

The application of economics to contemporary health issues

- Efficiency, for example the cost–benefit analysis of health policies and the cost-effectiveness of various medical treatments or value for money of health behaviours such as weight loss

- Funding for healthcare, for example insurance, co-payments, state funding or rationing
- Equity, for example prescribing and treatment in relation to need or postcode lottery
- Market systems in healthcare, for example private companies and state provision

---

Economics deals with two basic problems:

- the allocation of resources to production

- the distribution of the outputs of that production.

One way of dealing with these is for government to eschew any role at all, leaving everything to 'market forces' – essentially, the interaction between supply and demand. How much of any country's resources to allocate to the production of shoes, for example, and what mechanism to employ to distribute shoes are rarely issues to which governments pay much heed. If left alone, market forces do the job perfectly well. If any government feels that it is somehow wrong when poor people cannot afford shoes, the response is normally a welfare payment or some other form of income redistribution rather than any direct interference in the workings of the market for shoes.

Market forces and healthcare

The principle of market forces and the relationship between supply and demand are key concepts in economics. 'Demand' is defined as that quantity of a good for which consumers are willing and able to pay at any given price. Economic theory says that consumers will demand more at a lower price than they will at a higher price, as shown by the line 'd' in Figure 11.1. Similarly, supply is defined as that quantity producers are willing to offer for sale at a given price. The theory states that they will wish to supply smaller quantities when prices are low than when prices are high, as shown by the line 's' in Figure 11.1. There are textbooks full of theories to explain why this is the case, but for present purposes we will simply assume that such supply and demand behaviour makes intuitive sense.

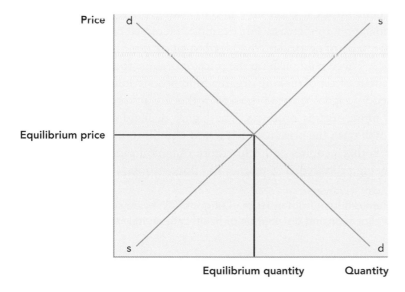

Figure 11.1 **Supply, demand and market equilibrium**

A market is where the exchange takes place, the price determining how much money changes hands for every unit of the good bought and sold. If the quantity that producers supply exceeds the quantity that consumers demand, there will be a pressure on prices to fall. The opposite occurs when demand exceeds supply – there will be a pressure on prices to rise. There is one price, the 'equilibrium price', at which supply and demand are equal and there is no pressure from within the market for the price to change. The quantity that is supplied and demanded at the equilibrium price is called the 'equilibrium quantity'.

This simple analysis shows how market forces have solved the first economic problem – the allocation of resources. Some level of resources is required to produce the equilibrium quantity, but no one has told producers how many resources to allocate to the production of this good: it just happened. The market has also dealt with the second economic problem – the distribution of output, since – by definition – only those consumers willing and able to pay the equilibrium price can consume the good. Price can therefore be seen as a rationing mechanism limiting the distribution of the good only to those who demand it at the equilibrium price.

Of course, markets do not settle down at an equilibrium and stay there for all time. Changes are occurring outside the market that cause supply and demand to change. On the demand side, people's incomes, tastes and preferences, as well as the prices of other goods, are constantly changing. On the supply side, production techniques and the cost of labour and materials are also constantly altering. Equilibrium is thus rarely reached, but what matters is that if demand and supply are not in equilibrium at any given moment, economic theory can predict what will happen to the price, which will in turn trigger a whole set of other predictable economic forces to come into effect.

Consumer demand for a good may initially cause prices to rise and also production and supply to increase. For example, increased concern about the possible health effects of pesticides could lead to an increase in the demand for organic produce. This would push up the price of organic foods, which would have the immediate effect of making organic food production more profitable. This would send a signal to producers to reallocate resources towards the production of more organic products. The higher demand and the resulting higher supply will push the price towards a new equilibrium. In this example, the end result is that people's desire for more organic food has led to more organic food being produced. The market has done its job.

? Is healthcare different from other market goods? Why do so few countries leave the allocation and distribution of healthcare entirely to market forces?

A number of economic assumptions have to be upheld for the free market to work in the way described. Donaldson et al. (2005) outline these as:

- consumers making their own choices – consumer sovereignty
- consumers being well informed – symmetry of information
- consumers' choices affecting only themselves – externalities
- competition between suppliers.

In a free market, no elite with some 'preferred' set of values tells consumers what they should or should not demand. Individuals are assumed to be the best judges of their own welfare, and economic theory shows how, subject to certain assumptions, perfectly competitive and unregulated markets produce socially optimum results. In the case of healthcare, however, the appropriateness of consumer sovereignty can be challenged. Is the patient necessarily the best judge of their own welfare? Does the patient necessarily want to be the judge? Many may prefer to be left out of the decision process altogether and leave it to the doctor, who 'knows best what's good for me'.

Market theory assumes that consumers are well informed and can judge how much utility (satisfaction) they get from consuming a good. In the case of healthcare, however, individuals will rarely be able to diagnose themselves, are unlikely to be aware of the range of available treatments, and cannot judge how much utility they will get from treatment even after consuming it, since they do not know what would have happened in the absence of any treatment. They have to rely on the doctor's superior knowledge, so there is an 'asymmetry of information' between supplier and consumer, with the doctor deciding the treatment the patient will demand and supplying it.

Many consumers considering buying a new car may, of course, be no more knowledgeable about cars than they are about healthcare, yet they are unlikely to leave the decision about which car to buy totally to the salesperson. Why not? The difference between these two cases is simply that the consumer of healthcare trusts the doctor – at least more than they trust the salesperson. Doctors are expected to act according to a code of medical ethics; car salespeople are not. But it is debatable whether an ethical code means that doctors will end up making the same consumption decisions that fully informed consumers would make if they had the medical knowledge. Factors such as attitudes to risk, aversion to pain, or personal circumstances (who will mind the children if I go into hospital?) can affect consumption decisions. Doctors are unlikely to have all this information and possibly would not take it into account even if they did.

Also implicit in the theory of how unregulated (or free) markets produce socially optimal results is the assumption that individuals' consumption decisions affect them and them alone. This may not, however, always be the case. Someone's decision to buy a guard dog that barks all night may well provide their neighbours with a great deal of negative utility. Where such 'externalities' (positive or negative) exist, it can be easily shown that unregulated markets will not produce socially optimal solutions. Healthcare arguably has externalities, both positive and negative. The decision to seek treatment for an infectious disease affects not only the treated individual but others too, in that their risk of catching the disease is reduced. It has also been argued that a 'humanitarian externality' may exist in healthcare if people derive positive utility from the knowledge that others are receiving the healthcare they need.

connections Chapter 12 discusses how codes of practice influence the work of health professionals and how philosophical activity can help to understand the balance of actions and effects.

For the market to work as described earlier, a number of assumptions are also needed on the supply side, chief among these being assumptions concerning the competitive behaviour of firms. In reality, private healthcare markets are rarely, if ever, characterized by many small hospitals competing with each other on grounds of price. Elements of monopoly powers normally exist together with many other features, which suggest that the free-market model does not describe what happens in the market for healthcare.

Healthcare is arguably different from other goods or services in the marketplace. Various forms of regulation have been introduced in different countries to overcome specific problems without taking the step of removing healthcare entirely from the marketplace and replacing it with publicly provided services. In the end, however, the issue of whether healthcare should be considered as a market good can only be settled by resorting to philosophy and ideology. In the UK, the decision to take healthcare (almost) completely 'off the market' by setting up the NHS was taken mainly because of a social consensus that access to healthcare should be regarded as a 'fundamental human right' – like access to the courts of justice – rather than as part of society's reward system. Unsurprisingly, in the US, where political ideology favours reward rather than rights, a far greater proportion of healthcare is delivered through private firms, with insurance being used to deal with the uncertainty as it is with regard to fires or car accidents.

connections Chapters 8 and 9 discuss the marketization of the NHS and how neoliberal political ideology is changing state provision in England.

The allocation and distribution of healthcare 'off the market'

If healthcare is taken off the market, some alternative means of allocation and distribution have to be found. On the allocation side, a committee deciding what proportion of total public expenditure will be spent each year on healthcare normally does this. On the distribution side, healthcare is provided to those who need it.

In 1948, healthcare was taken 'off the market' in the UK by the creation of the NHS. It was assumed that doctors would determine how much *need* there was and government would simply allocate the appropriate volume of resources to ensure that all needs would be met. This clearly has not happened. To explain why requires a deeper examination of what is meant by need.

thinking about In your view, should a person with a crooked nose be able to have NHS surgery to correct it? What criteria would you use to decide whether that person should have treatment?

To an economist, need means 'capacity to benefit' from treatment. Economists use the terms 'wants' and 'demands' to refer to consumer-based judgements and 'need' to refer to judgements made by some third party. In a private healthcare system, the consumer will be given a nose-straightening operation if they are willing to pay the money price. In a zero-priced public healthcare system, the doctor will judge whether or not the individual needs the operation – perhaps because of breathing difficulties. If there is no clinical need, the operation will be denied.

Defined in terms of capacity to benefit from treatment, need is clearly a dynamic concept. Every new medical development that allows the previously untreatable to be treated is increasing need. Similarly, any development that allows the previously treatable to be better treated also increases need. Not long ago, for example, nothing could be done to prevent very premature, low birth weight babies dying. Today, thanks to new technology and skills, those same babies have a need for, and benefit from, neonatal intensive care.

While the growth in new treatments that allow people to benefit more from healthcare is clearly a good thing, it also means that 'total need' is growing year on year – and at an increasing pace. So, while healthcare resourcing has also been growing, the rate of growth of resourcing has not matched the rate of growth of need. In other words, the gap between total need, which is what we would like to meet in an ideal world of infinite resources, and met need, which is what we can meet in the real world of scarce resources, has been widening year on year.

To an economist, need means 'capacity to benefit' from treatment. Chapter 12 discusses how the values we hold about health may influence views about entitlement to treatment.   **connections**

example 11.2

The relativity of need: the case of Viagra

Until the introduction of Viagra (sildenafil), erectile dysfunction in men had always been considered to represent a clinical need. Available treatments included:

- psychological management
- vacuum constriction devices
- intracavernous injection therapy
- transurethral drug delivery (Muse)
- a penile prosthesis
- surgery.

All were provided free on the NHS apart from vacuum pumps, which patients in some parts of the country had to purchase privately. The cost of meeting erectile dysfunction need was not an issue.

In 1997, Viagra was licensed by the US Federal Drug Administration. Prior to its launch, the sexual function disorder market in the US had total sales of $157 million, mainly on Muse (alprostadil). Within four weeks of Viagra being launched, the market increased to over 10 times its previous size, Viagra capturing a staggering 97.5% of the total market (IMS America, 1998).

In the UK, with its publicly funded, zero-priced healthcare system, it was estimated that Viagra could add £1 billion per annum to the NHS drugs bill (*Daily Mail*, 1998). The government quickly stepped in, setting specific criteria for who could and could not be prescribed Viagra on the NHS. Those who did not meet the criteria obviously did not 'need' Viagra. Moreover, the decision of whether or not there was a need was no longer to be left to doctors.

In 2013, the patent on Viagra expired, meaning that other pharmaceutical companies could produce and sell sildenafil at a fraction of the price charged when the patent was in place. It will be interesting to see if this influences the prescribing of sildenafil by doctors.

In a world of infinite resources, all men who could benefit from treatment would be prescribed Viagra, regardless of its patent status and price. In the real world of scarcity and choice, those at the less severe end of the sexual dysfunction continuum may continue to be judged not to need it.

? Why will resources for healthcare always be scarce?

Economists argue that even if health need were finite, it would still not be in society's interest to allocate sufficient resources to meet all health need. This somewhat provocative statement can be justified by focusing on the fact that society clearly has needs other than those relating to health, for example education, defence, transport and law and order. However, since the total amount available to spend on all these is also finite, spending in one area means having less to spend in another. Similarly, more public expenditure means higher taxes and thus less to spend on private consumption.

The balance between private and public expenditure and the distribution of the latter between the different public sector areas is driven by a fundamental economic principle known as 'diminishing marginal benefit'. This states that as any activity expands, the extra benefit produced by each extra unit of input gets progressively smaller. For example, a single nurse working in a community will focus their efforts on where the need is greatest. A second nurse will also produce benefits, but as the most pressing needs are already being met by the first nurse, the marginal (extra) benefit produced by the second will be less than that by the first. And so on.

If increased spending on health produces positive marginal benefits, this will be at the cost of benefits forgone elsewhere in the economy. If healthcare's relative share of total spending is increased, that of another area must be reduced. According to the above economic principle, the extra spending on health will produce decreasing marginal benefits, while reduced spending in the other area will incur increasing marginal sacrifices. If the marginal gain exceeds the marginal sacrifice, the total benefit from the shift in expenditure will increase, but this can go on for only so long. Eventually, the continually decreasing marginal benefits in health will no longer exceed the marginal losses elsewhere.

If society has a multiplicity of need, the socially optimal balance of expenditure will be at that point at which any further shifts will begin to make total benefit fall, that is, society will begin to be made worse off. Since the share of total societal resources devoted to health will always be less than the level at which all needs can be met, some form of rationing is inevitable.

Part 2 Theoretical and research approaches

example 11.3

Examples of research in health economics

- Economic evaluation: most health economics units have economic evaluation as part of their wider programmes of work. The Centre for Health Economics at the University of York (www.york.ac.uk/che) is an acknowledged leader in this area. An example of one of its recent evaluations is Griffiths et al. (2014), which examines the cost-effectiveness of a drug for treating chronic heart failure
- Public health: the Centre for Health Economics and Medicines Evaluation at Bangor University (http://cheme.bangor. ac.uk) has a programme of work in the economics of public health. A good example of its output is Edwards et al. (2011). This paper describes a study that looked at the cost-effectiveness of a programme to improve heating and ventilation as a means of producing health gains in children with asthma
- Schools/children: the School of Social and Community Medicine at Bristol University (www.bristol.ac.uk/social-community-medicine) is at the leading edge of evaluating schools-based trials aimed at improving children's health. An example of its output is Hollingworth et al. (2011). The paper describes the cost-effectiveness of a 'peer-led' intervention aimed at reducing the number of children who smoke
- Priority-setting: the Health Economics Research Unit at the University of Aberdeen (www.abdn.ac.uk/heru) has a long track record of using economics in priority-setting in health. An example of its recent output in this area is Watson et al. (2012), which applied an economic technique of preference elicitation to assist in priority-setting

Resources and money

'Resources' are defined as those things that contribute to the production of an output. Producing corn requires resources such as land, seeds, workers and tractors. No amount of money will produce corn unless it is used to buy land, hire workers and so on. Resources in healthcare include doctors, nurses, hospital buildings, bandages and drugs. Again, money pays for these resources, but, by the above definition, volunteers and informal carers are also resources even though they do not receive any monetary reward. The distinction between money and resources is thus important. More money normally means control over more resources, but this is not always the case. A shortage of nurses trained in intensive care will constrain activity in an intensive care unit regardless of the cash available.

For present purposes, money also has a second function in that it provides a common measure of value. Expressing resources in terms of a common measure allows them to be added together and compared with other combinations of resources. The same is true for outputs. By definition, all the outputs of healthcare are of value, and expressing each in terms of its monetary value allows different outputs to be added and compared.

> **thinking about** Do you think a monetary value can be put on health? Can you compare the life of a premature baby, whose life depends on intensive care, with the pain relief of thousands of older people achieved through simple hip replacements?

The output of healthcare

Economists have long argued that the principal output of the healthcare industry is 'health'. The inverted commas reflect the fact that many health services, for example palliative care of the terminally ill, are not intended to raise health status as such. However, if 'health' is perceived in the broad sense of wellbeing, all effective interventions will make people better off than they would otherwise have been.

The practical difficulties of viewing output in this way stem from the fact that health is notoriously difficult to define, measure and value. Broad definitions of health, such as that by the World Health Organization, as a 'state of complete physical, mental and social well-being' (WHO, 1946), are unhelpful when trying to compare the output of alternative therapies.

In practice, therefore, intermediate measures are often used as proxies for the final (health) outputs. This is acceptable as long as the link between the proxy measure and health is well established. Thus, evidence that a reduction in smoking prevalence will result in a reduction in smoking-related morbidity and mortality means that the 'number of quitters' is an acceptable proxy for the output of a smoking cessation programme, even though smoking is not a disease and quitting is not in itself a health gain. The less well established the link between the proxy and health, the less useful the proxy.

> **connections**   Chapter 3 discusses some of the problems of identifying outcomes from health interventions.

The economic notion of cost

To an economist, cost means sacrifice: an accountant will measure cost as the amount of money spent; an economist will look at what has been forgone. The term 'opportunity cost' is used in economics to emphasize this notion of an opportunity forgone. Within economics, 'cost' is used as shorthand for 'opportunity cost'.

A cost can thus be incurred without money changing hands. A new clinic that takes a nurse off a ward for one hour a week will not affect the nursing wages bill, but it will involve the sacrifice of the benefit that the nurse could have achieved in one hour on the ward. Similarly, freeing an hour of nurse time provides the opportunity to use that hour to produce benefits that could not otherwise be produced. The difference in benefits from exchanging the work done during the hour can be compared in economic terms, regardless of the fact that no money will be saved.

?   On what basis should resource allocation choices be made?

The principal criterion used in economics is **efficiency**, which maximizes the benefits from the available resources. It concerns the relationship between inputs and outputs, that is, most benefit being available at least cost. Being efficient means getting as much health as is possible from the available resources; being inefficient means getting less.

It is important to note, however, that whereas efficiency is a good rule to be guided by, it is never a substitute for decision-making (Drummond, 1981). Demonstrating that A is more efficient than B suggests that A should be pursued unless alternative criteria can be identified to argue otherwise. B may be justified, for example, on equity, public relations or political expediency grounds, and no economist would argue that these are not relevant alternative criteria. However, it becomes difficult to argue for the pursuit of inefficient B over efficient A on grounds such as the political power of the doctors involved, historical precedent, or who can get most public support by waving a shroud in front of a television camera – factors which, in part, explain the current pattern of resource allocation.

The cost–benefit approach

Figure 11.2 illustrates the cost–benefit way of thinking. The principle of weighing gains against sacrifices is the cost–benefit approach. In each situation, there are costs which mean that an alternative must be forgone. There will also be particular benefits that result.

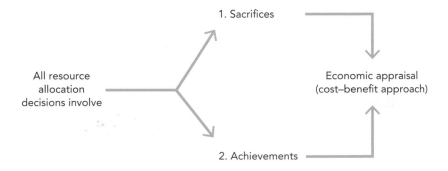

Figure 11.2 **The cost–benefit framework**

An intervention will fail the cost–benefit test if the benefits achieved are judged to be of lower value than the benefits forgone by not using the resources in other ways. In this case, the gains and sacrifices are both understood in terms of health. Failing the cost–benefit test does not mean that these health gains are not worth some amount of money – just that the health gains do not exceed the health sacrifices.

> **?** Is it ethical to make healthcare decisions on the basis of efficiency?

It is natural for doctors and other health professionals to want to do what is best for their patients, and it is important to stress that the cost–benefit approach is not being advocated at the level of decision-making relating to the individual patient. Doctors have always practised under a system of medical ethics that has conventionally focused on the two ethical theories of 'virtue' and 'duty' (Jonsen and Hellegers, 1987). These are individualistic ethics based on the doctor's responsibility for the individual patient, a guiding principle that it is unethical to do anything that does more harm than good.

connections   Chapter 12 discusses the guiding principles of beneficence and non-maleficence, which, in medical ethics, means that health workers should not take any action that does more harm than good.

Given that the first duty of doctors will inevitably be to their patients, their preference for making clinical decisions on the basis of clinical effectiveness rather than efficiency is understandable. It is still legitimate to take the costs that others will have to bear into account, but the patient in front of the doctor is a person with a name, a face, a family, a history. Efficiency is still relevant, but perhaps less important in this situation.

More recently, and due to an increasing awareness of the scarcity of resources, ethicists have begun focusing on a third ethical theory, that of the 'common good' (Mooney, 1992). This is a social ethic based on responsibility for the health of populations. In this, the guiding principle of only doing those things that do more good than harm still applies, but the terms now reflect a social perspective. On this basis, any intervention that yields only a small benefit to the patient but will mean a large sacrifice to other patients will, from a social perspective, be doing more harm than good. Those responsible for health policy-making and broad resource allocation decisions have to see their duty as being to the whole population – including the potential future consumers of healthcare.

A decision to put additional resources into developing neonatal intensive care units will be made before any of the babies who will benefit from them have been conceived. Similarly, it is not possible to identify the individuals who will benefit from increasing the level of resources going into mass screening or immunization campaigns. These are statistical lives without names, faces, families or histories. At this level of decision-making, efficiency is an important factor, since being inefficient means achieving less health than could have been achieved – and what is ethical about that?

thinking about Think about some health policy decisions that benefit individuals but may adversely affect populations.

example 11.4

The case of treatment for bone marrow cancer

In the UK, the National Institute for Health and Care Excellence (NICE: www.niceorg.uk) is the body that determines which new treatments should be recommended for use by the NHS. This is done on the basis of evidence of cost-effectiveness as well as clinical effectiveness and safety. Where a new treatment is shown to be more effective but more costly than the one it will replace, a decision rule is applied, based on how much extra the new treatment costs per unit of extra health produced – where 'health' is expressed in quality adjusted life years (**QALY**) (see below for a fuller explanation of QALYs). Currently, NICE is unlikely to recommend a new treatment for use on the NHS if the extra cost per extra QALY gained is above £30,000.

In 2009, NICE considered the case for bortezomib monotherapy for relapsed bone marrow cancer (multiple myeloma). Although bortezomib was shown to be effective in extending the lives of these patients, the initial NICE guidance was that bortezomib not be recommended for use in the NHS on the grounds that the extra cost per extra QALY gained was above this £30,000 threshold.

Unsurprisingly, organizations representing cancer patients responded angrily to this recommendation. While it is understandable that they should focus solely on potential benefits to cancer patients, NICE has a duty to all patients and therefore has to consider the sacrifices that others would have to bear if bortezomib were approved, that is, its opportunity cost. As NICE approvals are not accompanied by budget uplifts, the costs of providing approved treatments means reducing expenditure on services to other patients and hence denying other patients health gains they would otherwise receive.

The NICE (and health economics) way of thinking, however, is rarely promoted by the media. In this case, the *Daily Mail* not only introduced a campaign in support of bone marrow cancer patients, but raised £230,000 from its readers to support the legal cost of a challenge to the NICE recommendation through the courts.

In the end, a compromise was reached. Janssen-Cilag, the manufacturer of bortezomib, agreed to rebate the full cost of bortezomib for patients who, after a maximum of four cycles of treatment, had less than what had been defined as a 'partial response'. With this condition specified in its recommendation, NICE approved bortezomib for use in these patients (NICE, 2010).

Several messages emerge from this story:

- In a world of scarce resources and finite budgets, it is not possible to provide every treatment that is shown to be clinically effective, regardless of how small the benefit and no matter what sacrifices others will have to bear
- The sacrifices others will have to bear (opportunity cost) involve real people forgoing health benefits they otherwise could have had. If the value of these sacrifices exceeds the value of the benefit to patients receiving bortezomib, then a NICE approval raises interesting ethical questions

- Economic evaluation is an aid to decision-making and not a substitute for it. It would be wrong to blindly approve or reject treatments solely on the basis of cost-effectiveness
- Bortezomib is provided to bone marrow cancer patients in many other countries worldwide at list price. The NICE process, which led to the manufacturer's agreement that it would not charge for patients who did not respond to treatment, secured a better deal for the NHS.

Techniques of economic appraisal

All the techniques of economic appraisal fall under the broad umbrella of the cost–benefit approach. All are concerned with examining one or more interventions by comparing the resources needed against the effects produced. How they differ depends essentially on how these effects (benefits) are perceived, which in turn depends on the objective of the appraisal.

Cost–benefit analysis

The most comprehensive technique of economic appraisal is **cost–benefit analysis**. Its objective is to assess whether, or to what extent, something is worth doing. Cost–benefit analysis thus addresses *allocative* efficiency, in that it tells us whether or not (or how much) resources should be allocated to this programme. This involves weighing all the benefits of the programme (or the extra benefit from an expansion of the programme) against the total (or extra) cost of achieving them. This can only be done if all the costs and benefits are expressed in common units. Although similar to a financial appraisal, cost–benefit analysis is concerned with value of gains and losses rather than money spent and money received, which is the basis of financial appraisal.

In economics, costs are all the resources directly or indirectly used by the programme that have alternative uses, that is, which incur opportunity costs. Benefits are everything of value that results. Cost–benefit analysis normally adopts a 'social welfare' perspective, in that all costs are considered regardless of who bears them, and all benefits are included regardless to whom they accrue. Cost and benefit variables are identified, measured in appropriate physical or other relevant units and finally valued.

Where they exist, market prices are normally used to express the money value of costs and benefits. Where market prices do not exist, 'shadow prices' can be used. For example, the time of volunteers does not command a market price, but it is possible to impute a price to volunteers' time using the wages of paid workers who do roughly the same work as a proxy.

thinking about Do you think a monetary value can be put on health?

The valuation of health and other intangible benefits and costs is, however, no easy task. A variety of methods are available to do this, which will not be detailed here (see, for example, Fox-Rushby and Cairns, 2005). Nevertheless, many people find the very act of placing a monetary value on such things as pain relief or the extension of life to be at best distasteful and at worst immoral. According to the economic way of thinking, the values are always there – the only issue is whether they are to be explicit or implicit. Economic appraisal attempts to make valuations explicit in order to assist the pursuit of efficiency. For example, if an economic evaluation shows some new intervention to have a cost per life saved of £100,000 and a decision is taken not to introduce that intervention, it is implied that those lives are valued at less than £100,000. The rejection of a programme with a low implied value of a life would be difficult to defend if another programme is currently running with a much higher implied value of a life. Efficiency in terms of maximizing the number of lives saved from any given level of expenditure will be improved by making a marginal reduction in the latter programme in order to support the former.

Many people feel an understandable distaste at the idea on putting a monetary value on intangible health benefits – such things ought somehow to be above considerations of cost. Yet, if cost is perceived in terms of sacrifice, it is evident from individual behaviour and collective decision-making that this is clearly not the case. For example, the decision to reject a proposal to build a flyover at a dangerous intersection on the grounds of costs implies that the value of the anticipated lives saved and injuries avoided is less than the cost of building the flyover. The fact that preventable road deaths are tolerated shows that society does not put an infinite value on the lives that could be saved.

Cost-effectiveness and cost–utility analysis

Often, the issue is not whether or not to do something but more simply how to do it. For example, if the question is one of deciding how to treat people with raised blood pressure – given that a decision has already been taken to treat them – **cost-effectiveness analysis** can compare alternative blood pressure-reducing interventions in terms of their cost per unit reduction. Cost-effectiveness analysis addresses *technical* efficiency, in the sense that it can tell us the best way to do something but not whether or not that something is worth doing. That is an allocative efficiency issue that can only be dealt with by cost–benefit analysis.

Cost-effectiveness analysis is a simpler technique than cost–benefit analysis. By perceiving benefits more narrowly and measuring them only in physical units, it avoids the difficult task of benefit valuation. At the same time, it provides information that is much more limited since it can only compare alternative ways of pursuing the given objective – in this case to reduce blood pressure. It says nothing about how efficient any blood pressure reduction programme is compared with other programmes of healthcare.

Cost-effectiveness analysis can, however, be broadened by using more general benefit measures that are not unique to the programme in question. For example, since reducing blood pressure is expected to reduce mortality, the objective of a blood pressure reduction programme can be expressed in broader life-saving terms. By comparing alternative ways of reducing blood pressure in terms of cost per life year saved, the most cost-effective way of reducing blood pressure can then be compared with the cost-effectiveness of any other life-saving programme.

> **?** Why might it be difficult to assess the effectiveness of blood pressure reduction using broad measures?

Assessing cost per life year, however, involves a more complex appraisal than assessing cost per unit reduction in blood pressure. Whereas blood pressure can be accurately measured, translating today's reduced blood pressure into tomorrow's lives saved involves a greater use of assumptions and estimations. Moreover, this broader cost-effectiveness analysis will still be limited because it is restricted to comparing interventions that extend life and many healthcare interventions, for example hernia repair, do not affect length of life. It also has to assume that each year of life is of equal value regardless of the quality of that life.

This problem can be overcome by broadening the object to take in both life extension and quality of life improvements, or, stated more generally, to produce 'health'. The advantage of so doing is that the cost-effectiveness of all the interventions, whether preventive, curative or caring, can then be compared in terms of cost per unit of 'health' produced.

If 'health' is the output of healthcare, some means of measuring health is needed. Perfect measures of health will, however, never exist because health is multidimensional and value laden. People who are in pain, who suffer depression or have impaired vision or restricted mobility are all in a state of health that is less than perfect. Although each of the dimensions of ill health can be measured independently (more versus less pain, greater versus lesser visual impairment and so on), a measure of 'health' will have to combine all these into a unidimensional index. Who will have 'worse' health, the person with depression or the person in pain? Such a decision obviously involves a value judgement, but who should be the judge? The depressed person will quite rightly feel that depression is the worse state and will value an improvement from depression to perfect health more highly than an improvement from a state of pain to perfect health. The person in pain may, unsurprisingly, disagree. A 'perfect' health status measure therefore cannot exist until such problems are reconciled.

Nevertheless, economists have made considerable progress in measuring health by focusing on the idea that all interventions must either extend life, improve the quality of life, or achieve some combination of the two. Therefore, in principle, all effective interventions produce quality adjusted life years (QALYs). If the effectiveness of any programme is measured in terms of QALYs, a comparison of cost per QALY can indicate the most technically efficient ways of producing health.

Cost-effectiveness analyses that use QALYs (or similar value-based health measures) as the measure of effectiveness are often called 'cost–utility analyses', and these are increasingly being used worldwide to inform prioritization by helping to decide which interventions will be provided by healthcare systems or covered by health insurance plans.

The use of QALYs has become so commonplace in economic evaluation in recent years that it is easy to lose sight of some of the difficulties inherent in any attempt to measure quality of life. Example 11.5 explores how QALYs were developed.

example 11.5

The development of the QALY

In the early 1970s, Grogono and Woodgate (1971) attempted to prioritize patients in need of non-urgent surgery using an index based on 10 dimensions of ill health. The thinking behind this was that while treating people purely on a first-come, first-served basis may have its attractions, surgeons are unlikely to ignore factors such as how much pain patients are in, or whether or not their condition is preventing them going to work, when deciding priorities for treatment. If surgeons are therefore implicitly making judgements of need on the basis of undeclared criteria, would it not be possible, and more ethical, to make these criteria explicit? Grogono and Woodgate came up with the following list:

- ability to work
- ability to enjoy hobbies and recreation
- malaise, pain or suffering
- worry or unhappiness
- ability to communicate
- ability to sleep
- independence of others
- ability to eat/enjoy food
- bladder and bowel control
- sex life.

The idea was that, in the course of a normal consultation, it ought to be possible to give patients a score of 0, 0.5 or 1 according to whether they were normal, impaired or incapacitated on each of the dimensions. These figures could be added together: the higher the Grogono–Woodgate index score, the higher the patient's priority.

The problem with the Grogono–Woodgate index is that the dimensions are not weighted to reflect their relative importance. The absence of weighting implies that all are valued equally, which is clearly unrealistic. Most people would probably agree that someone with a score of 1 as a result of double incontinence is worse off than someone with a score of 1 resulting from an inability to participate in hobbies and recreation. If so, and assuming that effective interventions exist for both, the former has a greater need. But this is a value judgement rather than a clinical judgement.

Note that this approach was not an attempt to prioritize patients according to diagnosis, for example hernias versus ingrown toenails, but according to how the condition was affecting them in terms of pain or their ability to get out and about. The sought-after valuations occur between the dimensions of ill health rather than between diagnosed conditions.

In an early attempt to see whether there were such things as 'social values', Rosser and Kind (1978) identified 29 health states with different combinations of 'disability' (from 'none' to 'unconscious') and 'distress' (from 'none' to 'severe'). While everyone will prefer less pain/less disability to more pain/more disability, each of us will have our own preference for a health state with less pain/more disability over another with more pain/less disability. However, if 90% of a representative sample of the population indicate that they prefer one over the other, would such a consensus not allow us to say that 'society' prefers, that is, puts a higher value on, that one over the other?

Rosser and Kind (1978) took a sample of people representing doctors, nurses, patients and health individuals and asked them to rank each of the 29 health states, giving a score of 1 to the top-ranked state, which would inevitably be no disability and no distress, and 0 to the state judged to be equivalent to death. All other states were to be scored cardinally (0.8, for example, being 'twice as good' as 0.4), with negative scores permitted for states judged to be worse than death.

Although this exercise can be criticized on a number of grounds, for example that the sample was small and possibly unrepresentative and the method used to elicit preference values was crude, the fact that reasonably consistent scores were produced suggested that there is such a thing as 'social values'. Health gains could now be measured directly, with the difference in scores between a pre-treatment health state and a post-treatment health state representing the extent of the health gain, or, more accurately, the value or 'utility' associated with that health gain. More recently, social valuations of health states from much larger and more representative samples, and with values obtained using much more sophisticated methods, have been obtained (see, for example, www.euroqol.org).

Health states can be converted in QALYs by producing a graph that maps the 'utility' value of a patient (or the mean for a group) at given points in time on the vertical axis against time on the horizontal axis. This shows the time profile of utility values 'with treatment' and 'without treatment' or 'with different treatment'. The QALY gain from the treatment is the vertical difference between the treatment and the alternative plot, known as the 'area under the curve' method.

Economics is the study of trade-offs. It explicitly recognizes that health improvements are achieved at a cost, that is, by forgoing (trading off) the benefits of something else in exchange. Although this has been discussed in terms of choices regarding the distribution of healthcare, the same way of thinking can be applied to decisions made by individuals regarding their own behaviour. At first sight, this may seem odd, and indeed one of the reasons why health issues were ignored by economists for so long was the belief that health was so important that no individual would be willing to trade it off for anything else (Fuchs, 1972). It is, however, easy to show that this is not in fact the case.

Smokers who are aware of the associated health risks are trading off the risk of future illness or death against the present satisfaction and pleasure they get from smoking. Careful driving reduces risk but can mean longer journeys. As Cullis and West (1979) stated:

> Few people, if any, seek to maximize their health and life expectancy per se. To do so, involves sacrificing opportunities to eat, drink, play games, drive and so on that at the margin may be a greater source of utility than any additional (expected) minute or so of life.

Of all the disciplines that examine health, economics is perhaps unique by its focus on *optimum* health as opposed to *maximum* health. Optimum health is achieved when the marginal benefits of improved health (or the reduced risk of future ill health) are outweighed by the marginal opportunity cost. Optimum health is thus likely to be lower than maximum health. While maximum health is something everyone wants, it is clearly not something everyone demands (in the sense that demand equals willingness to pay for).

case study the use of QALYs in the treatment of obesity

In 2010, 35% of men and 44% of women were at high or very high risk of health problems based on their BMI and waist-to-hip ratio (NHS Information Centre, 2012). Orlistat (trade name Xenical) is a drug that has been shown to help reduce obesity by preventing absorption of fat in the intestines. It was licensed in 1998, but the issue remained as to whether or not it should be made available for use on the NHS.

As explained earlier, NICE is the organization that makes these sorts of judgements. NICE prefers evidence of cost-effectiveness to be on the basis of costs and QALYs and is unlikely to recommend a new treatment for use on the NHS if the extra cost per extra QALY gained is above £30,000. Orlistat was one of the first treatments to be considered by NICE. NICE began the process by commissioning a systematic review of the evidence of the clinical effectiveness and cost-effectiveness of orlistat in the management of obesity (O'Meara et al., 2001) and also took evidence from the drug's manufacturer. Perhaps unsurprisingly, there was a large difference in the evidence from the systematic review and that from the manufacturer. In the former case, the cost per extra QALY gained was £46,000 (range = £19,000–£55,000) compared with the manufacturer's estimate of £10,400 (range = £8,400–£16,000). The difference between the two was mainly due to differences in key assumptions, for example with regard to the effect of short-term weight loss on longer term illnesses.

NICE felt that the manufacturer's assumptions were overly optimistic, which had the effect of underestimating the true cost per QALY. Its overall best estimate suggested that orlistat would produce an extra incremental cost per QALY below the £30,000 threshold only if patients achieved a weight loss of about 5% of their body mass for each three months of treatment or showed a cumulative loss of at least 10% of body weight from the start of treatment over the first six months.

NICE guidance on the use of orlistat was issued in March 2001 (NICE, 2001). It recommended prescribing orlistat only to people who had demonstrated they were able to lose weight (had lost at least 2.5 kg by dietary control and increased physical activity alone in the month prior to the first prescription) and to continue maintaining them on orlistat only if they met the weight-loss conditions above. This recommendation was reviewed in 2006 as part of more general NICE guidance on obesity (NICE, 2006) and subsequently updated in 2010. Based on the best available evidence of clinical effectiveness and cost-effectiveness, the condition for adults being prescribed orlistat was now simply that they have a BMI of 30 kg/m^2 and the condition for continuation of therapy beyond three months was that they have lost at least 5% of their initial body weight since starting treatment. Despite these relaxations in conditions for initial and continued prescribing, the uptake of orlistat has been limited due to associated side effects (Mullard, 2012).

Summary

- The focus of health economics is on finding rational ways to allocate scarce resources to healthcare services

- In a period of scarce resources, priority-setting is important. Economics provides a framework for this to take place at broad policy level and in individual treatment decisions. Various techniques have been used to assess what type of value can be put on aspects of health

- Health economics uses different types of economic appraisal techniques to help to make more effective decisions: cost–benefit analysis is the process of weighing gains against sacrifices. Benefits need to be set against the cost, which means that an alternative is forgone

- Economics is not concerned with optimum health. The health improvements need to outweigh the benefits from doing something else

Questions for further discussion

1. Why is it important that health services operate efficiently?
2. Is it unethical to put a monetary value on human life and suffering?
3. Can there be any justification in disinvesting in programmes known to be effective?

Further reading

Donaldson, C., Gerard, K., Mitton, C. et al. (2005) *The Economics of Health Care Financing* (2nd edn). Basingstoke: Palgrave Macmillan.
Covers theoretical issues in an applied way, giving examples of how these economic issues are addressed in different healthcare systems.

Donaldson, C., Baker, R., Mason, H. et al. (2011) 'The social value of a QALY: raising the bar or barring the raise?' *BMC Health Services Research* 11: 8.
Assesses the role that QALYs can play in the allocation of healthcare resources and the value that might be placed on a QALY.

Drummond, M., Sculpher, M., Torrance, G. et al. (2005) *Methods for the Economic Evaluation of Programmes in Health Care* (3rd edn). Oxford: Oxford University Press.
Fox-Rushby, J. and Cairns, J. (2005) *Economic Evaluation*. Maidenhead: Open University Press.
Morris, S., Devlin, N. and Parkin, D. (2007) *Economic Analysis in Health Care*. Chichester: Wiley.
These three books explain the 'how' of economics and offer guidance to those wishing to undertake economic evaluations.

McGuiness, L. and Wiseman, V. (2011) *Introduction to Health Economics*. Maidenhead: Open University Press.
Mooney, G. (2009) *Challenging Health Economics*. Oxford: Oxford University Press.
Wonderling, D., Gruen, R. and Black, N. (2005) *Introduction to Health Economics*. Maidenhead: Open University Press.

These three volumes provide a good overview of the economic way of thinking and the range of issues addressed by the discipline. Deal with conceptual issues such the nature of the commodity of healthcare and whose values ought to be used in deciding how to use scarce healthcare resources.

Phillips, C.J. (2005) *Health Economics: An Introduction for Health Professionals*. Oxford: Blackwell Publishing.
Covers basic principles in the context of decision-making in the UK NHS.

References

Cullis, J.G. and West, P.A. (1979) *The Economics of Health: An Introduction*. London: Martin Robertson.

Daily Mail (1998) Health scare over online Viagra, 8 July. Available at www.dailymail.co.uk/health/article-25195/Health-scare-online-Viagra.html (accessed 4/11/2014).

Donaldson, C., Gerard, K., Mitton, C. et al. (2005) *The Economics of Health Care Financing* (2nd edn). Basingstoke: Palgrave Macmillan.

Drummond, M.F. (1981) *Principles of Economic Appraisal in Health Care*. Oxford: Oxford Medical Publications.

Edwards, R.T., Neal, R.D., Linck, P. et al. (2011) 'Enhancing ventilation in homes of children with asthma: cost-effectiveness study alongside randomised trial'. *British Journal General Practice* 61(592): e733–41.

Fox-Rushby, J. and Cairns, J. (2005) *Economic Evaluation*. Maidenhead: Open University Press.

Fuchs, V.R. (1972) 'Health care and the US economic system'. *Milbank Memorial Fund Quarterly* 50: 211–37.

Griffiths, A., Paracha, N., Davies, A. et al. (2014) 'The cost effectiveness of ivabradine in the treatment of chronic heart failure from the UK National Health Service perspective'. *Heart* 100(13): 1031–6.

Grogono, A.W. and Woodgate, D.J. (1971) 'Index for measuring health'. *Lancet* 2(7732): 1024–6.

Hollingworth, W., Cohen, D. Hawkins, J. et al. (2011) 'Reducing smoking in adolescents: cost-effectiveness results from the cluster randomised ASSIST (A Stop Smoking In Schools Trial)'. *Nicotine and Tobacco Research* 14(2): 161–8.

IMS America (1998) Viagra prescriptions continue to climb. IMS America Health Facts press release, 4 May.

Jonsen, A.R. and Hellegers, A.E. (1987) Conceptual foundations for an ethics of medical care, in L.R. Tancredi (ed.) *Ethics of Health Care*. Washington: National Academy of Sciences, pp. 3–20.

Mooney, G. (1992) *Economics Medicine and Health Care* (2nd edn). London: Harvester Wheatsheaf.

Mullard, A. (2012) 'Panel meeting prompts excitement for antiobesity drug'. *Lancet* 379(9819): 882.

NHS Information Centre (2012) *Statistics on Obesity, Physical Activity and Diet: England, 2012*. The Health and Social Care Information Centre. Available at www.ic.nhs.uk/pubs/opad12 (accessed 3/7/2014).

NICE (National Institute for Health and Care Excellence) (2001) Orlistat for the treatment of obesity in adults. Technology appraisal 22, www.nice.org.uk/ta22.

NICE (2006) Obesity: Guidance on the prevention, identification, assessment and management of overweight and obesity in adults and children. Available at http://guidance.nice.org.uk/cg43 (accessed 4/7/2014).

NICE (2010) Bortezomib monotherapy for relapsed multiple myeloma. Available at http://guidance.nice.org.uk/TA129/Guidance/pdf/English (accessed 4/7/2014).

OHE (Office of Health Economics) (2013) *Compendium of Health Statistics*. London: OHE.

O'Meara, S., Riemsma, R., Shirran, L. et al. (2001) *A Systematic Review of the Clinical Effectiveness and Cost Effectiveness of Orlistat in the Management of Obesity*. University of York/University of Maastricht: NHS Centre for Reviews and Dissemination.

Rosser, R. and Kind, P. (1978) 'A scale of valuations of states of illness: Is there a social consensus?' *International Journal of Epidemiology* 7(4): 347–58.

Samuelson, P.A. (1976) *Economics*. Tokyo: McGraw-Hill.

Watson, V., Carnon, A., Ryan, M. and Cox, D. (2012) 'Involving the public in priority setting: a case study using discrete choice experiments'. *Public Health* 34(2): 253–60.

WHO (World Health Organization) (1946) *Preamble of the Constitution of the World Health Organization*. Geneva: WHO.

Ethics and law

Overview   402

Introduction   402

Part 1 The contribution of ethics to health studies   404
Aristotelianism   405
Immanuel Kant and deontology   407
J.S. Mill and utilitarianism   408
Creating 'worthwhile lives': perspectives from ethics on 'the genetic
revolution'   409
The contribution of law to health studies   410
The sources of law   412

Part 2 Theoretical and research approaches   414
Theoretical and research approaches in ethics   415
Theoretical and research approaches in law   417
The relationship between ethics and law: Is what we *must* do the same as
what we *ought* to do?   421
Dealing with the *must–ought* 'gap': consent and professional conduct   423

Case study Banning 'junk food' advertising   424
Summary   427
Questions for further discussion   428
Further reading   428
References   428

Learning outcomes

This chapter will enable readers to:

- Understand the key concerns and principles of ethics and law
- Understand and describe how theory, debate and research in ethics inform and illuminate policy and practice in healthcare
- Understand and describe how theory, debate and research in law inform and illuminate healthcare policy and practice
- Understand and describe how and why ethical positions and judgements on the dilemmas posed by healthcare may differ substantially from legal positions and judgments

Overview

This chapter explores the central relevance of ethics and law to health studies. It exposes a range of dilemmas facing those involved in healthcare provision. These dilemmas relate to issues such as the nature and value of life (at its beginning and its end), the rationing of scarce healthcare resources, and the accountability of health professionals to the public they are supposed to serve. Is it possible to justify the actions of healthcare professionals who assist patients in committing suicide? Should economic priorities determine ability to access treatment? To what extent, if at all, should we allow healthcare professionals just to 'get on with their job' without the application of external monitoring or standards? These questions can only be properly understood and addressed through consideration of the disciplines of ethics and law. Furthermore, dilemmas are not simply confined to 'life and death' situations, but cover the whole span of healthcare activity from prevention and health promotion through treatment to rehabilitation. In Part 1, ethical theory is discussed and related to practical health and healthcare examples; then law, its nature and application to health and healthcare is explored. Part 2 moves on to expose and investigate difficulties in the relationship between ethics and law and asks the essential question: Is what we must do (our legal obligation) always the same, in healthcare, as what we ought to do (our ethical or moral duty)? The chapter closes with a case study on the dilemma posed by policy-makers' attempts to intervene in the food choices of children and young people and, in so doing, draws out the problems and possibilities attached to a consideration of healthcare through the lenses of law and, especially, ethics.

Introduction

Healthcare planners and workers are faced by major decisions concerning:

- life and death
- the power held by professions and the point at which the level of power becomes unacceptable
- priorities for the way in which public money is spent.

In addition, such decisions are relevant not only when we are talking about 'acute' treatment and care, they are of equal relevance for those concerned with the prevention of disease and the promotion of public health. In the area of healthcare rationing, for example, to what extent should we devote resources to population health promotion when this might result in some individuals being deprived of the treatment and care they acutely need?

| connections | Chapter 11 considers how economic principles can be applied with regard to healthcare and public health spending decisions. |

The following are examples of essential questions spanning the enterprise of healthcare, from prevention through to acute care:

- To what extent should a health professional use their power to 'persuade' someone to give up what the professional concerned believes is 'unhealthy' behaviour?

- Given medicine's increased ability to 'decide', in a technical sense, when life can end, does killing or assisting people towards death become acceptable in certain circumstances?

- Equally, from developments in the field of reproductive technology and the so-called genetic revolution (Glover, 2006), should we be concerned about the implications of medicine's technical capacity to decide whether and when life should begin, or even what kinds of lives are created in the first place?

A further question, always important, has assumed even greater urgency in present times: To what extent should economic priorities determine treatment (or the lack of it)? As expectations of health services rise, and as more people are helped to live longer, the burden on health services is increased. In the past few years, these expectations have coincided with a global economic crash and the 'austerity' response to this disaster on the part of many Western governments (Labonte, 2012). Consequently, to an even greater extent than previously, health service reforms have stressed the importance of limiting public expenditure while declaring that quality and clinical excellence in health services must continue to be driven forward (in relation to the English context, see, for example, DH, 2010a). The question above about economic priorities and healthcare access has thus become even more central and pressing.

Chapter 9 considers the influences on patterns of welfare in England and the emergence of efficiency as a driver.   **connections**

All these questions represent key dilemmas for healthcare. Such dilemmas can, of course, be helpfully investigated by disciplines such as sociology (in relation to, say, the understanding of professional–patient relationships and professional power) and economics (considering, for example, the financial cost of particular healthcare decisions). Doubtless, pathology, genetics, pharmacology and other medical disciplines would also have much to say about the 'life and death' dilemmas that have been brought up. But none of these dilemmas can be thought about simply through consideration of facts and empirical evidence. They all concern values – for example, the value of 'health for its own sake' as against the value of economic efficiency.

We often expect others to hold the same kinds of values as ourselves; for example, that killing is wrong. Such values can be thought of as normative, that is, we believe that the value concerned should be assumed and accepted without argument. We often believe that a certain value, such as 'killing is wrong', is so important that we establish prescriptive rules to prevent action contrary to the value, or to punish those who do act in such a way. So, laws are enacted, which society as a whole attempts to uphold and enforce. This is the territory of ethics and law, making a consideration of these two disciplines vital to the study and understanding of health.

Part 1 The contribution of ethics to health studies

example 12.1

The application of ethics and law to contemporary issues in health and healthcare

Ethics and law are important disciplines that can be applied to understanding, analysing and dealing with the complex issues and questions raised as a result of healthcare policy and practice:

- The capacity through healthcare technology and interventions to create certain kinds of lives (issues associated with the so-called genetic revolution) and hasten death (euthanasia)
- The financing, organization and delivery of healthcare – the legal frameworks within which the NHS was founded and operates, and controversies connected with this operation, which often possess ethical dimensions such as disagreement on provision or resource allocation

- The duties and responsibilities of individual healthcare professionals
- The collective responsibilities of governments and healthcare organizations for the health and welfare of the populations they are supposed to be serving
- The duties and responsibilities of the individual citizen of the state for their own health and wellbeing. What are or should be the rights and responsibilities with regard to how they are treated? To what extent should individuals be 'active citizens' in creating their own opportunities for health, preventing illness and disease, and participating in the development of better and more responsive health services? Within a democratic society, citizens cannot simply be passive; and in becoming and being active, they face choices that have ethical dimensions and quite possibly legal ones too

There are three main branches of philosophy, the discipline within which ethics lies:

- *epistemology:* enquiry into the nature and grounds of belief, experience and knowledge

- *metaphysics:* the study of the nature of being

- *ethics:* enquiry into how we ought to act and conduct ourselves.

Ethics is the branch of philosophy that has traditionally concerned itself with examining the worth or value of conduct, with developing and defending views on what might be meant by a 'worthwhile life' and how such a life could be led. Different ethical traditions have developed separate, and frequently conflicting, views on the purpose of ethics and the kind of conduct in which we should actually engage. In particular, Western philosophy has been profoundly shaped by three theories of ethics: Aristotelianism or virtue theory, deontology and consequentialism, the best known form of this being utilitarianism. Each of these three theories can be seen as essentially a product of the times in which it was originally born; they are all attempts by the philosophers concerned to answer questions about how those living in the society they were themselves part of should conduct themselves. These theories are based on trying to determine:

- what is meant by leading a good or virtuous life: the focus particularly of Aristotelianism

- what kinds of duties or obligations we owe each other: the focus especially of deontology

- how we might take account of consequences when deciding a particular course of action: the focus particularly of utilitarianism.

Aristotelianism

Aristotle (384–322 BC) was a Greek philosopher, whose *Nicomachean Ethics* is representative of those ethical theories that aim to work out what a good (moral) life might mean and how the development of such a life can be encouraged (Aristotle, 1955). Aristotle attempted to do this by looking at the nature of the world and the individuals within it in order to assess what being virtuous might mean. For this reason, Aristotle is frequently thought of as an empiricist, that is, his theory is based on observation and experience. In observing the world, he argued that we become virtuous by performing virtuous actions.

For Aristotle, the virtuous lies in moderate action, leading him to the famous 'doctrine of the golden mean' (Russell, 1979). Every virtue is a mean between two extremes (or vices). In Aristotelian terms, what is most important is not simply the identification of the mean (the virtuous) in all aspects of human action. It is the idea that, through reflection and contemplation, we should develop our lives so that we know how to act according to the mean; in other words, how to act virtuously (or morally). We thus become more morally expert, reflection and the consequent performance of virtuous action determining what it means to lead 'the worthwhile (good) life'.

example 12.2

The dilemma of life

Assisted suicide is, at present, illegal in the UK. Michael Irwin, a retired GP and campaigner for voluntary euthanasia, has,

it is claimed, provided help for at least nine people who wished to commit suicide (Beckford, 2010). These have included Patrick Kneen, who suffered from prostate cancer, May Murphy, a 75-year-old widow from

Glasgow who was afflicted with multiple systems atrophy, and Dave Richards, a 61-year-old former welder who had been diagnosed with Huntington's disease. Dubbed 'Dr Death' in the media, he has supported people in various ways towards their death. In Mr Kneen's case, Mr Irwin (the title 'Mr' follows his removal from the General Medical Council (GMC) register) travelled to the cancer sufferer's home on the Isle of Man with about 60 sleeping pills, enough to kill the patient. But Mr Kneen was too ill to take them and died a few days later in September 2003. Mr Irwin was later cautioned by the police for possession of a Class C drug and then struck off the GMC register for serious professional misconduct. Two years later, in August 2005, the retired GP travelled with Mrs Murphy to the Dignitas clinic in Zurich, Switzerland (where assisted suicide is legal) and was in the room with her and her son when she swallowed a fatal dose of barbiturates (Duncan, 2010). He also accompanied Mr Richards to Dignitas in November 2006, where the Huntington's sufferer committed suicide. In 2010, he was told that he would not face prosecution for his involvement in Mr Richards' death (Beckford, 2010).

The issue of assisted suicide is deeply contentious and controversial. In May 2006, peers blocked a bill introduced to the House of Lords by Lord Joffe to legalize assisted suicide in certain circumstances. Although not entirely clear, the distinction between assisted suicide and euthanasia lies in the former involving doctors giving patients the means to kill themselves, while the latter involves medical practitioners directly administering fatal doses of medication themselves. More recently, Lord Falconer made an attempt to amend the Coroners and Justice Bill so that helping someone to travel to a country such as Switzerland where assisted suicide is legal was not to be viewed as assisting their suicide (House of Commons, 2012). The amendment was defeated and the bill passed into law without containing it (Coroners and Justice Act 2009). An announcement was made in 2013 that Lord Falconer intended to introduce a private member's bill aimed at making assisted suicide legal in England and Wales (BBC News, 2013). The contentiousness of the issue is also demonstrated by the fact that in 2013 the Director of Public Prosecutions (DPP) in England and Wales was forced by the Court of Appeal to clarify whether he would prosecute healthcare professionals assisting suicide. (DPP guidance makes it clear that friends or family members are unlikely to be prosecuted for assisting in the suicide of a loved one.)

thinking about In your view, did Mr Irwin carry out virtuous acts in assisting or attempting to assist the deaths of those he was involved with?

Whether Mr Irwin did the right thing and acted morally may depend on our conception of the virtue of caring. It could be argued that Mr Irwin was acting virtuously and caring for Mrs Murphy because the requirement in this situation was to relieve the distress, pain and anguish she was suffering as she faced her death.

Much depends here on the intention of Mr Irwin's actions. While under current UK law he would have been culpable whether he had given Mr Kneen, Mrs Murphy and Mr Richards the means for suicide or actually killed them himself, if his motive was to care, then arguably he was acting morally. In Aristotelian terms, his actions were virtuous. It is necessary to emphasize the word 'arguably' because of the extremity of the separate situations and related actions. If the virtuous is the mean between two extremes, the virtue of caring lies somewhere in the middle between excessive 'caring' leading to dependency and loss of autonomy and not caring at all (or not caring in the 'right' way). Given that we do not usually understand caring as killing or even helping people to die, Mr Irwin's actions could only be seen as a 'mean' within a situation of enormous and distorted extremes. The guidance offered by Aristotelianism in these particular situations might therefore be somewhat limited, although it does allow for an interpretation of the actions. That interpretation is likely to become more substantial if we look beyond these particular situations, consider a range of others in which Mr Irwin had been involved, and from that try to determine whether he demonstrated 'caring' according to more usual conceptions. If this was possible, it could be suggested that Mr Irwin was leading the 'worthwhile (good) life'.

Immanuel Kant and deontology

Immanuel Kant (1724–1804) was a German philosopher who developed ideas representative of deontology; thinking based on the notion that we owe each other particular **duties** or obligations.

Kant claimed the existence of a reality independent of our experience. Part of his justification for this claim lay in his analysis of our experience as humans. We live in a world subject to scientific laws of causation, yet we retain freedom of will, having the capacity to act morally or otherwise. Our moral choices must therefore be framed within an independent reality. Kant argued that reason exists independently of experience and that the right use of reason is directed towards moral ends. Reason moves us to act out of duty for its own sake and independently of any thought about the consequences. This leads to Kant's famous statement of the categorical imperative: 'I ought never to act in such a way *that I cannot also will that my maxim should become a universal law*' (Paton, 1948).

example 12.3

Kant and the dilemma of life

At first glance, Kant's conception that we hold certain moral obligations independent of ideas about consequences seems to hold the possibility of definitive judgements in the cases of the patients with whom Mr Irwin was involved. We might say that helping people to die is always wrong; therefore, we should judge him to have committed acts of which we morally disapprove, even if (at least in the jurisdictions where they took place), they are legal. There is, however, a major difficulty at this point. We seldom act with regard to only one moral imperative: we usually have multiple ethical considerations. Mr Irwin would have known that in the UK at least helping people to die is legally wrong and that many people believe it to be morally so as well. But he would also have known that allowing suffering is wrong, or, framed more positively, that he had a duty to care for the patients concerned. If Mr Irwin had not helped Mrs Murphy and Mr Richards to die, they would have continued with their terrible suffering. The deontologist faces a problem at this point. There is either agreement that conflicting duties exist, in which case helping people to die may not always be wrong; or there is persistence in the belief that the overriding duty is to preserve life. We need to be clear, though, that not acting will result in continued suffering.

thinking about In your view, was Mr Irwin carrying out his duty?

How then, is the difficulty overcome? One way, which the strict deontologist could not accept, is to allow that consideration of consequences plays an important part in making moral decisions. This leads to the third ethical tradition to be considered – utilitarianism.

J.S. Mill and utilitarianism

John Stuart Mill (1806–1873) was a Scottish philosopher and probably the most famous advocate of the ethical theory known as **utilitarianism**. In this view, careful thought needs to be given to the consequences of any action, and if those consequences are likely to be adverse for some, the reason for the action must be robust. Put simply, the theory of utilitarianism seems appealing:

> Utility, or the greatest happiness principle, holds that actions are right in proportion as they tend to promote happiness, wrong as they tend to produce the reverse of happiness. By happiness is intended pleasure, and the absence of pain; by unhappiness, pain, and the privation of pleasure. (Mill, 1962, p. 257)

Utilitarianism, and consequentialist ethical theory in general, corresponds with a belief held by many that whereas there are important moral duties, action simply for the sake of duty, whatever the consequences, is problematic. In addition, deliberation about consequences may well include thoughts about the level of 'happiness' or 'unhappiness' likely to accrue from a particular course of action.

example 12.4

J.S. Mill and the dilemma of life

Mr Irwin's view might have been that helping the patients he was involved with to die would have been a merciful release for them and the end of much anguish for their families. But there are at least two difficulties in relying too heavily on consequences to determine moral decision-making:

1. How is it ever possible fully to know the consequences of any particular action? The self-administration by Mrs Murphy and Mr Richards of the lethal barbiturates might have resulted in considerable distress before their deaths. The choice may not have been a clear-cut one, between intolerable pain and peaceful deaths. It could have been the case that Mr

Kneen, who finally died without Mr Irwin's assistance, had a more peaceful death than Mr Murphy and Mr Richards, who he did help to die. Introducing the possibility that a complex set of possible consequences exists beyond the action concerned may make some people more likely to see Mr Irwin not as acting in his patients' best interests but instead as toying with the fates of vulnerable patients.

2. What if Mr Irwin's actions had resulted in members of the various patients' families being terribly distressed by their death, far more so than if their passing had been different, or had not involved him in some way?

Mr Irwin may not have intended this to be the case, but if either or both of these things had been the consequence of his actions, the end result could arguably have been more misery than if he had not acted. Utilitarianism contains the paradoxical possibility that someone can intend an action to be ethical, but for it to become unethical as it is mediated by circumstances. Even more problematic, of course, is the notion that someone can intend an unethical action but circumstances render it unexpectedly ethical. These difficulties all contribute to the view that a reliance solely on consequences as the measure of moral judgement makes ethics a rather haphazard business.

thinking about In your view, were the consequences of Mr Irwin's actions beneficial?

Creating 'worthwhile lives': perspectives from ethics on 'the genetic revolution'

Historically, the concern of ethics has been with understanding how lives already in existence can be 'worthwhile'. But the huge leaps in scientific understanding about the nature of life itself that have taken place since Crick and Watson's discovery of the structure of DNA in the 1950s (Watson, 1970) have led ethics into completely new territories. The so-called genetic revolution has made it possible for science to create and shape certain kinds of lives. These *technological* possibilities lead us immediately towards profound *ethical* problems.

Glover (2006) suggests that we need to consider the justifiability of the genetic and reproductive technologies used to minimize or eliminate the possibility of babies being born with disabilities or disorders. At first sight, such projects seem eminently justifiable; how could we not want for less babies who will suffer the pain and distress of being disabled or suffering from chronic ill health to be born into the world? But the issue is not as clear-cut as this. At its heart, it is an issue about the nature of 'the worthwhile life'. What causes us to believe that lives of disability and chronic ill health are less worthwhile than lives free of these things? We know that many people who are disabled or are living with a chronic disorder lead lives that are purposeful and worthwhile. Why should we deny the possibility of such lives? Where do we draw the line? If we agree that it might be reasonable to prevent the birth of people with a disability such as Down syndrome, why might we disagree that we should also prevent the birth of people with a sensory handicap such as deafness?

As Glover (2006) argues, if we are engaged in projects about limiting or eliminating lives of disability and disorder, what does this say about societal attitudes towards people currently living with these things? Surely they are entitled to 'equality of respect', a notion that does not seem very evident within projects designed to make everyone 'normal' (whatever that means). For many, this idea (contained within genetic engineering projects designed to reduce or eliminate disability and disorder or, even more contentiously perhaps, to create the kinds of lives desired by some parents, so-called designer babies) smacks of Nazi eugenics (Glover, 2006). The horrors of this particular project have reverberated through the second half of the twentieth century and into the present one (Burleigh, 2001). For this reason alone, it is hardly surprising that we have significant ethical worries about medicine's constantly developing technical capacity to create and alter particular kinds of lives.

example 12.5

The use of genetic and reproductive technologies

While the ethical focus on genetic and reproductive technologies often centres on issues around the creation of 'normal lives' (and the prevention or elimination of 'abnormal' ones), there are also questions related to their use in creating certain kinds of lives that we might consider likely to be 'problematic':

Sharon Duchesneau and Candy McCullough [a lesbian couple who are both deaf] used sperm donated by a friend with hereditary deafness to have a deaf baby. They took the view that deafness is not a disability but a difference. During her pregnancy, Sharon Duchesneau said, 'It would be nice to have a deaf child who is the same as us ... A hearing baby would be a blessing. A deaf baby would be a special blessing'. (Glover, 2006, p. 5)

thinking about Do you agree with the couple's course of action? If so, why? If you don't agree, why? Do you consider that your reactions and thoughts might be different here than in the case of a couple who were trying to use genetic and reproductive technologies to *avoid* giving birth to a baby who was deaf? If so, why do you think this might be the case?

The contribution of law to health studies

thinking about How would you define 'law' and what is its contribution to the study of health?

A fairly straightforward definition of law might be 'the development and study of a society's prescriptive laws and rules'. Given this, it is likely that law will (either actually or potentially) have a view on the kinds of health-care dilemmas I have described and discussed above. In the case of Mr Irwin, until he was finally cleared, he faced charges because his actions may have broken laws relating to the protection of life. At the other end of life, the law makes certain prescriptions with regard to the status and protection of fetuses and in what types of circumstances such protection can be legitimately neglected. Equally, there are laws relating to the provision of health services, which could inform or influence debates and dilemmas connected to healthcare rationing.

In addition, the study of law helps us to recognize the value placed by society on health and the expectations we have about the ways in which health workers and organizations conduct themselves. Between 2005 and 2009, as many as 1,200 patients may have died needlessly after they were routinely neglected at Stafford Hospital in the UK (Laurence, 2013). The Francis Inquiry, which investigated problems at the hospital following intense pressure from relatives and others in the local community to do so, discovered that 'for many patients the most basic elements of care were neglected' (Francis, 2010). Patients were left in soiled bed linen for hours, went unwashed for periods of up to a month, were not fed and were provided with pain relief late, if at all:

> I heard so many stories of shocking care. These patients were not simply numbers they were husbands, wives, sons, daughters, fathers, mothers, grandparents. They were people who entered Stafford Hospital and rightly expected to be well cared for and treated. Instead, many suffered horrific experiences that will haunt them and their loved ones for the rest of their lives. (Francis, 2010)

Among the factors responsible for the deeply substandard care were chronic staff shortages and low morale within the trust. There were also disturbing examples of staff showing lack of compassion. Staff who spoke up about the situation at the hospital were ignored, while others were prevented from doing so by an organizational culture of fear and bullying.

In April 2013, the first criminal investigation into a death at Mid Staffs, that of 66-year-old diabetic patient Mrs Gillian Astbury, was announced. Mrs Astbury had died in a hypoglycaemic coma after staff had forgotten to administer her regular injection of insulin. For some, Mid Staffs represents in large scale and with shocking detail the way in which healthcare professionals and organizations have the capacity not only to fail, but also when failure occurs to become closed and secretive cabals determined to prevent any meaningful investigation of their practices. The issues raised by Mid Staffs are just one example of deep-seated problems in healthcare organization and professional regulation that seem to require the attention of the law and its concern with prescribing rules for individual and social behaviour.

Chapters 9 and 10 refer to the Mid Staffordshire inquiry.   **connections**

The sources of law

Generally, regardless of the country in which it is applied, law has several possible origins, or sources:

- *precedent:* law evolves through cases, judgments on these and the application or otherwise of these judgments to later cases

- *customs:* the use of rules over a long period have given them the force of law

- *legislation:* the formal development of laws through deliberation and enactment by a legislative assembly or parliament

- *statutory interpretation:* the interpretation of such laws that have been placed on statute.

The laws governing those who live in the UK have historically had as their sources legislation (statute law) and precedent. Statute law has long been decided in the Westminster Parliament, but since the late 1990s, the devolution of government to a greater or lesser extent to national assemblies in Scotland, Wales and Northern Ireland has seen the emergence of other important places for legislative enactment. Law decided by precedent has mostly emerged through decisions made in particular cases by the courts and so is talked about as 'case law'. While the sources of law in all four UK countries comprise both statute and case, there are differences between them. In the case of Scotland, the differences are substantial not only because of relatively recent changes to statute-making assemblies (as has also been the case in Northern Ireland and Wales) but also because of long-standing differences in the legal system of that country itself (Ham, 2009).

Legislation (statute law)

Regardless of the nature and impact of political devolution, during the twentieth century and into the twenty-first, **statute law** has assumed great significance in all four UK countries. Taking the particular example of England, Acts of Parliament (statutes) are primary legislation and become law after both Houses of Parliament have passed them and royal assent has been received. A recent and important example of primary legislation directly affecting healthcare provision in England has been the Health and Social Care Act 2012, which ended its 15-month passage through Parliament when it was granted royal assent on 27 March 2012. The Act legislates for the reforms to the NHS set out in the White Paper, *Equity and Excellence: Liberating the NHS* (DH, 2010a). (White Papers establish government policy in particular areas and often, although not always, precede legislation related to the area concerned.) Among other things, the 2012 Act redefined the duties of the secretary of state for health with regard to the provision of healthcare, established new commissioning arrangements for NHS-funded health services, and restructured public health services in England (British Medical Association Parliamentary Unit, 2012).

As well as enacting primary legislation, Parliament has the ability to delegate the right to the relevant secretary of state (in the case of the legislation above, for health) to draw up regulations or orders dealing with details or future situations that cannot be included in the main act. This is known as 'delegated legislation'.

Case law

Case law is law that emerges from decisions made by the courts. Court decisions may be the only authority with regard to a particular issue, or they may be the authority charged with interpreting a particular piece of legislation. If, however, there is a conflict between case and statute, the latter must always be followed. If the outcome of this is not acceptable, it is the responsibility of legislators to consider changing the statute. Case law's essential ingredient is legal precedent, judges referring back to similar cases in order to make consistent decisions. Not all decisions made by the courts are binding on later cases. The court system in England and Wales is hierarchical, a decision made by a higher court becoming binding on lower ones. Since October 2009, the Supreme Court of the United Kingdom has been the supreme court in civil and criminal cases in England and Wales, as well as Northern Ireland. It has also been the supreme court in civil cases under Scottish law.

Note that criminal law is that under which the Crown (the state) has the right to prosecute individual offences, for example robbery or murder. Civil law involves action by an individual – the plaintiff, in legal terms – against another. The state takes no side in the action, although if necessary it will enforce the court's final judgment. Although it is necessary to make the distinction between criminal and civil law, it should be noted that some actions can be pursued both as criminal offences and as civil wrongs.

Case law is often applied in relation to healthcare, and often under civil law. Examples include:

- Anthony Bland, a case decided in 1993, in which the right to self-determination was given priority over the principle of sanctity of life

- Maureen Grogan, a 2006 case related to who should pay for continuing NHS care

- Pat Morris on behalf of 'Health in Trafford', another 2006 case about public involvement and consultation on the closure of Altrincham General Hospital.

These three examples demonstrate the breadth of application that civil case law has in the field of health and healthcare, which can be understood at least partly in terms of the frequent contentiousness of healthcare policy and practice, and the impact these things have on the lives of individuals and communities.

While statute decided by Parliament, together with case law, has historically been the source of law for England and Wales, recent years have seen European law become a further crucial influence over its development.

European law

The European Communities Act 1972 allowed for the application of European Community law within the UK. The essential purpose of applying European law to member states of what is now the European Union (EU) is to effect harmonization, frequently to support economic aims, for example the free movement of goods and labour. There is, however, a different kind of impact on UK domestic law emerging from Europe. Since October 2000, when the Human Rights Act 1998 came into force, the 1950 European Convention on Human Rights (ECHR) has been incorporated into UK law, meaning that rights under the convention are enforceable in the courts of England, Wales, Scotland and Northern Ireland (Ministry of Justice, 2013). Key articles of the ECHR that actually or potentially affect questions related to health and healthcare include:

- the right to life (Article 2)

- the right not to be subjected to inhuman or degrading treatment (Article 3)

- the right to liberty (Article 5)

- the right to marry and have a family (Article 12).

Part 2 Theoretical and research approaches

example 12.6

Examples of research in ethics and law and health

- Quality of care: for example analysis of patients' claims of negligence by health staff, tried in civil law courts, to determine societal expectations of healthcare
- End of life care: for example review cases of prosecution of those assisting the suicide of others, to identify underlying ethical and legal principles
- Access to care: for example review cases

where health reforms have been legally challenged by members of the public, to identify underlying principles of healthcare
- Professional practice: for example analysis of the grounds given for striking medical and health practitioners off professional registers, to determine the ethical principles underpinning professional practice
- Resource allocation: for example the criteria on which decisions are made regarding medications

As expectations of treatment and care rise and ever-increasing numbers of people live longer lives, the burden on health services is increased. Recent organizational reform of healthcare in a range of different countries has emphasized the importance of clinical excellence, individual choice in treatment decisions and participation in care. Moreover, the global financial crisis that began in 2007 has renewed concerns about the efficiency and affordability of health services in many so-called developed countries. For example, the World Health Organization, on behalf of the European Observatory on Health Systems and Policies, has published extensive research in this area (see Chevreul et al., 2010). There are also interesting perspectives on these issues, including and beyond the European context, in Nuffield Council on Bioethics (2007).

These kinds of strategic decisions, and the resource and other implications that they carry, can in part be understood as being made on the basis of empirical evidence (cost–benefit, cost-effectiveness, a knowledge of the total financial package available to the healthcare systems concerned and so on).

> Chapter 11 considers this economic basis on which resource allocation is made and argues this is an ethical process.
>
> **connections**

There often comes a point, however (and there may *always* come a point), at which decisions get whittled down to being about competing values, for example economics versus health and wellbeing. The theoretical and research approaches adopted in ethics and law support our analysis of the range of values related to health and represented within healthcare.

Theoretical and research approaches in ethics

The territory of ethics – the examination and discussion of the values underpinning conduct – is largely conceptual, and in the case of many of the concepts discussed in ethics, there is a large degree of dispute, or contestedness.

Some philosophers have attempted to argue that certain values, and judgements based on these, have what is known as 'normative' status. By this is meant that the values and judgements are ones that we would want everyone to hold. So, for example, asserting that 'killing is wrong' expresses both a value (the sanctity of life) and a judgement related to it (breaching that sanctity through causing the death of another is wrong).

> **thinking about** Should everyone hold such a value and what might be the consequences of a judgement related to that value?

Classical and contemporary philosophers have attempted to develop ethical theory that assumes and attempts to justify normative ethical judgements. Aristotle, Kant and Mill are all trying to develop and defend normative theories. More recently, contemporary philosophers concerned with the ethics of healthcare have argued that there are important normative values and principles that should underpin healthcare provision. Beauchamp and Childress (2013) argue that the following four principles are particularly important for healthcare workers:

1. Respect for **autonomy**: the obligation to respect the autonomy of others, for example patients or clients, to the extent that this is compatible with the autonomy of all who are likely to be affected by the action concerned

2. **Beneficence**: the ethical commitment in healthcare to produce benefit for patients or clients

3. **Non-maleficence**: the obligation not to harm patients or clients, closely linked to the previous principle, because any given action has the potential to result in benefit and harm. The obligation on healthcare professionals is to ensure that the balance is always in favour of benefit in any given situation

4. **Justice**: the obligation to act fairly when dealing with competing claims to do with, for example, resources or rights.

---

example 12.7

Conceptual and theoretical examination in ethics

Research in ethics is approached through conceptual and theoretical examination, which in part involves the application and development of particular examples. (A helpful resource is Shafer-Landau (2013), a large, edited collection of papers employing the conceptual-analytical approach.)

Setting the value and judgement expressed in the statement that killing is wrong against separate classical theories comes up with different perspectives on what might have seemed like a clear normative position:

1. Aristotelian theory would state that killing might be generally wrong but we could conceive of some circumstances in which killing, for example compassionate or 'mercy' killing, actually promotes the virtuous life.
2. Kantian theory would hold that we always have a duty to uphold the sanctity of life and therefore killing *must* always be wrong.

However, we would then be faced (as in the examples involving Mr Irwin) with the possibility that keeping someone alive at all costs might lead to terrible consequences for that person and their loved ones. Thus, we might be forced to alter our normative judgement from 'killing is wrong' to 'killing is wrong but may sometimes be right depending on the consequences', which is quite a different kind of statement.

3. The four principles of Beauchamp and Childress applied to the judgement that killing is wrong would suggest that not killing will produce benefit, although what exactly is understood by 'benefit' here is unclear, as is the question of who might be the beneficiary. But the principle of beneficence will directly conflict with the principle of respect for autonomy, because Patrick Kneen, along with Mr Irwin's other patients, actually *wanted* to die.

Beauchamp and Childress, and other advocates of the four principles, recognize this difficulty. Importantly, the four principles are presented as prima facie (literally, 'at first sight'), which is interpreted as meaning that each is binding unless it conflicts with another. When this happens (as in the conflict between beneficence and respect for autonomy), a choice must be made between the competing principles about which one should be followed. Those who support the four principles argue that whereas they cannot yield a definitive ethical judgement in all healthcare situations, they do provide a framework for considering, and reasoning about, obligations.

This section necessarily ends with a note of caution. Study and research in ethics cannot provide us with quick or easy answers to extremely difficult questions and situations. Such answers simply don't exist. However, an awareness of moral theory and ethical principles, together with an appreciation of the conceptual-theoretical and analytical 'tools' of ethics can offer real help in understanding and dealing with the complex problems posed by healthcare policy and practice.

thinking about Identify an example from your own practice or potential practice in the field of health and healthcare, which you consider holds ethical difficulties (many everyday activities in health and social care hold difficulties, such as giving advice, arranging routine care, supporting those who are attempting to change aspects of their health behaviour and so on). What exactly are they? Why are they present? Is your way of understanding the difficulties the only way of doing so or might others understand them differently? If so, how and why? What conclusions about dealing with the example are you led to? If others have different understanding (which is more than likely), what conclusions might they reach in dealing with it?

Theoretical and research approaches in law

Similar to ethics, law is an analytic enterprise. Those engaged in the development and understanding of legal theory, and in legal research, frequently work with written statutes and recorded cases. Such work is often with the purpose of discovering whether legislation or existing precedent is sufficient to apply to a new case or whether a new precedent will have to be set. To this extent, there will always be, either actually or potentially, a particular legal perspective (a judgment) on a situation. Analysis in law in this respect, and using these methods, differs from ethical analysis, in that the former yields more absolute conclusions, although as will be discussed in the following section, this does not mean that we cannot question some of the conclusions the law makes.

A further aspect of research in law is an attempt to understand the theoretical foundations of law and its nature. This particular field of the study of law is known as 'jurisprudence' and has different focuses. One of these embodies efforts to understand how and why a particular legal system is constructed as it is. A wider (and arguably more problematic focus) is to try and understand how and why law is constructed as a social institution within a larger political system. Here, to some extent, law presents methodological dilemmas similar to those encountered in the wider social sciences: for example, can we argue that law is an expression of objective truths; or is it something that is simply a social construction, so making claims of its objectivism fundamentally mistaken? Hart (1997) provides a classic account of the problems contained in the study of jurisprudence.

The ambiguities and complexities inherent in delivering healthcare expose some of the limitations of law as an analytic enterprise and its relative weakness in dealing with the problems raised by healthcare policy and practice. One way of demonstrating this is to point to the conflict that sometimes occurs when an individual or population has certain expectations of healthcare and for whatever reason these are not met. The role of law in helping to resolve such conflict is often limited and difficult.

Although probably expressed in different ways, states generally consider that they possess duties towards the health of their citizens. In the UK, this duty is partly expressed through the provision of the NHS. Since 1948, although it has been weak at times, there has generally been a broad political consensus and commitment to provision of a comprehensive healthcare service, free at the point of delivery and funded by general taxation (Webster, 2002). Despite recent deep political debate and anxiety, the secretary of state for health in England continues to have a duty for:

> the promotion in England of a comprehensive health service designed to secure improvement –
>
> (a) in the physical and mental health of the people of England, and
>
> (b) in the prevention, diagnosis and treatment of physical and mental illness. (HM Government, 2012, p. 2)

Yet, although there is a continuing commitment to a comprehensive health service, there is frequently no legal right to insist that particular services are available. Courts are reluctant to scrutinize decisions made by health service organizations that have denied patients access to the services they want.

In this area, the law's position is difficult. It might be generally accepted that individuals have a *right* to healthcare, but statute allows the nature of that right to be decided by those controlling healthcare. In addition, unless a right can be acted on, it is hardly a right at all. There are two main ways in which individuals can attempt to enforce their **rights** to healthcare, both with their roots in the civil law. These are:

- the public law action for *judicial review*, which allows a challenge to be made to the decisions of public bodies on the basis that they have been irrational, illegal or procedurally improper

- claims for compensation on the basis of the right to healthcare having been breached.

example 12.8

Judicial review and Lewisham Hospital, London

Judicial reviews have taken place in relation to a wide range of healthcare issues, from access to individual treatment through to wider questions of service organization and access. An example of the latter is the case of Lewisham Hospital (then part of Lewisham NHS Trust) in southeast London. In 2012, after a long period of severe financial difficulty, Matthew Kershaw was appointed as a Trust Special Administrator (TSA) to run the services of the neighbouring South London Healthcare NHS Trust and to establish a means of returning health services in the area to solvency.

Mr Kershaw proposed that as part of the cost-cutting measures necessary to revive services, facilities at Lewisham Hospital (including its A&E department) should be reduced. In January 2013, Jeremy Hunt, the secretary of state for health, accepted these proposals. Lewisham Hospital was extremely well regarded in the local area and a 'Save Lewisham Hospital' campaign was established, supported by, among many others, the area's local authority, Lewisham London Borough Council. The campaign organizers petitioned for a judicial review. In July 2013, Mr Justice Silber in the High Court ruled in favour of the campaigners. His judgment was based on the opinion that Mr Kershaw as TSA had no legal power to substantially reconfigure NHS services and bodies beyond the boundaries of the South London Healthcare NHS Trust, which he had specifically been appointed to administer (*The Queen on the application of London Borough of Lewisham and Save Lewisham Hospital Campaign Ltd v. Secretary of State for Health*). In August 2013, it was announced that the secretary of state for health was preparing to appeal against the High Court's decision (www.savelewishamhospital.com), an appeal that was subsequently lost.

? What does this example illustrate about the ethical dilemmas about 'rights' to healthcare and the role of the law?

The difficulties relate to:

1. Disputability over what 'rights' to healthcare we actually possess. We would probably want to assert that people in Lewisham had a right to good quality healthcare, but do they have a right for it to be provided from a particular source?

2. The restrictions law faces in deciding between different conceptions of healthcare rights. The secretary of state's conception on the one hand, and that of the campaigners on the other cannot be described in purely legal-technical terms; they also involve values and ideologies, things that are not easily dealt with through judgments of law.

The law, as well as its involvement in establishing or limiting healthcare rights, also attempts to express societal expectations of how healthcare professionals should conduct themselves and the obligations they have to clients or patients. Professionals owe those whom they serve a general duty of care. If this is breached, the professional has acted not only unprofessionally, but also negligently. If patients' or clients' expectations of the duty of care are not met, they may wish to seek redress in civil law through a negligence action – from patients' perspectives, to achieve compensation in some way for the wrong believed to have been done.

So it seems reasonable, in legal terms, to talk about individual *expectations* of healthcare professionals. There is an expectation that they hold a duty of care, and if there is a failure in this respect, there is an equal expectation that they should be subject to redress. This is perhaps optimistic because the legal system is in practice so complex, and its use so costly, that individuals often have little chance of fulfilling the complete 'expectation equation'.

The basis of the duty of care in English law was laid in a judgment in 1932 by Lord Atkin (*Donoghue* v. *Stevenson*). He judged that someone must take reasonable care to avoid actions or omissions in action that could reasonably be foreseen to cause injury to someone directly affected by those acts. (This is quite different from an obligation to act for the *benefit* of another, which generally does not exist in English law.) Breaching this duty and causing harm is negligence; a civil liability has thus been created, so compensation can be claimed. If a negligence action is to be successful, three things must, on the balance of probability, be established:

- The plaintiff (the person pursuing redress) must establish that the defendant (the person defending the action) owes them a duty of care

- This duty has been breached

- The result of the breach has been that the plaintiff suffered foreseeable harm.

If healthcare professionals consider the duty of care, it is likely that they will want to ask a number of questions:

1. To whom do they owe a duty?
   The law would usually deem that they owe duty to their patients and probably their patients' relatives, as well as to their colleagues.

2. When would a duty be regarded as having been breached?
   The law would probably take the view that the duty has been breached if the required standard of care has not been met. The 'Bolam test' (based on the judgment resulting from *Bolam* v. *Friern Hospital Management Committee*, 1957) indicates that healthcare professionals would breach the standard of care if they failed to meet the standards of their peers. This is not a simple test, however, at least in part because the law is less likely to take a judgment on 'acceptable care' provided by some professional groups in healthcare than others.

3. What is the extent of proof required that the damage or harm done was actually caused by negligent professional behaviour?

In the case described in *Barnett* v. *Chelsea and Kensington Hospital Management Committee* (1968), a night watchman was turned away from a hospital A&E department, later to die of arsenic poisoning. It was judged in this case that there is an obligation to provide care to someone presenting at an A&E department. However, it was also judged that the factors causing death in this case were not within the capacity of a medical practitioner to treat, and therefore the doctor who turned the patient away could not be held liable for his death.

The relationship between ethics and law: Is what we *must* do the same as what we *ought* to do?

When we approach healthcare professionals, we generally do so because we need help and have an expectation and confidence that those we approach can offer us such assistance. We believe (or hope we can believe) that they will take their duty of care towards us seriously, will respect our confidentiality, inform us of what they intend to do on our behalf and why, and only go ahead and do it if we consent to their proposed actions.

Yet healthcare practice, and the relationships between professionals and patients, is frequently messy and difficult. We are right to expect the possibility of redress when things go wrong. The law might to some extent be able to provide such redress as part of its role in 'formally' expressing societal expectations of both the healthcare systems operating on our behalf and the individual professionals working within them. However, when we seek help from healthcare professionals, our expectations are not simply that they will operate within relatively narrow and legalistic conceptions such as those of 'negligence' and 'duty of care'. It has been argued, for example, that in law, the duty of care rests on the requirement to avoid actions or omissions that are likely to result in injury or harm and not on an obligation to produce benefit. Would we seek the help of a practitioner simply because we knew they had an excellent reputation for avoiding harm, which is largely all the law requires them to do?

This is moving towards the idea that there is a difference between what we *must* do (what the law requires us to do) and what we *ought* to do; what, for want of better words, our personal and professional moral character obliges us to do. In addition, it may be the healthcare professional who does what they ought to do (rather than simply what must be done) whom we would regard as a 'good' or 'moral' practitioner (Lesser, 2002; Duncan, 2010).

In the cases of assisted suicide involving Mr Irwin, it could be argued that he did what he felt he ought to do in supporting the relief of the pain and suffering of Mrs Murphy and others. Yet Mr Irwin was struck off the GMC register for his involvement in these cases, as well as facing the prospect of criminal prosecution. In other cases of assisted suicide, for example the 2008 case of Daniel James, whose parents assisted him to die at the Dignitas clinic in Zurich, it was decided that prosecution of the parents was not warranted (House of Commons, 2012).

> **thinking about** In these two cases, different judgments were made relating to the responsibility and actions of healthcare professionals versus those of families. Why might this be?

There is an unevenness of judgment where there is a difference between who is providing the assistance in cases of assisted suicide.

Another example where expectations of care have fallen short is the case of Stafford Hospital. The inquiry into this case argued that the appalling practices and the fact that they were allowed to continue for such a prolonged period was because corporate self-interest and supposed organizational priorities (for example, cost control) allowed the practices in the first place and then let them continue (Francis, 2010). The weakness and delay in investigation and eventual criminal prosecution (in relation to the particular case of Mrs Astbury) arguably suggest that legal action and redress in this kind of case are slowed or supplanted by competing social priorities.

We can also reasonably argue that, in the case of Mid Staffs, what *must* be done and what *ought* to be done should be indistinguishable from one another, in a way that is indisputable and unlike the other situations we have reviewed. We *must* have protection to ensure that those who are charged with taking care of our fundamental wellbeing are competent to undertake the task, and those who perform that task (and others who regulate them) *ought* to ensure that this is the case. Despite this indisputability, Mid Staffs was allowed to happen and it was allowed to continue. This state of affairs seems to suggest that what we might consider is the moral duty to professional competence that healthcare professionals should hold might not be matched by equally rigorous laws. Even with the regulatory strengthening that has been one of the fundamental health-related concerns of recent UK governments, we might be doubtful about its ultimate effect on individual practice. After all, Mid Staffs was one in a line of healthcare 'scandals', each of which has exposed the difficulty in ensuring professionals do what they ought and what they must do.

> **?** What are the advantages and disadvantages of a professional group, for example nursing, regulating itself?

It could be argued that it is professionals themselves, by virtue of their technical expertise and moral commitment, who stand the best chance of dealing with the *must–ought* 'gap', of understanding not simply what they have to do but also what they should do. We might say that although cases such as Mid Staffs are catastrophic, thankfully they are relatively rare. Given such rarity, why don't we simply allow healthcare professionals to get on with their jobs and think for themselves about issues of what must and should be done?

Dealing with the *must–ought* 'gap': consent and professional conduct

One of the ways in which professional groups have attempted to deal with this gap is through the development of **codes of conduct**. Nurses, midwives and specialist community public health nurses in the UK, for example, are bound to practise according to the duties set out in a code of conduct (NMC, 2008). A commitment to the code of conduct seems to bind these professionals to do certain things they *ought* to do (the code being an expression of moral commitments), and what they *must* do (the professional being likely to be sanctioned if the commitments are neglected or breached).

Article 13 of the code declares that the practitioner must: 'Ensure that you gain consent before you begin any treatment or care' (NMC, 2008, p. 3). This is rather a broad statement, although slightly more specific directives and advice supplement it. However, if we accept what has just been said, it is clear that the professional ought to and must engage in processes aimed at achieving informed consent on the part of their patients.

> **?** What difficulties do you think there might be with the concept of informed consent?

Informed consent is a reasonable obligation and expectation. The difficulty comes when we start going beyond generality and think about what it might mean in practice. Informed consent involves two processes; informing and consenting (Gorovitz, 1985). The end result of informing should be understanding, yet there are many possible barriers to understanding, particularly in the healthcare context:

- Patients or clients are frequently in a critical state in which their ability to understand is limited

- Individuals have different capacities with regard to understanding

- Informing has a cost, in that it is time-consuming and demanding of skills that health professionals have in different measures.

Moreover, some people do not want to be informed and understandably dread 'bad news'. Consenting should also be regarded not simply as one instance of a patient or client acquiescing, but an ongoing process, with a healthcare practitioner's duty perhaps being continually to nurture and confirm understanding and awareness.

Teasing out the complexities of informed consent as a moral obligation and a professional duty for the health worker raises at least two problems for the NMC code of conduct:

1. The complexity of informed consent exposes the generality of the code, which makes it more difficult to decide when it is being breached. There will be many circumstances in which professionals are 'pushed' to achieve informed consent; at what point is it possible to step in and suggest that duty has been breached? This problem relates particularly to the 'must' side of the gap. Professionals generally know what they must do, but is it possible to blame them when they cannot do it?

2. By delving deeper into this article of the code, we are made aware of how much commitment a health worker must have in order to practise according to its general requirements. This problem relates especially to the 'ought' side of the gap. The health worker must be involved in a continuous process of self-deliberation, and possibly of negotiation and agreement with clients or patients. Is it reasonable to expect this sort of commitment from nurses and other professionals?

It appears, then, that seeing codes of conduct as devices to close the gap between must and ought in the actions of healthcare professionals is simplistic. By themselves, codes are at once too general and too intimidating. We can probably expect health workers broadly to work according to the particular code that governs their activity, and it is right to demand sanctions for those who grossly offend against that code. However, such cases are, by and large, exceptional and do not help most practitioners who are involved in the messy and complicated business of everyday healthcare. Understanding this requires using, but extending beyond, the kind of prescriptive ruling contained in codes of conduct, and engaging in the development and exploitation of other 'tools' for ethical reasoning and action. These include critical reflection and careful discussion with colleagues (Duncan, 2010).

case study banning 'junk food' advertising

Recent years have seen an increasing concern in the UK (as in other developed countries) with rising levels of obesity in childhood and the risk this poses to the future health of the nation (DH, 2010b).

This concern has led to experts and politicians pursuing a range of strategies to address the problem. One of these is efforts to ban junk food advertising within children's TV programming. In 2007, the regulator Ofcom banned the promotion of foods high in fat, salt and sugar (HFSS), as defined by the Food Standards Agency, during children's TV programmes. In a final review of the ban, published in July 2010, which was being enforced by the Advertising Standards Authority (ASA), Ofcom estimated that since its introduction, children had seen around 37% less HFSS advertising.

However, a report published in February 2012 by researchers at Newcastle University appeared to draw contradictory conclusions to Ofcom (Adams et al., 2012). It said that children were now watching *more* junk food adverts than before the ban. This was partly because children were watching adult programmes, within which the restriction of HFSS food advertising scheduling did not apply. In addition, there have recently been concerns about children's online exposure to HFSS food adverts. While the ASA has a non-broadcast advertising code, which applies to internet content, there are difficulties in this area with monitoring and enforcement. Concerned especially about children's exposure as a result of watching adult programmes, NICE called for the advertising ban on HFSS foods to be extended to all programmes screened before the so-called 9 pm 'watershed' (the point after which broadcasters are allowed to transmit 'adult' programmes) (Bailey, 2012).

Underlying this state of affairs and the often intense debate that has taken place in relation to the issue in recent times, there are important ethical questions: Should we be restricting this kind of advertising? What is the moral justification for such action? This question might seem strange to some people. There is a growing incidence (some experts have referred to it as an 'epidemic') of childhood obesity. There is also strong evidence that obesity is connected to problems of health and wellbeing in childhood and in later life. It would not be unreasonable to suggest that obesity trails behind it a huge burden of morbidity and premature mortality. The widespread availability of junk food – HFSS foods with little nutritional value – and consequent changes in dietary behaviour have been linked to the increased incidence of obesity (Bailey, 2012). So if junk food leads to obesity and obesity leads to health problems (even death), then surely those concerned about health and its protection and promotion should be unequivocal in their support for any measure likely to reduce the consumption of unhealthy foods?

Perhaps this is true. This chapter has argued that issues and questions of healthcare centrally involve values. As a consequence, there is a need for us to develop our skills of moral reflection and our ethical intuition. If the arguments of this chapter are accepted, we cannot take for granted the position on the banning of junk food advertising outlined above. We need to subject it to further examination and critique. One way

of undertaking this is to examine the action of banning advertising in relation to the four principles of healthcare ethics described earlier: beneficence, non-maleficence, respect for autonomy and justice.

Banning junk food advertising and the principle of beneficence

At first sight, the case here seems clear. After all, the 'commonsense' position outlined above on the matter (ban advertising, reduce obesity and prevent suffering through ill health and early death) is one that resonates with many. How can bans *not* produce benefit and do good? This position depends, though, on at least two further things being the case:

- that there is a causal relationship between the advertising ban, reduction in junk food consumption and lowering of obesity levels
- that bans, and in particular what is included and excluded from them, are carefully constructed.

With regard to the first point, while we might be able to claim some relationship between the ban, food consumption and obesity levels, we cannot claim that it is causal. There are two reasons for this. First, childhood obesity is causally complex and involves broader aspects of lifestyle beyond simply eating behaviour (NHS Centre for Reviews and Dissemination, 2002). We not only eat in different ways than we have done previously, we also work and play and generally live our lives in different ways, too. So, while we could say that banning junk food advertising might play a part in the eventual reduction of childhood obesity, which might, in itself, be enough to convince us of the worth of such a ban, the nature and extent of this role are relatively unclear.

In relation to the second point, there is considerable fluidity and consequent difficulty in formulating controls and boundaries. Advertising of HFSS foods was banned from children's TV programming but children still saw it sandwiched between adult programmes. Moreover, the importance of the internet to children means that sources of advertising highly influential to them may be problematic to police. This raises the question about the effectiveness of the ban and thus its capacity to produce benefit. It is also important to note that this dispute goes no further than considering whether or not children see HFSS food advertising and does not even address the issue of whether not seeing it has actually resulted in changes of dietary behaviour.

Banning junk food advertising and the principle of non-maleficence

If benefit emerging from banning HFSS food advertising could be contested, this underlines the importance of assessing it in terms of not producing harm. (We may be less prepared to concede harm, even of a limited nature, if we are less clear about benefit.) It might be possible to construct an argument for the ban causing harm in terms of the social context to which it is applied. In banning junk food advertising, some might believe that those who continue to buy HFSS foods are engaging in harmful behaviour. The child buying a MacDonald's 'Happy Meal', say, becomes demonized; they turn into an object of ridicule and fun. This might be exacerbated by the fact that they are already overweight and subject to potential difficulties of self-image. In this demonization of junk food, its consumers also become vilified and so harm is caused to them.

The other side of this coin is the economic effect of the ban on junk food producers and advertisers. The Ofcom ban has already been recognized as contributing to a fall-off in sales of some junk foods (especially takeaway fast foods) and wider bans extending beyond children's to adult TV programming may well hasten this decline still further. In addition, there is the adverse impact on TV advertising revenue itself. While we might be less inclined to sympathy for supermarket and takeaway overlords and TV moguls, there is a need to recognize the effect of changing patterns of consumption on the employees who work for them.

Banning junk food advertising and the principle of respect for autonomy

For many considering the ethics of this case study, the principle of respect for autonomy is of crucial importance. Why should the 'nanny state' (albeit indirectly through advertising restrictions) try and direct the preferences and wishes of individuals? Can't we allow children and young people (and their parents) to make up their own minds about HFSS foods and their consumption? Here, there are important questions of vulnerability and capacity. There are strong traditions in the UK of legislative and other protection for children and young people, including protection from harms to health. Smoking and drinking are banned for children and young people because we believe they do not necessarily have the awareness of harm and capacity for self-protection from it that most adults possess. Such vulnerability might make us more inclined to believe that in this kind of case, restrictions on autonomy could be justified. Moral philosophers often refer to such restrictions as 'paternalistic', with some finding it relatively easy to defend 'soft' or 'weak' paternalism (Wikler, 1978).

On the other hand, a cherished goal of health promoters is the empowerment of those they work with (Green and Tones, 2010), because this is likely to lead to more authentic action, including action for health. If we deliberately coerce and restrict (even if only weakly), to what extent are we providing children and young people with models of how we would like them to behave as they become adults, that is, as individuals in charge of their own destinies and carefully deliberating on the choices available to them?

Banning junk food advertising and the principle of justice

There are a number of areas that are potentially relevant for healthcare-related ethical thought in relation to the broad principle of concern for justice. The most obvious in this case is distributive justice – the fair adjudication between competing claims to the scarce resource of healthcare. We know that there is a relationship between childhood obesity and morbidity. Treating illness costs the NHS money, so we need to do what we can to reduce the incidence of obesity and banning junk food advertising might contribute to this. So, an analysis of banning junk food advertising using the principle of distributive justice might reasonably come to the conclusion that the economic burden presented by unchecked obesity is unfair for those who have to bear it (taxpayers). It would also be unfair to those with other conditions who might be denied treatment as a result of scarce resources being devoted to dealing with severely overweight people.

However, this conclusion again depends on a strong relationship between banning the advertising of HFSS foods and the reduction in obesity incidence. It is not possible to claim such a relationship in an unproblematic way, simply because this intervention cannot be controlled for; it is only one of a myriad things that may or may not affect the dietary choices that children make. This difficulty of controlling for effect applies not only in this case but also to a wide spectrum of public health and health promotion interventions. So, any argument for the ethical worth of the intervention based on distributive justice needs to be carefully balanced with arguments for and against its worth in relation to the other principles.

This short analysis of the ethics of banning advertising of HFSS or junk food does not necessarily lead to definitive conclusions. Principles alone cannot support ethical reasoning and decision-making; we also need an awareness of theory and a capacity to reflect on how theory and principles connect with our own ethical intuition and 'moral sense'. However, this kind of analytical exercise can begin, in a very real way, to expose the complexity and difficulty inherent within health-related interventions and actions that appear, on the surface, to cause little problem.

Summary

- The study of ethics is conceptual enquiry, largely concerned with trying to understand how people ought to behave towards one another. It involves clarifying the meaning of concepts such as 'benefit' or 'duty'

- The study of law is an analytical enquiry into the development of society's prescriptive rules or laws, and establishing whether legal statute or precedent applies in a particular situation

- Ethics tries to describe what we 'ought' to do. The law prescribes what we 'must' do

- The study of ethics and law can help to identify the value placed on health over and above other values, the guides or limits to professional conduct, and the scope of obligations held by healthcare workers

- Neither ethics nor law can provide a definitive 'solution' to contemporary health dilemmas (these simply don't exist); but their study can provide a framework for considering key questions. Reflecting on ethical and legal principles and dilemmas may help in forming consistent judgements and the search for a moral life

Questions for further discussion

1. Does the law's concern with prescription and attempts to establish definitive judgements help or hinder those striving to be good (moral) health workers?

2. Consider a health dilemma you are personally aware of, or have become aware of through the media. Can the application of ethical principles clarify what should be done in this situation?

Further reading

Beauchamp, T. and Childress, J. (2013) *Principles of Biomedical Ethics* (7th edn). Oxford: Oxford University Press.
These authors developed the 'four principles' of healthcare ethics, and here their ideas are most completely expressed. Detailed and technical, it offers many helpful points of reference, including extensive signposts to further literature.

Duncan, P. (2010) *Values, Ethics and Health Care*. London: Sage.
Explores many of the issues raised in this chapter in more detail, concentrating on ethical problems confronted by those who engage in everyday ('ordinary') healthcare.

Glover, J. (2006) *Choosing Children: The Ethical Dilemmas of Genetic Intervention*. Oxford: Clarendon Press.
Beautifully written book by a leading moral philosopher, based on a series of lectures exploring the dilemmas faced by a society in which genetic and reproductive technology is radically changing the nature of life's beginnings.

Nuffield Council on Bioethics (2007) *Public Health: Ethical Issues*. London: Nuffield Council on Bioethics.
Report of a working group of experts on the ethical problems encountered in engaging in public health work; careful and detailed in its appraisals.

References

Adams, J., Tyrrell, R., Adamson, A.J. and White M. (2012) 'Effect of restrictions on television food advertising to children on exposure to advertisements for "less healthy" foods: repeat cross-sectional study. *PLoS One* 7(2): e31578.

Aristotle (1955) *The Ethics of Aristotle*, trans. J.A.K. Thomson. London: Penguin.

Bailey, C. (2012) *Food Advertising on Television*. London: House of Commons Library.

BBC News (2013) 'Labour peer Lord Falconer to table assisted dying bill'. BBC News, 15 May. Available at www.bbc.co.uk/news/uk-22535334 (accessed 15/8/2013).

Beauchamp, T. and Childress, J. (2013) *Principles of Biomedical Ethics* (7th edn). Oxford: Oxford University Press.

Beckford, M. (2010) '"Dr Death" Michael Irwin has helped at least nine people end their lives'. *Daily Telegraph*, 31 June. Available at www.telegraph.co.uk/news/uknews/law-and-order/7854549/Dr-Death-Michael-Irwin-has-helped-at-least-nine-people-end-their-lives.html (accessed 15/8/2013).

British Medical Association Parliamentary Unit (2012) *What We Know So Far: Health and Social Care Act 2012 at a Glance*. London: BMA.

Burleigh, M. (2001) *The Third Reich: A New History*. London: Pan Macmillan.

Chevreul, K., Durand-Zaleski, I., Bahrami, S. et al. (2010) 'France: health system review'. *Health Systems in Transition* 12(6): 1–291.

DH (Department of Health) (2010a) *Equity and Excellence: Liberating the NHS*, White Paper. London: TSO.

DH (2010b) *Healthy Lives, Healthy People: Our Strategy for Public Health in England*. London: TSO.

Duncan, P. (2010) *Values, Ethics and Health Care*. London: Sage.

Francis, R. (2010) *Independent Inquiry into Care Provided by Mid Staffordshire NHS Foundation Trust January 2005 to March 2009*. London: TSO.

Glover, J. (2006) *Choosing Children: The Ethical Dilemmas of Genetic Intervention*. Oxford: Clarendon Press.

Gorovitz, S. (1985) *Doctor's Dilemmas: Moral Conflict and Medical Care*. New York: Oxford University Press.

Green, J. and Tones, K. (2010) *Health Promotion: Planning and Strategies* (2nd edn). London: Sage.

Ham, C. (2009) *Health Policy in Britain* (6th edn). Basingstoke: Palgrave Macmillan.

Hart, H.L.A. (1997) *The Concept of Law* (2nd edn). Oxford: Clarendon Press.

House of Commons Library (2012) *Assisted Suicide*. London: House of Commons Library.

HM Government (2012) *Health and Social Care Act 2012*. London: TSO.

Labonte, R. (2012) 'The austerity agenda: How did we get here and where do we go next?' *Critical Public Health* 22(3): 257–65.

Laurence, J. (2013) 'First criminal probe into patient death at scandal-hit Mid-Staffs Hospital'. *The Independent*, 11 April. Available at www.independent.co.uk/life-style/health-and-families/health-news/first-criminal-probe-into-patient-death-at-scandalhit-midstaffs-hospital-8569410.html (accessed 15/8/2013).

Lesser, H. (2002) An ethical perspective: negligence and moral obligations, in J. Tingle and A. Cribb (eds) *Nursing Law and Ethics*. Oxford: Blackwell, pp. 90–8.

Mill, J.S. (1962) *Utilitarianism and Other Writings*. Glasgow: Fontana.

Ministry of Justice (2013) Human Rights. Available at www.justice.gov.uk/human-rights (accessed 29/8/2013).

NHS Centre for Reviews and Dissemination (2002) *The Prevention and Treatment of Childhood Obesity*. York: NHS Centre for Reviews and Dissemination.

NMC (Nursing and Midwifery Council) (2008) *The Code: Standards of Conduct, Performance and Ethics for Nurses and Midwives*. London: NMC.

Nuffield Council on Bioethics (2007) *Public Health: Ethical Issues*. London: Nuffield Council on Bioethics.

Paton, H.J. (1948) *The Moral Law*. London: Hutchinson.

Russell, B. (1979) *A History of Western Philosophy*. London: Unwin.

Shafer-Landau, R. (ed.) *Ethical Theory: An Anthology* (2nd edn). Chichester: Wiley.

Watson, J.D. (1970) *The Double Helix*. London: Penguin.

Webster, C. (2002) *The National Health Service: A Political History*. Oxford: Oxford University Press.

Wikler, D. (1978) 'Persuasion and coercion for health: ethical issues in government efforts to change lifestyles'. *Millbank Memorial Fund Quarterly* 56(3): 303–38.

Glossary

Administration the practice of being accountable for carrying out the decisions of others. Involves initiating action within defined limits of authority, and monitoring and recording progress, outcomes and events. It is an essential component of, particularly, a bureaucratic organization

Aetiology concerns assigning a cause to a given outcome. For example, the aetiology of coronary heart disease might involve smoking, a high cholesterol level, obesity and a stressful lifestyle

Association an identifiable relationship between exposure to a risk factor and disease. Causation implies there is a mechanism that leads from exposure to disease

Attitude the feelings an individual has about an object or action. There are three aspects to a person's attitudes to an issue – cognitive (knowledge and information), affective (their emotions, likes and dislikes) and behavioural (their skills and competences)

Attribution the perceived or reported reason given for an action, event or feelings

Attribution theory attributions are perceived or reported causes of actions, events or feelings. Attribution theory concerns the beliefs that individuals possess about the causes of events

Autonomy the capacity to be in charge of your own actions and your own destiny. The principle of respect for autonomy asserts that we have a moral obligation to allow this capacity to individuals to the extent that it does not infringe on the equal rights of others

Beneficence the production of good, or benefit. This is frequently regarded as a moral obligation that ought to be held by healthcare workers

Bias the result of any process that causes observations to differ from their true values in a systematic way (as opposed to chance, which is defined as random variation). Bias may be introduced into a study at its inception (e.g. when selecting the sample), during its course or during the analysis

Biomedicine the application of the principles of natural science (biology and physiology) to the human body. Focuses on the biological causes and treatment of ill health and disease

Body	the physical body, a concept encompassing not only the experience of living within our bodies, but also the meanings we attach to the body
Built environment	includes all human-constructed components of the environment we live in, such as buildings, roads, bridges, dams and farms
Bureaucracy	a term describing particular features of organizations in which structure, role relationships and procedures are specified in writing and are followed impartially and without deviation over long time periods, irrespective of the individual's personality or the personal preferences of the role occupants
Cells	the smallest self-contained living units in the body. Some, like those in the blood, are separate; others are connected to each other to form tissues
Citizenship	the possession of civil, political and legal rights, for example free speech and voting. In social policy, the possession of social rights, for example to economic security, is also regarded as a precondition to citizenship
Class	the division and ranking of groups of people according to occupational role, which arose during the growth and development of capitalism. Social class refers to status and power as well as to income
Cloning	involves the transfer of a nucleus from a body cell to a denucleated egg. No fertilization by sperm is involved
Code of conduct	an attempt to prescribe the ways in which members of an occupational or professional group ought to behave. Such attempts are frequently made by representatives of that occupational or professional group itself
Cohort	a group that can be followed or tracked over time
Collectivism	the general responsibility of all members of society to meet the needs of individuals, for example services funded through taxation
Community	a contested term that is usually taken to refer to a group of people living in a defined geographic area, but may also refer to those sharing a common culture or values
Compliance	behaving in line with that which has been suggested, such as taking medication, eating more healthily or attending a health check. Also known as adherence
Consumption	the way in which cultural artefacts are used or purchased, and the way in which we take meaning from them
Cost–benefit analysis	a technique of economic appraisal that assesses allocative efficiency by comparing the monetary value of all the costs of a policy, programme or intervention against the monetary value of all the benefits

Cost-effectiveness analysis	a technique of economic appraisal that assesses technical efficiency by comparing the money value of the costs of a policy, programme or intervention against a single, non-monetary measure of its effectiveness, for example number of life years gained
Culture	may be portrayed as monolithic, implying that all members of society share a common language, religion, traditions and customs. Culture is, however, increasingly pluralistic, different cultures interacting and influencing each other
Deduction	the converse of induction, whereby a specific inference or prediction is made from a generalization
Demography	the study of human populations and the patterns of population growth. Demographers are interested in the factors that affect the structure of human population, such as fertility and mortality
Discipline	a field of study with a bounded area of knowledge and agreed areas of interest and methods of inquiry
Discourse	can be used in the sense of language to refer to talk or writing. It can also be used to describe a set of ideas and norms about a topic
Disease	a biological definition sees disease as an alteration in the state of the body or some of its organs that changes it from its 'normal' state, interrupting or disturbing the performance of the vital functions. It can be used to refer to a specific, medically diagnosed condition with distinctive, recognized symptoms, which may cause pain or sickness. The concept of disease can also be seen as relative and has been differently defined historically and culturally
Duties	things that we morally or legally ought to do. Duty is usually distinguished from obligation. We incur obligations because of specific circumstances, but duty is something of longer standing and primarily connected with role. A nurse, for example, has a duty to care in a long-standing and general sense because they are a nurse. Nurses also incur obligations to care in a much more short-term sense and with regard to particular people (patients) by virtue of placing themselves in situations in which caring is required
Efficiency	achieving outcomes in the most economic manner possible
Empiricism	the view that knowledge is based on experience, not theory. Knowledge can therefore be proven to exist, because it is tested in real-life experiences. Empiricism is the basis of scientific knowledge

Empowerment	a process through which individuals and groups are able to recognize and express their needs and take appropriate action to meet them
Environmental change	refers to environmental changes that have resulted as a direct consequence of human activity, such as climate change
Epidemiology	the study of how diseases are distributed among different groups of people and the factors that affect this distribution
Epistemology	the philosophical study of the nature of knowledge and its production
Equity	being fair and just. This may involve targeting specific services for those most in need rather than providing the same blanket service for everyone
Ethnicity	characteristics of social life, such as culture, religion, language and history, which are shared by groups of people and passed on to the next generation. Often used instead of 'race', which focuses on physical differences and thus has been largely discredited
Eugenics	the process of using selective breeding for the goal of improving the human race
Evidence	that which tends to prove or disprove something. Used legally, data presented to a court or jury in proof of the facts in issue
Evidence-based practice	the conscientious, explicit and judicious use of current best evidence in decision-making
Experiment	characteristic of science as a way of testing a hypothesis. The aim is to reduce the number of factors that may affect the results so that the procedures are reproducible
Feminism	the theoretical perspective focusing on gender inequality and the role of women in society. This theory stresses the social and historical origins of women's inferior position in society
Functionalism	the theoretical perspective that sees institutions and processes as having specific social functions, which may differ from their overt function and which contribute to social continuity and consensus
Gender	the social role that is attached to being biologically male or female
Genes	a section of genetic material (DNA) that codes for a protein, that is, instructs the cell how to assemble amino acids into proteins. As there are thought to be about 100,000 proteins in humans, there are about 100,000 genes
Globalization	the increasingly interdependent social and economic relationships that span different countries around the world

Health	a contested concept that is variously defined according to place and time. Health is defined by the WHO (1946) as 'a state of complete physical, mental, and social well-being, not merely the absence of disease or infirmity' and, more recently (WHO, 1986), as the extent to which 'an individual or group [is] able ... to realize aspirations, to satisfy needs, and to change or cope with the environment. Health is, therefore, seen as a resource for everyday life, not the objective of living. Health is a positive concept emphasizing social and personal resources, as well as physical capacities.'
Health behaviours	acts that relate to health, such as eating, drinking or wearing a seat belt
Health beliefs	the opinions or thoughts that a person has concerning an object or action, for example the belief that potatoes are fattening
Hegemony	domination of one group or set of ideas over others through political means
Holism	from the Greek *holos* (whole), it is a theory that the parts of any whole cannot exist and cannot be understood except in relation to the whole. In health terms, holism refers to the view that the body cannot be separated from the emotions or mind
Homeostasis	the relatively constant and optimal internal environment, or conditions within organizations or cells, or the physiological processes that maintain these conditions
Hypothesis	a proposed explanation for a phenomenon
Identity	can be signified by the way in which we consume culture in order to convey a certain image
Ideology	a framework of concepts and values, similar to an intellectual paradigm, that shapes a view of the world, for example liberalism, feminism
Illness	commonly understood as the subjective experience of ill health or disease. Illness perceptions are constructed by the social, cultural, historical and geographical contexts which we inhabit
Incidence	the number of newly diagnosed cases during a specific time period
Induction	in science is the process of reaching a generalization or law from many individual specific observations
Interactionism	the theoretical perspective that emphasizes the meaning of social life. Meanings emerge from social interaction and interpretation and are conveyed via language, labels and signs
Interdisciplinary	the relationships both between and among disciplines that enable different perspectives on an issue

Internal market	the introduction of a commercial culture into health services in which different agencies (for example GP practices, hospitals and health authorities) seek to provide or purchase services in managed competition with the intention of increased efficiency
Interpretivism	a paradigm that views the world and knowledge as socially constructed. Typical questions for exploration include: Why? What is the lived experience? How does the person understand?
Justice	fairness in terms of one or other (or more) of resource allocation (distributive justice), meeting natural rights (rights-based justice) and the law (legal justice)
Lay health beliefs	non-professional interpretations of what causes health and illness. Lay beliefs may contrast with biomedical interpretations of cause
Lifestyle (conducive to health)	a way of living based on identifiable patterns of behaviour. Lifestyle is often presumed to be a matter of personal choice. However, lifestyles are determined by the interplay between an individual's personal characteristics, social interactions, and socioeconomic and environmental living conditions
Locus of control	refers to an individual's generalized expectations concerning where control over subsequent events resides – internal locus of control being the belief that control over future events resides primarily in oneself, while external locus of control is the expectancy that control is outside oneself – either in the hands of powerful others or due to fate/chance
Marxist and political economy perspectives	see medicine as a tool of capitalism and economic growth, stressing the conflict inherent in capitalism, characterized by opposing classes with different interests
Materialism	the theoretical perspective that emphasizes the importance of material resources and access to resources such as income and education. This theory focuses on social inequality
Medicalization	the process by which medicine has increased its power in society. This includes the use of medical technology and the professional power of doctors to make decisions about social and ethical problems
Methodology	the theoretical analysis of methods belonging to a specific discipline or branch of knowledge, for example 'the methodology used in this psychosocial research project is qualitative and social constructionist'. Also used to refer to a body of practices or the overall orientation of a piece of research, for example 'the study's methodology employed qualitative methods including questionnaires and observation'

Methods	the means to achieve something. In research, methods refers to specific means of collecting and analysing data, for example interviews and content analysis of interview scripts
Mixed economy of welfare	the provision of welfare through a mixture of state, private, voluntary and informal services. Sometimes referred to as welfare pluralism
Model	an abstract construction presenting possible relationships between phenomena, for example health belief model
Morbidity	the state of being diseased, usually measured by the number of cases of people with a medical condition in a given population at a given time
Mortality rate	the number of deaths in a population. Thus, the crude mortality rate is the total number of deaths in the population divided by the total population size. Specific mortality rates refer to particular subpopulations, for example the rate of deaths in males of social class I
Multidisciplinary	the study of a subject that applies the methods and approaches of several disciplines. It may also be used to describe a planning approach that includes professionals from different disciplines
Natural environment	all naturally occurring parts of the landscape that comprise the environment we live in, including air, water, flora and fauna
Need	a socially constructed and highly contested concept related to want. It may be publicly expressed by individuals or groups, or be professionally defined (normative needs)
Neoliberalism	a political movement of the 1980s espousing the free market and resisting state interference as a means of promoting economic development and securing political liberty. Critics see it as a means of sustaining inequalities
Non-maleficence	doing no harm. This is frequently regarded as a moral obligation that ought to be held by healthcare workers and is closely connected with beneficence
Null hypothesis	a prediction that there is no causal relationship between two factors. This hypothesis is then tested, by examining the likelihood that any observed relationship between the factors could have arisen by chance. Disproving the null hypothesis means that there is a strong possibility that a cause-and-effect relationship between two variables (which is very unlikely to happen by chance) has been discovered
Ontology	ways of constructing reality and the way things are; for example, in a positivist paradigm, there is an objective reality that can be discovered through the laws by which it is governed

Organizational culture	a set of collectively held, relevant, distinctive and shared meanings, values and assumptions, which operate unconsciously and define an organization's (unchallenged) view of itself, its environment and its mission. It also defines and governs the expected behaviour of its members
Organs	are composed of tissues that form a structure such as the heart, stomach, liver or skin tending to restore the status quo (in this case, raising the body temperature again)
Paradigm	in an intellectual discipline, this refers to a framework comprising the assumptions, concepts, theories and values within which the search for knowledge is conducted, for example a scientific paradigm
Paradigm shift	a term first used by Kuhn to describe the process by which one way of thinking is replaced by another through a series of 'revolutions', for example Keynesian economics replaced by monetarism
Partnership	two or more individuals, teams or organizations working collaboratively towards the achievement of agreed goals and targets. A partnership for health is a voluntary agreement between two or more partners to work cooperatively towards a set of shared health outcomes
Pathogenic	the presence of disease caused by a pathogen – a disease-causing agent such as a virus or bacteria
Policy	goals, decisions and purposeful actions generally associated with governments but also with a range of other organizations
Positivism	a paradigm that views only that which can be scientifically verified or capable of proof. Typical questions for exploration include: What causes? How much?
Postmodernism	an umbrella term referring to the rejection of modernism, linear progress and essential truths in favour of fragmentation, plural discourses and relativism
Prevalence	refers to disease rates in populations. The prevalence of disease X refers to the number of people with disease X alive on a certain date
Primary care or primary healthcare	healthcare that is located in communities and is the first point of call
Proteins	large (macro) molecules made of smaller subunits called amino acids. In living organisms, there are about 20 amino acids that can join together in a number of combinations to make many different proteins. Amino acids are formed from groups of chemicals similar in structure and composition to ammonia. The breakdown product of amino acids is ammonia, which gives urine

	its particular characteristic. The proteins formed from amino acids have a variety of functions, such as structural products (e.g. collagen), enzymatic products (e.g. the enzymes catalase, amylase) or transport products (e.g. albumin, haemoglobin)
P value	the probability that the data under consideration would have occurred by chance (that is, just due to sampling variation). The p value is crucial in deciding whether or not two variables are likely to be causally related. Quantitative research commonly tests a null hypothesis, that is, a statement that there is no relationship between two variables. If the p value is small, then the null hypothesis is more likely to be rejected, because the data under consideration are unlikely to have occurred by chance. A common threshold p value is less than 0.05, which means that the data could have arisen by chance (that is, without a causal relationship) in only 1 in 20 instances. When the p value is 0.05 or less, it is commonly accepted that a causal relationship between the two variables being considered exists
QALY	quality adjusted life year. A measure of health output that captures both length of life and quality of life
Quality of life	an individual's perception of their position in life. May include an assessment of physical health, psychological state, level of independence, social relationships, physical environment and personal beliefs
Randomized controlled trial	an experimental study in which subjects are randomly allocated to receive or not receive an intervention
Rationing	a mechanism to reconcile an excess of demand over supply. In competitive markets, consumption is rationed by price; that is, only those willing and able to pay the market price can consume the goods. With public provision, consumption is rationed using more explicit methods such as waiting lists, limited prescribing lists and so on. Often euphemistically referred to as 'prioritization'
Reductionist	a scientific approach of seeking explanation and understanding by focusing on smaller and smaller units, for example seeking to understand disease processes by focusing on cellular changes
Representation	how cultural artefacts are portrayed, discussed and given symbolic meanings
Rights	inalienable properties of all human beings, as in the right to independence and autonomy. Rights are often derived from moral and ethical frameworks, and may be protected by national or international legal frameworks

Risk factors	are those that make an individual or population susceptible to a disease or illness. They may be environmental (e.g. exposure to asbestos), related to lifestyle (e.g. drinking alcohol) or genetic (e.g. a familial history of breast cancer)
Risk groups	used in epidemiology to describe groups vulnerable to certain diseases or conditions, whether because of their behaviour or their economic, environmental or social characteristics
Science	from the Latin *scientia* (knowledge), science comprises two main fields – the natural sciences, which study natural phenomena such as the human body, and the social sciences, which study human behaviour and societies
Scientific method	a systematic way of gathering data through observation and experimentation, and the formulation and testing of hypotheses. The scientific method, and resulting knowledge, is often viewed as more rigorous and dependable than alternative forms of gathering knowledge, for example reflection
Screening	the presumptive identification of a disease or condition through the use of tests (e.g. blood tests in newborns to detect phenylketonuria) or examinations (e.g. the use of chest X-rays to detect tuberculosis)
Self-efficacy	the belief relating to the degree of confidence an individual has in whether a behaviour can be performed
Sick role	Parsons' theory that ill people enter into the sick role, which confers both rights and obligations. The sick role legitimates and regulates illness and hence minimizes the disruption caused by illness
Social capital	the degree of cohesion that exists in communities, characterized by networks of belonging and trust, linked to social participation and access to resources
Social constructionism	the theoretical perspective suggesting that all knowledge and discourse (as well as ideology and representations) are socially constructed within a context in which different groups of people have differing interests and priorities, and therefore represent only a partial truth
Social environment	all the facets of an individual's surroundings that relate to interactions with other people. The social environment includes the political, cultural, social and economic environments
Social inequalities	inequalities in income, access to resources, power and status that are produced, reproduced and maintained by social processes and institutions

Social justice	the concepts of rights and fairness in the distribution of resources
Statute law	a law made by a sovereign or legislative authority
Structuralism	a term covering theoretical perspectives arguing that the social world is shaped by underlying forces such as economic structure and the role of language
Target	a formalized goal set by an individual, team or organization. Health targets state, for a given population, the amount of change (using a health indicator) that could be reasonably expected within a defined time period. Targets are generally based on specific and measurable changes in health outcomes, or intermediate health outcomes
Team-building	an essential component of organizational development, whereby the needs and roles of individual group members and team objectives are identified and clarified, and responsibilities are negotiated and assigned. Team-building can take place both 'off the job' through facilitated training exercises and also through work-related activity, innovation and feedback on work performance
Theory	a logical and plausible explanation of why systems or people behave in observed ways, for example why people adopt protective health behaviours. A theory is capable of predicting future occurrences and being tested through experiment or otherwise falsified through empirical observation, for example theory of planned behaviour
Transdisciplinary	the development of conceptual frameworks that use concepts, methods and questions that transcend traditional disciplinary boundaries to answer key issues
Universalism	benefits and services available to all within a society, regardless of ability to pay
Utilitarianism	the moral theory asserting that we always ought to do what will produce the greatest good
Values	things that are valuable. Value may be subjective (something is valued simply because it is wanted), instrumental (something is valued because it has a useful function) or intrinsic (something is valued because it has fundamental and irreducible importance). It is, of course, possible for something to be valuable in more than just one of these separate senses
Welfare	the conditions necessary to secure the wellbeing of individuals in any society

Index

Page numbers printed in **bold** type refer to figures; those in *italic* to tables. An asterisk (*) before a page number indicates a glossary entry

A

abnormality 5, 34, 87–8, 90, 251
administration 335, 336, *431
advertising 244, 284–6, 326
  banning, for junk food 424–7
  tobacco 177
aetiology 79, 199, *431
AIDS 35, 42, 115, 134
air pollution 59
alcohol 130
almanacs 68–9
anthropology, contribution to health studies 229–30, 249
anxiety, affecting pain perception 130
appraisal 137
Aristotelianism 405–7
Aristotle 23, 274, 405
artefact explanation, for health inequalities 161–2
association 99, *431
attitude 17, *431
  towards behaviour 139
attribution 119, *431
attribution theory 118–19, *431
autonomy 296, 348, 416, 426, *431

B

behaviour
  change 141
  theory of planned behaviour 138–40
behaviourists 114
behaviours 117–18
  see also health behaviours
beliefs
  about causality and control 118
  about confidence 122
  about health 118
  about health and illness 126
  health professionals' beliefs 126
  impact on behaviour 138
    case study 147–9
  impact of, on health 154–5
  lay health beliefs 126, 240–3, *436
beneficence 415, 425, *431
Bevan, Aneurin 269, 321

Beveridge Report 300
bias 37, 92, 96, 97, 98, 102, 103, *431
biobanks 33
biological psychology 114
biology, contribution to health studies 24–33
biomedical model of health 34, 115–17, 250
biomedical model of medicine 115
biomedicine 52, 53, 63, 235, 238, *431
biopsychosocial model of health and illness 116, **116**
Black Report 159, 161–3, 183
BMI (body mass index) 2, 12, 44, 104–7, 325, 397
body 5, 25, 29, 35, 55, 67, 115, 182, 232, 235, *432
  as a machine 63–4
  sociology of 180–1
body fat 44, 45
breastfeeding across cultures, case study 212–15
bureaucracy 340, 341, 359, *432

C

cancer
  bone marrow 391
  bowel 118
  breast 32, 203
  colon, obesity as risk factor *107*
  lung 117, 201
  ovarian, obesity as risk factor *107*
  prostate 84–5, 203
  risk factors 151
  skin, cause-and-effect relationships 99
care
  duty of 419–21
  informal 297–8
care management 308
Cartesian dualism 5, 157, 235
case control studies 102–3, **102**
causality, beliefs about 118–19, 125, 239
cause-and-effect relationships 98–9
causes of disease, germ theory 35, 82
cells 25-6, **26**, *432

change
  managing 357
  stages of change model 140, **141**
chaos (complexity) theory 368
childhood obesity 85, 106, 256, 326,
    369–70
  junk food case study 424–7
citizenship 272–3, 296, *432
civil law 413
class 159, *432
clinical trials 41, 84, 99
  double-blind 41
  RCTs 99–101, **100**, *101*
cloning 37, *432
code of conduct 423, *432
cognitive hypothesis model 124, *124*
cognitive psychology 114
cohort 101, *432
cohort studies 101–2
collectivism 299, 300, *432
communication, in health settings 124–7
community 266, 272, 281, *432
comparative welfare 314–16, *315*
complexity (chaos) theory 368
compliance 124–9, 146, *432
  Ley's model of **124**
congruency model of organizational
    behaviour 366, *366*
consequentialist ethical theory 408
conservatism 275–6
  New Right 276
consultations 125, 167
consumerism 304, 311
consumption, health as item of 181, 231,
    *432
content theories 362–3
contingency theory 362
control
  beliefs about 118–19
  locus of 119, *436
  self-control and stress 121
coping 137–8, 142, 143–4
coronary heart disease 33, 137, 165, 170,
    183
cost
  in economics 388
  opportunity cost 388, 391
cost–benefit analysis 12, 380, 392, *432
cost–benefit approach 389–92, **389**
cost-effectiveness analysis 393–5, *433
cost–utility analyses 393–5
cultural studies 228–65
  application to health studies 230–3
culture 229, *433
  vs ethnicity 170
  food as 233–4

health and illness across 235–40
illness conceptualization 156
organizational 347, *348*, *349*, 350–1,
    411, *438

D
death see mortality
decision-making
  on basis of efficiency 389–90
  ethical 408–9
  in organizations 348–50
deduction 38, *433
demographic transition model 205–7, **205**
demography 83, 204, *433
deontology 405, 407–8
descriptive epidemiology 80
diabetes see type 2 diabetes
diet 55–6
  inequalities in, social causation of 183–5
  obesity and 147–9
disability 395–6, 409–10
discipline(s) 1, 4–6, 8–10, 13, 17, 19, *433
discourse(s) 253–5, *433
  the body as 180–1
  medical 254
  public service 254
discourse analysis 253–4
disease(s) 31–2, 85–6, *433
  causes of 92–3
  classification 93
  cycle **201**
  diagnosis 34, 89
  germ theory 35, 82
  historical definitions 54
  infectious 64, 82–3, 202–3, 205
  natural history of 92–3
  web of causation 98
  see also ill health; illness; sickness
doctors 51, 66, 97, 119, 126, 174, 175,
    176, 253–4, 383, 390
duties 405, 408, *433
duty of care 420, 421

E
economic appraisal
  cost–benefit analysis **389**, *432
  cost-effectiveness analysis 393–5, *__433__
  techniques of 392–5
economic evaluation, and obesity, case
    study 397
economics 378–99
efficiency 380, 389–90, *433
  in economics 392–3
empiricism 5, 37, *433
empowerment 311, *435
empowerment model 174–5

environment 198
　　built 206–10, *432
　　　obesity and, case study 219–21
　　natural 200–6, *437
　　sociocultural 210–13
environmental change 46, 202, 283, *434
　　and dengue fever 203–4
environmentalism 283–4
environmental justice 208–10
epidemiology 5, 79–109, *434
　　lay 85–7
　　medical/clinical 87–9
　　social 89–91
epistemology 9, *434
equity 277, 296, *434
ethics 402–28
　　autonomy 416, 426, *431
　　beneficence 416–17, 425, *431
　　consequentialist theory 405
　　deontology 405, 407
　　justice 207–9, 276, *278*, 296, 426–7,
　　　*436
　　non-maleficence 416, 426, *437
　　relationship with law 421–3
　　utilitarianism 418–19, *441
ethnicity 159, 169–70, *434
ethnography 251–2
eugenics 39, *434
evidence 68, *434
evidence-based practice 83–4, *434
experiment 37, 40–1, *434
experimental studies 98–101

F
feminism 281–2, *434
food 11–12, **14–15**, **70–2**, 147–8
　　as culture 233–4
food industry, dietary inequalities and
　　285–6
food insecurity, social causation of 183–4
food safety, case study 70–1
Francis Report 310, *346*, 350, 355, 411,
　　422
functionalism 173–4, *434

G
Galen of Pergamum 57–8, 62, 69
gate control theory of pain 128–9, **129**
gender 158, *434
　　and health 165–7
　　and inequalities in health 167–9
　　life expectancy and 160
　　and obesity 105
genes 26, 30–2, *375
　　propensity to obesity 44–5
genetic disorders 31

genetic screening 32
genomes 30
geographic information systems (GIS)
　　216–19
geography 14, 196–227, **198**, **199**, **208**
　　health geography 199
　　medical geography 199–200
germ theory of disease 82
globalization 12, 213, 222, 316–17, 270,
　　277, 287, *434

H
Hawthorne experiments 360
healers 62, 238–40
healing, traditional 238–9
health 2–4, 5, 9, *435
　　biomedical model of 34, 250
　　biopsychosocial model of 116, **116**
　　mapping of 214–16
　　pathogenic model 35
　　patriarchy and 282
　　political nature of 270–3
　　representations of 243–8
health behaviours 118, 134, *435
health belief model 135–6, **135**
health beliefs 14, 69, 117–18, 126, 252,
　　*435
　　lay 126, 240–3, *436
　　see also beliefs
healthcare
　　expenditure 305, 378
　　and New Labour 302–5
　　rights to 418–19
　　spatial access to 212–13
　　see also rationing; resources
health determinants 271–2
health economics 377–400
　　see also economics
health inequalities 159–64, 271–2, 279,
　　280, 303
health policy, changes in **303**
health professionals
　　beliefs 124
　　duty of care 419–21
health promotion 6, 13–17, 244
health psychology 113–54
　　see also psychology
health services 316, *345*, *348–9*
　　clinical commissioning groups 270, 306,
　　　341, **342**, 346, 351
　　commissioning *345–6*, 352, 412–13
　　evaluation of 94, 371
　　planning 83, 94, 352, 336, 369–70
　　use of 160, 167
health studies 1–3
　　employability skills 19

interdisciplinary 13, *435
multidisciplinary 4, *437
transdisciplinary 5, *441
hegemony 269, 275, *435
Hippocrates/Hippocratic 56–7, 58, 59, 61,
    63, 80, 198
history, contribution to health studies 50–77
HIV/AIDS 174, 211, 212
    and discourses 254–5
    gender and 169
    and the internet 246
holism 35, *435
homeostasis 29–30, *435
human rights 273
    approach to health 278
humours 5, 56–8, 61, 63
hypertension 107, 124, 237
hypothesis 39–40, 126–7, *437

I
identity 122, **142**, 179, 232, *435
ideology 249–50, 275, *435
    see also political ideologies
ill health
    biological model of 25, 33
    material causes of 163
    socioeconomic conditions and 85–6
    see also disease(s); illness; sickness
illness 34, 35, 36, *435
    beliefs about 122–3
    as biographical disruption 180
    biopsychosocial model **116**
    cultural concepts 162
    definition 89–90
    social construction of 90, 156
    see also disease(s); ill health; sickness
incidence 104, *435
induction 38, *435
inequalities
    dietary 183–4
    gender 167–9
    social 85, 159–61, 163, *440
    see also health inequalities
infant feeding across cultures, case study
    256–8
informed consent 33, 100–1, 423–4
interactionism 179, *435
    symbolic interactionism 179
interdisciplinary perspectives 1, 2, 4, 13–17
internal market 301, *436

J
judicial review 418
    and Lewisham Hospital 419
junk food
    banning advertising, case study 424–7

justice 296, 416, 426–7, *436
    environmental 208–9, 210
    social 209, 276, 296, 278, *441

K
Kant, Immanuel 407–8
Keogh Review 310, 346, 352, 355
knowledge, theory of 9

L
law
    contribution to health studies 410–12
    relationship with ethics 421–3
    theoretical and methodological
        approaches 414–24
lay epidemiology 86–7
lay experts 240
lay health beliefs 126, 240–3, *436
lay knowledge 240–3
leaders and leadership 354–7
legislation (statute law) 412–14
liberal democratic ideology 275
liberalism 276–8
life expectancy 159, 160, 161, 164, 166
lifestyle, conducive to health 165, 233,
    *436
limiting long-standing illness (LLSI) 161,
    166
locus of control 119–20, *436
longitudinal studies see cohort studies

M
management
    of change 295
    consensus management 352
    see also organization and
        management
market forces 380–2
Marx, Karl 67, 70, 274
Marxism 67, 177, 187, 249
Marxist perspectives 231
materialism 67
materialist conception of history 67
media 17, 68, 158, 229, 243–9, 284,
    286
    SARS and the 247–8
medical anthropology 230, 249
medical discourse 247
medical history 33, 51, 52, 54, 66, 127,
    239
medical model 35, 52, 89
medicine 5, 18, 25, 34, 37, 51–3, 63–6,
    87–9, 115, 116, 156–8, 174–6, 198,
    231, 240, 273
    scientific 156–7, 174
    as threat to health 176

mental health 67, 167
    cultural perceptions of 236
methodology/ies 9–10, 96, 251
    quantitative vs qualitative 10
    see also under individual topics
methods 10, *437
Mill, J.S. 285, 408–9
mixed economy of welfare 297–8, *437
model 206, 243, 250, 314, *437
modelling *see* social learning
morbidity 160, *437
mortality
    behaviour and 118
    causes of death 117
    rate 103, *437
    standardized mortality ratio 103
motivation 308, 309
motivation theories 136–9, 362–5
multiprofessional working 18, 20

N
National Health Service *see* NHS
nationalism 280–1
need(s) 278, 296, 361–3, 365, *437
    competing 386
    of individuals 296, 302
    Maslow's hierarchy 363
    relativity of 385–6
neoliberalism 276–7, *437
NHS
    Commissioning Board 319
    funding of treatments 385–6, 391–2
    internal market 301
    judicial review 419
    leadership 355–7
    legislation 412–13
    marketization of 7–8
    organization of 335–45
    organizational change 345–6
    politics of 268
    rationing 307–8
    reforms before 2010 303
    reforms since 2010 302, 305, 306
    structure **342**
NICE (National Institute for Health and
    Clinical Excellence) 83, 107, 109, 301,
    303, 391, 397
noncompliance 124, 134
non-maleficence 416, 426, *437
non-naturals 58, 59–63
normality 87–8
null hypothesis 39, *437
nutrients 42, 43
nutrition 11–12, 56, 70
    obesity, food and, case study 43–6
nutritional medicine 61

O
obesity 11–13, **14–15**
    associated diseases *107*
    biological explanations for 43–6
    built environment and, case study
        219–22
    calculation/measurement of 44, 104
    childhood and, case study 424–7
    factors for rise in levels of 44, 104–6
    genetic propensity to 45
    health effects of 106–7, *107*
    impact of beliefs on behaviour 147–9
    increasing 11, 104–7
    politics and, case study 284–8
    prevalence 105–6, **105**
    QALYs in treatment of, case study 397
    social policy, case study 325–8
    strategy for, case study 369–71
    trends in, case study 104–8
    WHO definition 11, 104
obesogenic environment 16, 219–21, 326
observational studies 101–3
    case control studies 102–3, **102**
    cohort studies 101–2
    prevalence (cross-sectional) studies 103
older people 106, 184, 241, 307–9,
    313–14
ontology 9, *437
operant conditioning, effect on pain
    perception 130, 133
opportunity cost 388, 389, 391
oral history 69
organisms 25, 29, 31, 200–2
organizational behaviour, congruency
    model 366, **366**
organizational culture 347–51, *348, 349,*
    *438
organizational structure 339–42
organization and management
    contribution to health studies 337–57
    theoretical and methodological
        perspectives 357–69
organs 25, 27–8, **28**, 41, *438

P
pain 127–34
    accounts of 243
    gate control theory of 128–9, **129**
paradigm 9, 30, 40, *438
    scientific (positivistic) 96
paradigm shift 5, 40, *438
partnership 17, 18, *438
    between organizations 351–2
pathogenic 35, 64, 199, *438
patriarchy 282
PESTLE analysis 343, *344*

philosophy, branches of 404–5
philosophy, political 275
physiology 23 4, 87
planned behaviour, theory of 138–9, **138**
policy 16, *438
policy analysis, levels of 320–1
policy-making 323–4
policy process 321–3, *321*
political economy 176–8
political economy perspectives 177, 182
political ideologies 275, 275–84
political science 266–89
    contribution to health studies 267–70
    theoretical and methodological
        approaches 274–83
politics
    definition of 266–7
    and the NHS 269–70
positivism 9, *438
postmodernism 232, 250, *438
power 177, 211–12
    of leaders 354
    politics as 267
prevalence, definition 103, *438
prevention 13
primary care 107, *438
priority-setting, in healthcare 387
profession, definition 17, 18, 178–9
professional competence 422
professionalization, of medicine 52
professionals, roles of 17–19
prospective studies see cohort studies
protection motivation theory 137–8, **137**
proteins 31, 32, *438–9
psychology 113–55
    biological 114
    branches of 114
    cognitive 114
    contribution to health studies 115–27
    social 114
    see also health psychology
public health 5, 79, 82, 160, 200, 284, 302,
    306, 347
public service discourse 254
p values 98, *438

Q
QALYs (quality adjusted life years) 391,
    394–6, *439
    use of in treatment of obesity, case study
        397
quality of life 134, 338, *439

R
'race' 169–70
racism 171

randomized controlled trials (RCTs) 99–101,
    100, *101*, 107, *439
rates, in epidemiology *103*
rationing, of healthcare 7, 307, 382, 387,
    402, 411, *439
reductionism 36, 250
reductionist 35, 157, *439
religion 60, 250, 276
representation 229, *439
research
    bias in, see bias
    confirmatory 10
    exploratory 10
resources 335–6, 378–9, 382
rights 3, 173, 272, 273, 418–19, *439
risk
    beliefs about 120–1
    identifying 93
    increased, for the obese *107*
    lay interpretation of 86
    understandings of 242
risk factor(s) 13, 97, *440
    obesity as 11, 13, 101–2, 107, *107*
risk groups 93, 254, *440

S
science 24, *440
    basic/applied 24
    hypothetico-deductive method 40
    theoretical and methodological
        approaches 36–41
scientific management 358–9
scientific medicine 156–7, 174
scientific method 40, *440
scientific paradigm, in medicine and
    epidemiology 96, *438
screening 32, 93, 145, 116, 118, 136, 140,
    144, 390, *440
screening tests 84–5, **95**
self-efficacy 121–2, 136–7, *440
self-help groups 241
self-regulatory model 141, **142**, 146
semiotics 255
sexual health 168
sickness 89, 211
    see also disease(s); ill health; illness
sick role 89, 173–5, *440
smoking 98–9, 117–19, 121, 125, 136, 140,
    160, 305, 388
    ban 323–4
    see also tobacco
Snow, John 35, 81, 96, 199, 207, 214, 217,
    218
social capital 164–5, *440
social class, mortality rates 159, 162–3
social cognition models 144–7

LIBRARY, UNIVERSITY OF CHESTER

social constructionism 9, 67, 250, *440
social control 175, 313
social democracy 278–9
social epidemiology 80, 90–1
social history 66–7
social inequalities 85, 159–61, 163, *440
socialism 278–80
social justice 278, 279, *441
social learning 147
social policy
    contribution to health studies 293–333
    research methods in 318–25
social psychology 114
social selection, explanation for health
    inequalities 162
socioeconomic conditions, and ill health
    78, 80–1
socioeconomic factors 6, 82, 171
sociology
    contribution to health studies 155–72
    theoretical and methodological
       approaches 72–182
Stafford Hospital 310, 350, 411, 422
stages of change model 140, **141**
statute law 412, *441
stress 98, 121–2, 134
structural explanations
    for gender inequalities in health 167
    for racial health inequalities 171
structuralism 231, *441
surveillance 182
    in epidemiology 83, 94–5
Sydenham, Thomas 55, 63
symbolic interactionism 179
symptoms 34
    perception of 46, 142–3 , 236, 243
systems theory 366–7

T
target 145, 370, 369, *441
team-building 352, 370, *441
teams
    classification of 353
    stages of development 353–4

theory of planned behaviour **138**, 138–49
theory of reasoned action 138
tobacco
    advertising, state regulation 271, 297
    smoking 98, 117, 119–21, 125, 136,
       139–40, 160, 162, 303, 305, 388
    smoking ban in workplaces 323–4
traditional healers 238–40
    and people with epilepsy 239
transtheoretical model of behaviour see
       stages of change model
type 2 diabetes, obesity as risk factor 13,
       44, 45, 106–7, 107

U
universalism 299, *441
    as NHS principle 300–1
utilitarianism 405, 408, *441

V
values 326–7, 347–9, 396, 403, 415, *441
    social values 395–6

W
water 34, 57, 70–1, 81, 198, 204–5, 217
web of causation 98
welfare 277, 279, 294–301, 312–15, *441
    challenge to state welfare 301–2
    changing role of state welfare 298–300
    comparative welfare regimes 318
    dependency 296
    materialist critiques 238
    mixed economy of 297–8, **298**, *437
    organization of 296–8
    regimes 314–16, 315
    residual systems of 312–13
    responsibility for provision of 300
    vs risk 235
    as social control 313
welfare state 7, 269, 297, 299–301,
       312–13
World Health Organization (WHO)
    definition of health 3, 52, 388, *435
    definition of obesity 106

LIBRARY, UNIVERSITY OF CHESTER